The
Frontal Lobes
and
Neuropsychiatric Illness

The
Frontal Lobes
and
Neuropsychiatric Illness

Edited by

Stephen P. Salloway, M.D., M.S.
Paul F. Malloy, Ph.D.
James D. Duffy, M.B., Ch.B.

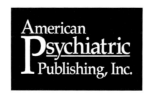
American Psychiatric Publishing, Inc.

Washington, DC
London, England

This book was developed and updated from material originally published as a special issue, "The Frontal Lobes and Neuropsychiatric Illness," in *The Journal of Neuropsychiatry and Clinical Neurosciences,* Volume 6, Number 4, 1994.

Copyright © 2001 American Psychiatric Publishing, Inc.
ALL RIGHTS RESERVED
Manufactured in the United States of America on acid-free paper

04   03   02   01   4   3   2   1
First Edition

American Psychiatric Publishing, Inc.
1400 K Street, N.W.
Washington, DC 20005
www.appi.org

Library of Congress Cataloging-in-Publication Data
The frontal lobes and neuropsychiatric illness / edited by Stephen P.
Salloway, Paul F. Malloy, James D. Duffy.-- 1st ed.
        p. cm.
Includes bibliographical references and index.
      ISBN 0-88048-800-X (alk. paper)
   1. Neurobehavioral disorders. 2. Frontal lobes--Pathophysiology.
      [DNLM: 1. Frontal Lobe--physiopathology. 2. Brain
Diseases--physiopathology. 3. Mental Disorders--physiopathology. WL
307 F9348 2001] I. Salloway, Stephen. II. Malloy, Paul. III. Duffy,
James D.
   RC386.2 .F76 2001
   616.8'047--dc21
                                                      00-046472

British Library Cataloguing in Publication Data
A CIP record is available from the British Library.

About the cover:
Top left: The medial orbitofrontal cortex–basal ganglia loop.
Top right: T_1-weighted midline sagittal magnetic resonance imaging scan showing marked segmental atrophy of the frontal lobe in a 56-year-old man with disinhibition and violent outbursts.
Bottom left: Sagittal and axial PET scans showing decreased metabolism in the fronal lobes in depressed patients with Huntington's disease (*top*) compared with nondepressed patients with Huntington's disease (*bottom*).

*This book is dedicated to the memory of
Per Mindus, M.D., whose premature death in
1998 deeply saddened us. Per participated in the
development of this book from its inception. He
was a tireless worker who pioneered the
introduction of gamma knife capsulotomy,
bringing relief and new hope to patients disabled
by refractory obsessive-compulsive disorder.*

Contents

Contributors

Michael P. Alexander, M.D.
Staff Scientist, The Rotman Research Institute, Baycrest Centre for Geriatric Care, University of Toronto, Toronto, Ontario, Canada; Associate Clinical Professor, Neurology, Harvard Medical School, Behavioral Neurology Unit, Boston, Massachusetts

Karen F. Berman, M.D.
Chief, Unit on Integrative Neuroimaging, Clinical Brain Disorders Branch, National Institute of Mental Health, Bethesda, Maryland

John J. Campbell III, M.D.
Director of Geriatric Psychiatry and Neuropsychiatry, Department of Psychiatry, Henry Ford Health System, Detroit, Michigan; Medical Director, Kingswood Hospital, Ferndale, Michigan

Jeffrey L. Cummings, M.D.
Augustus Rose Professor of Neurology, Professor of Psychiatry and Biobehavioral Sciences, Director of the UCLA Alzheimer's Disease Center, UCLA School of Medicine, Reed Neurological Research Center, Los Angeles, California

James D. Duffy, M.B., Ch.B.
Medical Director, Huntington's Disease Program, University of Connecticut Health Center; Associate Professor of Psychiatry, University of Connecticut School of Medicine, Farmington, Connecticut; Director, Psychiatric Consultation Services, Hartford Hospital, Hartford, Connecticut

Barry S. Fogel, M.D., M.S. (Management)
Clinical Professor of Psychiatry, Harvard Medical School, Boston, Massachusetts; Adjunct Professor of Community Health, Brown Medical School, Providence, Rhode Island; Attending Neuropsychiatrist and Behavioral Neurologist, Behavioral Neurology Group, Brigham and Womens Hospital, Boston, Massachusetts

Elkhonon Goldberg, Ph.D., A.B.C.N.
Clinical Professor, Department of Neurology, New York University Medical Center, New York, New York

Patricia S. Goldman-Rakic, Ph.D.
Professor, Department of Neurobiology, Yale University, New Haven, Connecticut

Suck Won Kim, M.D.
Associate Professor, Department of Psychiatry, University of Minnesota, Minneapolis, Minnesota

Marilyn F. Kraus, M.D.
Associate Professor of Psychiatry and Neurological Surgery, Stritch School of Medicine; Director, Neuropsychiatry Program, Loyola University Medical Center, Department of Psychiatry, Maywood, Illinois

Harvey S. Levin, Ph.D.
Professor, Departments of Neurosurgery, Physical Medicine, and Rehabilitation, Baylor College of Medicine, Houston, Texas

Christer Lindquist, M.D., Ph.D.
Consultant Neurosurgeon and Director, Cromwell Hospital Gamma Knife Centre, London, England; Associate Professor of Neurosurgery, Karolinska Hospital, Stockholm, Sweden

Mark Lovell, Ph.D.
Director, Sports Medicine Concussion Program, Department of Orthopedics, University of Pittsburgh Medical Center, Pittsburgh, Pennsylvania

Paul F. Malloy, Ph.D.
Associate Professor, Department of Psychiatry and Human Behavior, Brown University; Director of Psychology, Butler Hospital, Providence, Rhode Island

Helen S. Mayberg, M.D., F.R.C.P.C.
Professor, Psychiatry and Medicine (Neurology), University of Toronto; Sandra Rotman Chair in Neuropsychiatry, Rotman Research Institute, Toronto, Ontario, Canada

Michael S. Mega, M.D., Ph.D.
Assistant Professor of Neurology, UCLA School of Medicine; Director, Memory Disorders Clinic, Laboratory of Neuroimaging, Reed Neurological Research Center, Los Angeles, California

A. Meyer-Lindenberg, M.D., Ph.D.
Doctor of Medicine, Research Fellow, Unit on Integrative Neuroimaging, Clinical Brain Disorders Branch, National Institute of Mental Health, Bethesda, Maryland

Per Mindus, M.D., Ph.D.†
Professor of Psychiatry, Psychology, and Neurosurgery, Karolinska Institute, Stockholm, Sweden

George Noren, M.D., Ph.D.
Associate Professor of Neurosurgery, Director, New England Gamma Knife Center, Rhode Island Hospital, Providence, Rhode Island

Terence W. Picton, M.D., Ph.D.
Staff Scientist, The Rotman Research Institute, Baycrest Centre for Geriatric Care; Professor of Medicine (Neurology) and Psychology, University of Toronto, Toronto, Ontario, Canada

Kenneth Podell, Ph.D.
Director, Division of Neuropsychology, Henry Ford Health System, Detroit, Michigan

Steven A. Rasmussen, M.D.
Associate Professor of Psychology and Human Behavior, Brown University; Medical Director, Butler Hospital, Providence, Rhode Island

Emily D. Richardson, Ph.D.
Assistant Research Professor, Associate Director, Raimy Training Clinic, Department of Psychology, University of Colorado, Boulder, Colorado

Stephen P. Salloway, M.D., M.S.
Associate Professor of Neurosciences and Psychiatry of Human Behavior, Brown University School of Medicine; Director of Neurology and the Memory Disorders Program, Butler Hospital, Providence, Rhode Island

Donald T. Stuss, Ph.D.
Vice-President Research and Director, The Reva James Leeds chair in Neuroscience and Research Leadership, The Rotman Research Institute, Baycrest Centre for Geriatric Care; Professor of Psychology and Medicine (Neurology, Rehabilitation Science), University of Toronto, Toronto, Ontario, Canada

David H. Zald, Ph.D.
Assistant Professor, Department of Psychology, Vanderbilt University, Nashville, Tennessee

†Deceased.

PART 1

Introduction

The Frontal Lobes and Neuropsychiatric Illness

Stephen P. Salloway, M.D., M.S., Paul F. Malloy, Ph.D., James D. Duffy, M.B., Ch.B.

The frontal lobes have held great fascination for those who are interested in human behavior. The frontal lobes make up approximately one-third of the total cortical area and mediate critical social functions such as planning, regulation of behavior, and drive. For years neuroscientists regarded productive investigation of the prefrontal association cortex as impractical because of its vast size and varied functions. However, recent advances in neuroimaging, molecular biology, neuropharmacology, neurophysiology, and neuropsychological assessment have given clinical researchers and neuroscientists new investigative tools. Carefully designed studies are now beginning to bear fruit, and earlier pessimism is giving way to a sense of guarded optimism.

This book is intended for psychiatrists, neurologists, psychologists, basic and clinical neuroscientists, and trainees from each of these disciplines. The chapters cover a broad range of topics related to advances in our understanding of normal and abnormal frontal lobe functions and are written by experts in clinical neuropsychiatry, neuropsychology, neuroscience, and neuroimaging.

This book was first inspired by symposia on the frontal lobes and neuropsychiatric illness presented at Brown University and at the 146th annual meeting of the American Psychiatric Association and in a special issue of *The Journal of Neuropsychiatry and Clinical Neurosciences* devoted to the frontal lobes and neuropsychiatric illness.

The second chapter, an introduction by Dr. Fogel, puts frontal systems dysfunction in perspective. He describes frontal lobe dysfunction as a common pathway leading to social and occupational disability. As our population ages, a decline in executive cognitive abilities will have a major effect on health policy. He challenges clinicians, researchers, and health policy specialists to include the evaluation of executive cognitive functions in the care of patients, in the evaluation of new medications, and in the determination of eligibility for disability income and support services.

The editors thank Jeffrey Cummings, M.D., for his thoughtful comments in manuscript review and Sarah-Kate Giddings of Brown University for her assistance in preparing the manuscript.

The second part of the book is devoted to delineating the anatomical structures and neurochemistry of the extended frontal systems underlying neuropsychiatric illness. Drs. Mega and Cummings offer an in-depth review accompanied by colorful illustrations of three key prefrontal-subcortical circuits that are involved in many neuropsychiatric disorders. Drs. Zald and Kim provide a colorful, well-illustrated description of the functional organization and connections of the orbitofrontal cortex, an area intimately involved with the integration of sensory processing and behavioral control. They use this anatomical framework to describe obsessive-compulsive behavior as a breakdown in behavioral control by the orbitofrontal cortex.

Working memory systems allow us to hold information "on-line" and update information on a moment-to-moment basis. In a series of landmark studies, Dr. Goldman-Rakic has carried out intracellular recordings during cognitive testing in nonhuman primates to map specific aspects of working memory to areas of the prefrontal cortex. Her recent work has focused on the intricate pharmacology of working memory systems. Her contributions on working memory have wide applicability to understanding the pattern of deficits seen in schizophrenia and other frontal lobe disorders.

Dr. Podell and colleagues discuss the lateralization of prefrontal cognitive functions and propose the intriguing theory that the right hemisphere is primed to process novel cognitive stimuli and the left hemisphere is specialized for mediating activities that require adherence to predetermined motor and cognitive engrams. Drs. Stuss, Picton, and Alexander provide a framework for understanding the role that the prefrontal cortex plays in consciousness and self-awareness. In their hierarchical model, the frontal lobes are at the highest levels of conscious processing, with the right prefrontal cortex carrying out a critically important part in self-awareness.

The third part is designed to improve our understanding and treatment of prefrontal syndromes seen in clinical practice. Clinicians often describe patients with a wide variety of abnormal behaviors as having a "frontal lobe syndrome" without careful classification of the presenting symptoms. Drs. Duffy and Campbell offer a conceptual scheme for understanding the clinical features of three specific prefrontal syndromes. Their model of a dorsolateral dysexecutive syndrome, an orbitofrontal disinhibited syndrome, and a mesial frontal apathetic syndrome corresponds closely to the anatomical systems described by Mega and Cum-

mings and by Zald and Kim. Their conceptual framework is a positive step forward from the current level of clinical obfuscation, but their work needs to be validated and modified by careful clinical and epidemiological investigation.

Psychiatry and neurology have recently embraced the discipline of neuropsychology without providing a program of formal instruction for practitioners. Drs. Malloy and Richardson address this problem by providing a practical overview of the assessment of frontal lobe functions with guidelines for bedside and formal neuropsychological examination. Dr. Salloway describes the common problems encountered in diagnosing and treating frontal lobe disorders, and he offers suggestions for overcoming some of these pitfalls. Dr. Campbell and colleagues close this section by offering comprehensive treatment strategies for patients with complex frontal disorders.

We can learn a great deal about prefrontal systems from studies in specific neuropsychiatric syndromes. The fourth part of the book covers the role of the frontal lobes in major neuropsychiatric disorders. Dr. Mayberg summarizes the evidence from a series of carefully designed functional imaging studies showing prefrontal and anterior temporal hypometabolism in primary and secondary depression. Drs. Meyer-Lindenberg and Berman provide an extensive review of anatomical, imaging, and neurochemical studies in schizophrenia. They provide further evidence for frontal lobe impairment in schizophrenia and discuss the relation between frontal lobe and medial temporal lobe abnormalities in this disorder. They expand on their theory of how dopaminergic hypofrontality can lead to positive symptoms by causing subcortical dopaminergic hyperactivity. Drs. Kraus and Levin describe the neuropsychological and neuropsychiatric sequelae of closed head injury, work that will eventually lead to the development of more effective cognitive rehabilitation and pharmacological treatment for closed head injury. Drs. Richardson and Malloy summarize a large body of work on the neurological substrates related to interesting and often dramatic cases of content-specific delusions. The right hemisphere and dysfunctional frontal monitoring systems appear to play an important role in the formation of these delusions.

The last chapter builds directly on the constructs laid out in Parts 2 and 3. Dr. Mindus and colleagues report on the stereotactic neurosurgical treatment of refractory obsessive-compulsive disorder and its implications for understanding frontal lobe function. Small lesions in the base of the anterior limbs of the internal capsule interrupt connections to the prefrontal cortex and may ameliorate obsessive-compulsive disorder symptoms in refractory patients.

This book shows that the frontal lobes are no longer the *terra incognita* of the brain and that careful study of neuropsychiatric disorders provides valuable tools for understanding frontal lobe function. This volume is not meant to be comprehensive in scope but rather to suggest the importance of the work that has begun and to build anticipation about the advances still to come.

2

The Significance of Frontal System Disorders for Medical Practice and Health Policy

Barry S. Fogel, M.D., M.S. (Management)

Since the famous case of Phineas Gage,[1,2] behavioral syndromes due to frontal lobe damage have been recognized as examples of how major changes in personality, behavior, and social competence can result from brain lesions that spare not only basic motor and sensory functions but also many gross cognitive functions. Twentieth-century experiences, including missile brain injuries and therapeutic frontal lobotomies, have underscored the behavioral importance of the frontal lobes.[3] Neuropsychological studies of patients with frontal lobe damage led to an appreciation of an array of executive cognitive functions (ECFs) for which adequate function of particular frontal regions was a necessary condition. These executive functions include planning, organization, and execution of complex goal-directed behavior; accurate self-awareness; flexible response to changing environmental contingencies; persistence in a task or maintenance of a response set despite distraction; and creative problem solving.[4,5] New imaging methods and neuropsychological techniques have enabled the demonstration of frontal lobe functional abnormalities in patients who

do not have gross localized lesions, such as those with schizophrenia.[6–8] Neuroanatomists have established the reciprocal connections of the frontal lobes with the thalamus and basal ganglia as well as the basis for the occurrence of "frontal lobe" cognitive and behavioral syndromes from subcortical lesions.[9] These developments have now made it possible and attractive to conceive of frontal dysfunction, especially loss of ECFs, as a common component of a range of neurobehavioral syndromes with diverse etiologies, including schizophrenia, traumatic brain injury, multiple sclerosis, vascular dementia, Huntington's disease, and hydrocephalus.[10]

The thesis of this chapter is that medical practice, clinical research, and health policy can make good use of a unifying concept of executive cognitive dysfunction as a dimension of impairment that cuts across disease categories and has crucial relevance to disability, particularly occupational and social disability. In developing this thesis, I refer to ECFs, recognizing that no consensus exists on precisely which cognitive functions are executive and that not all executive dysfunction originates in the frontal lobe, or even in regions that are monosynaptically connected to the frontal lobe. For clarity, I assert here that the ability to develop and execute plans for complex goal-directed behavior is an executive function, as is the ability to conform one's behavior to social contingencies. Some cognitive deficits associated with frontal lesions often accompany impairment in ECF and help confirm a frontal system dysfunction, even though they are not ECF deficits in themselves. Impaired verbal fluency and impaired abstract reasoning offer two excellent examples.[4] Another syndrome of frontal system dysfunction that will figure in the discussion is apathy, as defined in the synthesis by Marin et al.[11–13] This syndrome, which is treatable in some cases,[14] may result either from anatomical lesions of the frontal lobes[15] or from disorders such as Parkinson's disease or depression, which alter levels of neuromodulators that affect frontal cortical activity.[11,16] Frontal system dysfunction as discussed here comprises ECF disorders, apathy, and other cognitive deficits, such as impaired fluency, that frequently accompany prefrontal lesions.

FRONTAL SYSTEM DYSFUNCTION AND CLINICAL MEDICINE

The concept of frontal system dysfunction is useful in capturing a dimension of functional heterogeneity within psychiatric and neurological diagnostic categories that is especially relevant to the instrumental and social functions of everyday life. One person with schizophrenia may work productively, whereas another with similar mental symptoms may be unable even to live independently. One person with mild Alzheimer's disease may be safely left alone, whereas another with the same Mini-Mental State Exam (MMSE) score may be in danger without supervision. The crucial difference between the more and less independent patient usually is in the ECFs. Neither schizophrenia symptom scales nor general cognitive scales such as the MMSE measure these functions and cannot therefore be used to distinguish them. On the other hand, as Royall and his colleagues[17,18] have shown, a bedside measure of ECF can distinguish levels of disability in both schizophrenia and dementia. In a similar way, measures of ECF may capture disability-relevant impairment in Parkinson's disease, traumatic brain injury, substance abuse, AIDS, and mood disorders.

The notion of impaired ECF as a cause of disability also sheds light on the concept of frailty or vulnerability among older people with multiple chronic diseases. A phenomenon often observed by geriatricians is the failure of older patients to cope with the demands of managing their diseases—including accurately self-administering medications, adhering to a diet or exercise regimen, keeping appointments, and coping with the paperwork associated with health care in America. Family members are called on to help, or social workers or other case managers become involved to manage the complexities. Many of these patients may have mild to moderate impairments of ECFs that leave them able to handle the instrumental functions of everyday life but unable to respond to the extraordinary demands of managing their own health care. Evidence for this hypothesis was reported by Gurland,[19] who demonstrated in a large population sample that failure to self-administer medications accurately was one of the earliest, most reliable, and most culturally independent signs of mild dementia.

Executive cognitive dysfunction affects not only self-management of health conditions but also daily instrumental tasks such as shopping, cooking, driving, using public transportation, and handling personal finances. One regularly encounters older people with chronic somatic diseases who give up some of these functions to spouses or other family members, attributing the change to a physical condition such as arthritis or congestive heart failure. However, frontal system dysfunction due to an often-undiagnosed central nervous system (CNS) condition may be decisive in these cases of functional change. For example, Fogel et al.[20] found that in a geriatric assessment clinic population, a measure of ECF was correlated better with declining physical and instrumental function than was the Cumulative Illness Rating Scale, a standard measure of somatic disease burden.

Furthermore, specific aspects of ECF have been shown to relate to different failures in real-world functioning in the elderly. The Frontal Lobe Personality Scale (FLOPS)[21] is a questionnaire designed to measure apathetic, disinhibited, and dysexecutive frontal syndromes. Research has shown that elevations on the FLOPS Apathy scale are related to failures in instrumental activities of daily living (ADLs) in both nondemented and demented elderly patients.[22,23] Frontal behavioral changes, including apathy and disinhibition, are also a common source of caregiver burden.[24]

Indeed, frontal lobe dysfunction may account for much of what makes a person with a mental disorder into a "mental patient"—that is, someone with manifestly abnormal behavior or beliefs. For example, consider two patients with severe depression. The first holds the delusional belief that her bowels have turned to concrete; the second complains bitterly of constipation and says that she feels as if her bowels have turned to concrete. The difference between the two patients may be their frontal lobe functions of abstract attitude and self-monitoring. The modulating influence of executive cognition on mental illness is borne out by Jaeger et al.,[25] who summarized evidence that social and occupational function in people with chronic schizophrenia was better correlated with measures of ECF than with symptom severity. Differences in effects on ECF have been advanced as the reason that patients who are given atypical neuroleptics show better social and occupational function than those who are given typical neuroleptics.[26–28]

The clinician should suspect impaired executive cognition in any patient who shows functional impairment in excess of what one would expect from his or her physical, sensory, or gross cognitive deficits. Sensitivity to the presence of the executive cognitive deficits may lead to the identification of previously unrecognized neurological disease and the implementation of effective compensatory treatment strategies. Even when the dysfunction cannot be remedied, the recognition of the problem may have implications for the appropriate choice of a treatment environment. Patients with ECF impairments have increased environmental responsiveness, so they will do better with cues and supervision than they will spontaneously. Identification of ECF deficits leads to the provision of supports that might not be seen as necessary if the assessment stops with evaluation of grosser cognitive functions, which might well be within normal limits.

IMPLICATIONS FOR CLINICAL RESEARCH

Given the vital role of frontal system functions, particularly motivation and ECF, in supporting real-world performance, measures of those functions should be routinely incorporated in psychopharmacological research and in the toxicological assessment of drugs with potential CNS side effects. When frontal system functions are measured, they can offer a different perspective on why drugs do or do not produce functionally relevant improvements or why patients do not like a drug despite the absence of gross CNS distur-

bance. For example, tacrine, when it is effective for Alzheimer's disease, may produce a greater improvement in maintenance of attention and in verbal fluency—frontal system functions—than in memory.[29] In my own work on clinical correlates of medication use in nursing home residents, I found that cimetidine was significantly more likely than ranitidine to be associated with apathy. The residents taking cimetidine were not more likely to be clinically depressed, delirious, or psychotic—they were just less likely to get up in the morning spontaneously or to participate in the life of the facility.[30]

Drug trials for Alzheimer's disease generally have used the Alzheimer's Disease Assessment Scale[31] (ADAS). This test samples and combines several cognitive and behavioral domains in 40 items. However, it does not permit the clear differentiation of drug effects on frontal functions,[32] and it is possible that clinically relevant improvements in ECF would show up only in the noncognitive section of the test. If the cognitive items of the ADAS were the primary endpoint of a drug study, a potentially valuable drug could be rejected as ineffective. Indeed, many caregivers would gladly live with their relative's amnesia if insight, judgment, and impulse control were preserved. The MMSE is also commonly used as an outcome measure in such trials, but research generally has shown a lack of sensitivity of the MMSE to ECF.[33] Hence, it is important that future trials include both cognitive and behavioral measures of frontal systems dysfunction as outcome measures.[34,35]

Disability from chronic diseases is a major challenge for all developed countries; if it is to be minimized, the reasons for variation in disability must be better understood. The evaluation of the role of subtle cognitive impairment in disability from systemic diseases may therefore be a valuable course for research in chronic disease epidemiology. The incorporation of measures of frontal system function into national epidemiological studies would enable more comprehensive modeling of the influence of cognitive impairment on disability. Because some cases of frontal system dysfunction are treatable, such models would be of more than academic interest.

RELEVANCE FOR HEALTH POLICY

A measure of ECF that worked well as a disease-independent index of mental disability would have evident application to determining eligibility for long-term care benefits, both public and private. Policymakers and advocates appreciate that basing long-term care benefits on physical disabilities alone fails to provide for the substantial needs of many people disabled by CNS disorders such as schizophrenia, severe mental retardation, dementia, or the late effects of traumatic brain injury. This point was underscored at a 1993 conference on mental disability held by the U.S. Department of Health and Human Services Assistant Secretary for Planning and Evaluation. It was noted that various disabilities described in terms that initially appear different may in fact share a common substrate of impaired ECF. Although consensus criteria for any large-scale benefit program would be likely to preserve some behavioral and disease-specific elements, a measure of ECF would be a useful adjunct and might also serve as a *primary* criterion for patients with less common neuropsychiatric disorders.

People with frontal system dysfunction may have difficulty in organizing and implementing their own medical care plans. The concept of frontal dysfunction, especially ECF and apathy, may help answer the question of who needs a care manager—whether an informed relative or a trained professional. A care manager may be needed when the complexity of care needs exceeds the capacity of the patient's ECF, motivation, and energy. Measurement of executive cognitive dysfunction and apathy permits estimation of how complex a plan of care a patient can accommodate. If the plan of care is too complex, one must either simplify it; add cues or incentives to enhance performance; improve ECF, motivation, or energy by medical treatment; or delegate part or all of the care management task. Patient education has mixed effects. Although it usually functions to simplify care, it can on occasion add complexity, with an adverse outcome. For example, if pharmacists inadvertently give patients instructions regarding medications that are discordant with physicians' advice, the patient with impaired executive function may simply follow the last advice given.

The definition of the appropriate clinical roles of specialists in caring for patients with frontal system dysfunction is relevant to the planning of health care reform. Assessment and management of frontal system dysfunction is at present a specialized task. Although generalists are now expected to diagnose and treat depression,[36] they are not expected to do a fine dissection of abnormal behavior or cognition. A con-

ventional view would hold that the specialist should do a specialized examination and make a diagnosis, then have the primary care physician, a generalist, provide subsequent care. The problem is that patients' frontal system problems may continually influence their reporting of symptoms and their ability to adhere to plans, and the severity of frontal dysfunction may vary over time because of disease course or treatment effects. Ongoing reevaluation of neurocognitive status, coupled with continual adaptation of the treatment, is often needed. If the patient has substantial ECF deficits, family members or other caregivers are involved, and they must be advised on how to actively modify the environment and how to respond to episodes of unacceptable behavior. Furthermore, the tasks and treatments involved in managing patients' other, nonneurological, illnesses often need thoughtful integration into the treatment plan. Even when a generalist physician or other specialists supply many components of the treatment, a neuropsychiatric specialist may be the only physician involved who knows how to actually get the patient to adhere to the desired plan. Until these issues are better understood, health plans should not put up structural and financial barriers to neuropsychiatric specialists providing principal care or care coordination for patients with frontal system dysfunction.

Similar issues apply to nonphysician clinicians in the care of patients with impaired frontal system function. One of the core skills of geriatric nurse specialists on Alzheimer's disease special care units is the management of behavior caused by impaired executive function. Such specialists know how to employ cueing and environmental modification strategies to manage behavior problems without the use of restraints or drugs. Social workers with sophisticated knowledge of the social and family consequences of frontal system dysfunction are better able to deal with families' frustrations and help them deal with their loved one's challenging behavior without anger or condescension. Knowledge of the frontal syndromes will help physical and occupational therapists design rehabilitative programs that are realistic given patients' problems with persistence and task organization.[37] Although physical therapists and occupational therapists working in brain injury settings may be experts in this activity, those working with elderly hip fracture patients may not fully appreciate the effect of coexisting executive deficits on rehabilitation, especially if those patients do not have obvious impairment of memory and orientation.

CONCLUSIONS

The development of magnetic resonance imaging (MRI), single photon emission computed tomography (SPECT), and positron-emission tomography (PET) has enabled the identification of frontal system damage or dysfunction in patients without gross frontal lesions. At the same time, advances in psychometrics and functional assessment have confirmed a strong linkage between impairment in prefrontal functions and impaired performance in goal-directed behavior in natural environments. Prefrontal dysfunction is now recognized as an important cause of disability in schizophrenia and in traumatic brain injury. Increasingly, it may be seen as an important mediating or modifying factor in the relation between disease and functional impairment in a wide range of chronic diseases. In some cases, the disease itself will cause impairment of frontal system functions, as in cerebrovascular atherosclerosis,[38] Huntington's disease,[39] and Lewy body dementia.[40] In other cases, such as osteoarthritis, the disease will not directly affect the brain, but another condition, such as preclinical dementia, could affect the executive functions necessary for coping effectively with the medical condition.

The future holds the promise of neuroprotective treatments that may prevent some kinds of frontal system damage; neuropharmacological agents that may restore or enhance frontal system function; and more rigorously designed and tested environmental and behavioral interventions to mitigate the adverse effects of frontal system dysfunction. These prospects make the understanding of frontal system function and dysfunction relevant not only to neurobehavioral specialists but also to all health care professionals who care for people with chronic diseases.

REFERENCES

1. Harlow JM: Passage of an iron bar through the head. Boston Medical and Surgical Journal 39:389–393, 1848
2. Harlow JM: Recovery from the passage of an iron bar through the head. Publications of the Massachusetts Medical Society 2:327–347, 1868
3. Benton AL: The prefrontal region: its early history, in Frontal Lobe Function and Dysfunction. Edited by Levin HS, Eisenberg HM, Benton AL. New York, Oxford University Press, 1991, pp 3–26
4. Damasio AR, Anderson SW: The frontal lobes, in Clinical Neuropsychology, 3rd Edition. Edited by Heilman KM, Valenstein E. New York, Oxford University Press, 1993, pp 409–460
5. Fogel BS: A neuropsychiatric approach to impairment of goal-directed behavior, in American Psychiatric Press Review of Psychiatry, Vol 15. Edited by Dickstein LJ, Riba MB, Oldham JM. Washington, DC, American Psychiatric Press, 1996, pp 163–173
6. Randolph C, Goldberg TE, Weinberger DR: The neuropsychology of schizophrenia, in Clinical Neuropsychology, 3rd Edition. Edited by Heilman KM, Valenstein E. New York, Oxford University Press, 1993, pp 499–522
7. Velakoulis D, Pantelis C: What have we learned from functional imaging studies in schizophrenia? The role of frontal, striatal and temporal areas. Aust N Z J Psychiatry 30:195–209, 1996
8. Weinberger DR, Berman KF: Prefrontal function in schizophrenia: confounds and controversies. Philos Trans R Soc Lond B Biol Sci 351:1495–1503, 1996
9. Cummings JL: Frontal sub-cortical circuits and human behavior. Arch Neurol 50:873–880, 1993
10. Salloway S, Cummings J: Subcortical disease and neuropsychiatric illness. J Neuropsychiatry Clin Neurosci 6:93–97, 1994
11. Marin RS: Differential diagnosis and classification of apathy. Am J Psychiatry 147:22–30, 1990
12. Marin RS, Biedrzycki RC, Firinciogullari S: Reliability and validity of the Apathy Evaluation Scale. Psychiatry Res 38:143–162, 1991
13. Marin RS, Biedrzycki RC, Firinciogullari S: The sources of convergence between measures of apathy and depression. J Affect Disord 28:7–14, 1993
14. Marin RS, Fogel BS, Hawkins J, et al: Apathy: a treatable syndrome. J Neuropsychiatry Clin Neurosci 7:23–30, 1995
15. Neary D, Snowden JS: Dementia of the frontal lobe, in Frontal Lobe Function and Dysfunction. Edited by Levin HS, Eisenberg HM, Benton AL. New York, Oxford University Press, 1991, pp 304–317
16. Weinberger DR, Berman KF, Chase TN: Cortical dopamine and human cognition. Ann N Y Acad Sci 537:330–338, 1988
17. Royall DR, Mahurin RK, True J, et al: Executive impairment among the functionally dependent: comparisons between schizophrenic and elderly subjects. Am J Psychiatry 150:1818–1819, 1993
18. Royall DR, Mahurin RK, Gray KF: Bedside assessment of executive cognitive impairment: the executive interview. J Am Geriatr Soc 40:1221–1226, 1992
19. Gurland BJ: The Fifth Annual Sidney Katz Lecture in Geriatrics/Gerontology: Early detection of dementia: quality of life considerations. Presented at the Center for Gerontology and Health Care Research, Brown University Medical School, Providence, RI, May 18, 1993

20. Fogel BS, Goldscheider F, Royall D, et al: Cognitive dysfunction and the need for long-term care: implications for public policy. Washington, DC, Public Policy Institute, American Association of Retired Persons, 1994

21. Grace J, Stout JC, Malloy PF: Assessing frontal behavioral syndromes with the Frontal Lobe Personality Scale. Assessment 6:269–284, 1999

22. Cahn-Weiner D, Malloy PF, Boyle P, et al: The prediction of functional status from neuropsychological tests in community-dwelling elderly individuals. The Clinical Neuropsychologist (in press)

23. Norton L, Malloy PF, Salloway S: The impact of behavioral symptomology on activities of daily living in patients with dementia. Am J Geriatr Psychiatry 9:1–8, 2001

24. Marsh NV, Kersel DA, Havill JH, et al: Caregiver burden at 1 year following severe traumatic brain injury. Brain Inj 12:1045–1059, 1998

25. Jaeger J, Berns S, Tigner A, et al: Remediation of neuropsychological deficits in psychiatric populations: rationale and methodological considerations. Psychopharmacol Bull 28:367–390, 1992

26. Gallhofer B, Bauer U, Lis S, et al: Cognitive dysfunction in schizophrenia: comparison of treatment with atypical antipsychotic agents and conventional neuroleptic drugs. Eur Neuropsychopharmacol 6 (suppl 2):S13–S20, 1996

27. Meltzer HY, Thompson PA, Lee MA, et al: Neuropsychologic deficits in schizophrenia: relation to social function and effect of antipsychotic drug treatment. Neuropsychopharmacology 14:27S–33S, 1996

28. Tollefson GD, Sanger TM: Negative symptoms: a path analytic approach to a double-blind, placebo- and haloperidol-controlled clinical trial with olanzapine. Am J Psychiatry 154:466–474, 1997

29. Alhainen K, Helkala EL, Reikkinen P: Psychometric discrimination of tetrahydroaminoacridine responders in Alzheimer patients. Dementia 4:54–58, 1993

30. Fogel BS, Mor V: Long-term care outcomes: influence of drug prescription practices: data needs for outcomes research in long-term care. Proceedings of symposium sponsored by Geriatric Drug Therapy Research Institute, American Society of Consultant Pharmacists, Research and Education Foundation. Washington, DC, American Society of Consultant Pharmacists, 1993, pp 63–80

31. Rosen WG, Mohs RC, Davis KL: A new rating scale for Alzheimer's disease. Am J Psychiatry 141:1356–1364, 1984

32. Bagne CA, Nunzio P, Crook T, et al (eds): Alzheimer's disease: strategies for treatment and research, in Treatment Development Strategies for Alzheimer's Disease. Madison, CT, Mark Powley Associates, 1986, pp 585–638

33. Malloy PF, Cummings JL, Coffey CE, et al: Cognitive screening instruments in neuropsychiatry: a report of the Committee on Research of the American Neuropsychiatric Association. J Neuropsychiatry Clin Neurosci 9:189–197, 1997

34. Cummings J: Changes in neuropsychiatric symptoms as outcome measures in clinical trials with cholinergic therapies for Alzheimer disease. Alzheimer Dis Assoc Disord 11 (suppl 4):S1–S9, 1997

35. Gauthier S, Panisset M: Current diagnostic methods and outcome variables for clinical investigation of Alzheimer's disease. J Neural Transm Suppl 53:251–254, 1998

36. AHCPR Depression Guideline Panel: Depression in Primary Care, Vol 1: Detection and Diagnosis. Clinical Practice Guideline No 5 (AHCPR Publ No 93-0550). Rockville, MD, U.S. Department of Health and Human Services, Public Health Service, Agency for Health Care Policy and Research, 1993

37. Robertson IH, Manly T, Andrade J, et al: 'Oops!': performance correlates of everyday attentional failures in traumatic brain injured and normal subjects. Neuropsychologia 35:747–758, 1997

38. Salloway S, Malloy P, Rogg J, et al: MRI and neuropsychological differences in early and late-life onset geriatric depression. Neurology 46:1567–1574, 1996

39. Paulsen JS, Stout JC, DelaPena J, et al: Frontal behavioral syndromes in cortical and subcortical dementia. Assessment 3:327–337, 1996

40. Londos E, Passant U, Brun A, et al: Clinical Lewy body dementia and the impact of vascular components. Int J Geriatr Psychiatry 15:40–49, 2000

PART 2

Functional Organization of Prefrontal Lobe Systems

3

Frontal Subcortical Circuits

Anatomy and Function

Michael S. Mega, M.D., Ph.D., Jeffrey L. Cummings, M.D.

Frontal subcortical circuits represent an organizational system central to brain-behavior relationships. Circuits unite functional regions of the frontal cortex with the basal ganglia and thalamus in networks mediating motor activity, eye movements, and behavior.[1] Disruption of the circuits originating in the prefrontal cortex results in a variety of cognitive and neuropsychiatric disorders.[2] The circuits are the subject of intensive study, and information is available concerning their precise anatomy and chemoarchitecture. In this chapter, their anatomy, chemoarchitecture, and behavioral relevance are described. The three frontal subcortical circuits most involved in mediating behavior are emphasized.

OVERVIEW OF FRONTAL SUBCORTICAL CIRCUITS

Five circuits have been identified and named according to their function or cortical site of origin.[1] The motor circuit, originating in the supplementary motor area, and the oculomotor circuit, originating in the frontal eye fields, are dedicated to motor function. The dorsolateral prefrontal, lateral orbitofrontal, and anterior cingulate circuits subserve executive cognitive functions, social-governed behavior, and motivation, respectively. The orbitofrontal lobe is divided into a medial division concerned with processing appetitive urges and assisting in the control of the organism's internal state and a lateral division concerned with integrating object feature analysis with emotional associations. Each circuit has the same member structures, including the frontal lobe, striatum, globus pallidus, substantia nigra, and thalamus. All circuits use the same transmitters at each anatomical site. The anatomical position of the circuits are segregated in each circuit structure; thus, the dorsolateral prefrontal cortex projects to the dorsolateral region of the caudate nucleus, the lateral orbitofrontal region projects to the ventral caudate area, and the anterior cingulate cortex

This project was supported by a National Institute on Aging career development award (K08AG100784) to M.S.M.; a National Institute on Aging Alzheimer's Disease Research Center grant (P50 AG16570), an Alzheimer's Disease Resources Center of California grant, and the Sidell-Kagan Foundation.

connects to the medial striatal/nucleus accumbens region. Similar anatomical arrangements are maintained in the globus pallidus and thalamus, at which progressive spatial compaction occurs.

Circuits originate in the frontal lobes with excitatory glutaminergic fibers terminating in the striatum (caudate, putamen, and ventral striatum). These striatal cells then project inhibitory γ-aminobutyric acid (GABA) fibers both to neurons in the globus pallidus interna/substantia nigra pars reticulata (direct loop connection) and to neurons in the globus pallidus externa (indirect loop connection). In the indirect loop, the external globus pallidus projects to the subthalamic nucleus via inhibitory GABA fibers; the subthalamic nucleus then connects with the globus pallidus interna/substantia nigra pars reticulata through excitatory glutaminergic fibers.[3,4] The direct pathway uses substance P with its GABA projection to the pallidum and expresses dopamine D_1 receptors, whereas the indirect loop combines enkephalin with GABA and receives its dopaminergic influence via D_2 receptors.[5] The globus pallidus interna/substantia nigra pars reticulata then projects inhibitory GABA fibers to thalamic targets that complete the circuit by sending a final excitatory gultaminergic connection to the cortical site of the circuit's origin in the frontal lobe (Figure 3–1).

Each circuit is a closed loop; dedicated neurons remain anatomically segregated from the parallel chains of neurons in the other circuits. There are, however, open elements in each circuit. Reciprocal connections between the cortical source of each circuit and regions outside the circuit modulate the circuit's activity. These reciprocal, as well as unreciprocated afferent and efferent, connections unite regions that share functions with each specific circuit. Circuits mediating limbic function connect to other limbic regions, whereas those involved with executive function interact with regions subserving cognition. Thus, the circuits integrate information from anatomically disparate but functionally related brain regions.

The anatomical segregation of each circuit supports the concept of circuit-specific behaviors. The dorsolateral prefrontal subcortical circuit mediates executive function; the lateral orbitofrontal subcortical circuit mediates socially critical restraint and object-affect associations; the medial portion of the orbitofrontal circuit's anatomy suggests greater involvement with mood, emotion, and appetitive urges; and the anterior cingulate subcortical circuit mediates motivation. Executive dysfunction, disinhibition, and apathy are the respective marker behaviors for dysfunction in these

circuits. The numerous structures and various transmitters, receptors, and modulators involved in these circuits account for the observation that lesions in different brain regions may have similar behavioral effects and that a variety of pharmacological interventions may have similar effects on behavioral disturbances.

Growing refinement of the brain's connectional anatomy is derived from nonhuman primate tracer studies, and all cortical anatomy described in this review is extrapolated from the Walker's areas in nonhuman primates to their homologous Brodmann's[6] areas on a human brain image. Many areas are homologous, but some are not—the orbitofrontal cortex is such an example.[7,8] In cases in which homology is not present, we interpret the animal connectional data with reference to the human clinical lesion data to locate the cortical regions. Future detailed clinical and functional imaging analysis will continue to refine the functional anatomical models described here.

Dorsolateral Prefrontal Circuit

The dorsolateral prefrontal subcortical circuit originates in Brodmann's areas 9 and 10 on the lateral surface of the anterior frontal lobe (Figure 3–2A). Neurons in these regions project to the dorsolateral head of the caudate nucleus.[9] From there, a projection is sent to the lateral aspect of the mediodorsal globus pallidus interna and rostrolateral substantia nigra pars reticulata via the direct pathway.[10] The indirect pathway connects the dorsal globus pallidus externa with the lateral subthalamic nucleus[11]; fibers from there target the globus pallidus interna/substantia nigra pars reticulata. Output from these two structures terminates in the parvocellular portions of the ventral anterior and mediodorsal thalamus, respectively.[12,13] The mediodorsal thalamus closes the circuit by projecting back to the circuit's origin in areas 9 and 10 of the dorsolateral frontal lobe.[14,15] Figures 3–2 and 3–3 illustrate the segregated anatomy of the circuits.

Functionally, the dorsolateral prefrontal circuit subserves executive function.[2] Executive functions include the ability to organize a behavioral response to solve a complex problem (including learning new information, copying complicated figures, and systematically searching memory), activation of remote memories, self-direction and independence from environmental contingencies, shifting and maintaining behavioral sets appropriately, generating motor programs, and using verbal skills to guide behavior (Table 3–1).

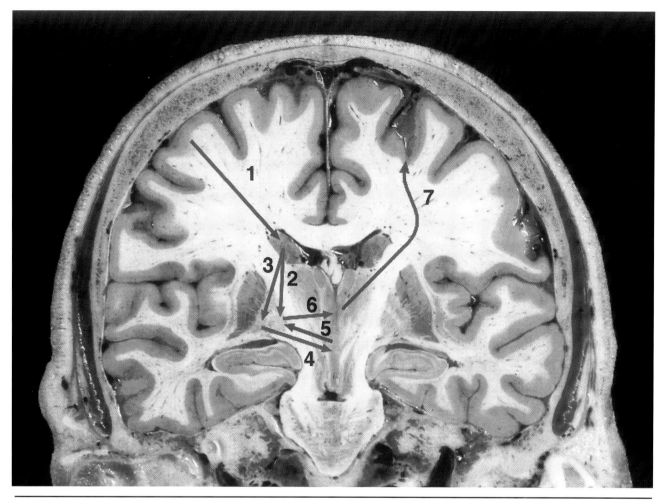

FIGURE 3–1.   Direct and indirect frontal subcortical loops (red arrows indicate excitatory connections; blue arrows indicate inhibitory connections).

1=Excitatory glutaminergic corticostriatal fibers.

2=Direct loop's inhibitory γ–aminobutyric acid (GABA)/substance P fibers (associated with D_1 dopamine receptors) from the striatum to the globus pallidus interna/substantia nigra pars reticulata.

3=Indirect loop's inhibitory GABA/enkephalin fibers (associated with D_2 dopamine receptors) from the striatum to the globus pallidus externa.

4=Indirect loop's inhibitory GABA fibers from the globus pallidus externa to the subthalamic nucleus.

5=Indirect loop's excitatory glutaminergic fibers from the subthalamic nucleus to the globus pallidus interna/substantia nigra pars reticulata.

6=Basal ganglia inhibitory outflow via GABA fibers from the globus pallidus interna/substantia nigra pars reticulata to specific thalamic sites.

7=Thalamic excitatory fibers returning to cortex (shown in contralateral hemisphere for convenience).

Damage to the dorsolateral frontal lobe produces deficits in executive function. Not all executive skills are reduced with all lesions; a spectrum of severity, as well as variation in the abilities compromised, is evident among patients with dorsolateral prefrontal dysfunction. Successful performance of the Wisconsin Card Sorting Test (WCST) requires several of the functions mediated by this brain region, including set shifting and maintenance, strategy generation, and organization of information.[16] The WCST has proved to be particularly sensitive to dorsolateral prefrontal abnormalities. Reduced verbal and design fluency, poor organizational strategies in learning tasks, and impoverished strategies on complex constructional tests are also observed.[17,18] Impairment of sequential motor tasks, such as alternating and reciprocal sequences, is

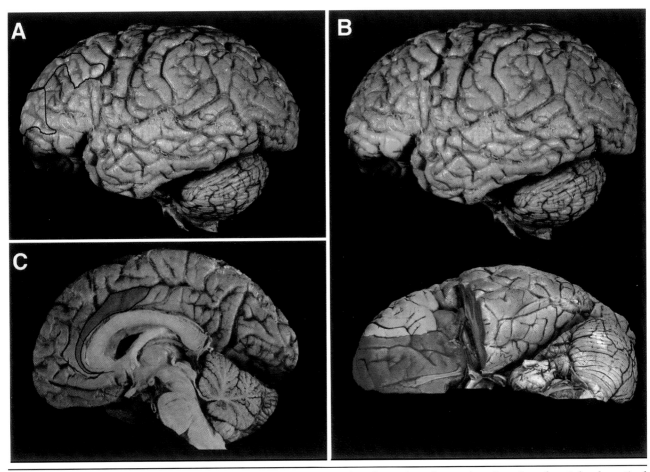

FIGURE 3–2.   Cortical sites of origin for the dorsolateral, orbitofrontal, and anterior cingulate frontal subcortical circuits.

A: Origin of the dorsolateral circuit. Brodmann's areas 9 and 10 are colored blue on the superior and inferior dorsolateral prefrontal cortex.   **B:** Origin of the orbitofrontal circuit. The medial division is in red and includes Brodmann's area 14 and the medial portion of areas 11 and 13 in monkeys—all equivalent to the gyrus rectus and medial orbital gyrus of area 11 in human. The lateral division is in green and includes the lateral portion of Brodmann's areas 11 and 13 and all of 12 in monkey—all equivalent to the lateral orbital gyrus of area 11 and the medial inferior frontal gyrus of areas 10 and 47 in human. The insula is shown in purple.   **C:** Origin of the anterior cingulate circuit. The anterior portion of Brodmann's area 24 is colored red on the medial frontal cortex.

characteristic of dorsolateral prefrontal dysfunction.[19] Executive function requires the integration of prefrontal and subcortical activity. Thus, similar behavioral changes are noted with lesions of the dorsolateral prefrontal cortex and subcortical structures linked to this region or from white matter lesions that disconnect circuit members. Neuropsychiatric disturbances include depression and anxiety with dorsolateral prefrontal strokes[20,21] and depression with caudate dysfunction in stroke and basal ganglia disorders.[20,22]

Orbitofrontal Circuit

The orbitofrontal cortex has two major subdivisions in monkeys: a lateral division containing the lateral por-

tion of areas 11 and 13 and all of 12 and a medial division comprising area 14 and the medial portion of 11 and 13.[23] Inferior portions of area 25 in the medial posterior prefrontal region and areas 24 and 32 in the inferorostral cingulate gyrus share connectional similarities with the medial orbital division.[24] The lateral orbitofrontal circuit sends projections to the ventromedial caudate[9] from its source in the ventral portion of areas 10 and 47 and the lateral portion of area 11 (interpreted as homologous to the lateral portions of areas 11 and 13 and all of area 12 in macaques—Brodmann did not find cytoarchitectural equivalents for areas 12 and 13 in humans) shown in Figure 3–2B. The ventromedial portion of the caudate projects directly

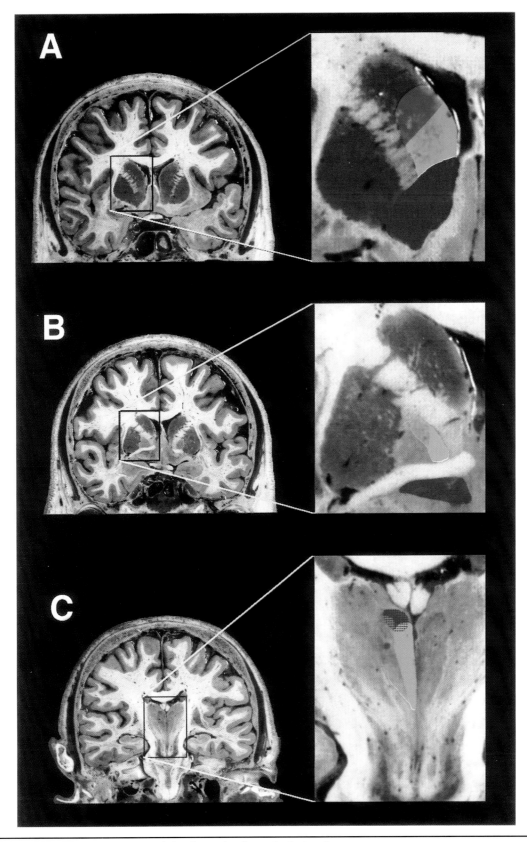

FIGURE 3–3. Segregated anatomy of the frontal subcortical circuits.

The general segregated anatomy of the dorsolateral (blue), lateral orbitofrontal (green), and anterior cingulate (red) circuits in the striatum **(A),** pallidum **(B),** and mediodorsal thalamus **(C).**

TABLE 3–1. Summary and classification of executive cognitive dysfunctions associated with disorders of the dorsolateral prefrontal cortex

Classification	Impaired functions
Poor organizational strategies	Segmented drawings
	Impaired organization of material to be learned
	Poor word list generation
	Reduced design fluency
	Poor sorting behavior
Poor memory search strategies	Reduced word list generation
	Poor recall of remote information
	Poor recall of recently learned information
Stimulus-bound behavior/environmental dependency	Poor set shifting
	Concrete interpretation of abstract concepts and proverbs
	"Pull" toward high-stimulus objects
	Imitation behavior
	Utilization behavior
	Reduced design fluency
	Impaired reciprocal programs
	Poor go/no-go performance
	Poor response inhibition (Stroop Color Word Test)
Impaired set shifting and maintenance	Impaired card sorting
	Poor alternation between concepts
	Perseveration on multiple loops, alternating programs, reciprocal programs, go/no-go test, Luria serial hand sequences
Verbal-manual dissociation	Impaired Luria serial hand sequences

Note. Items appear several times when they have multiple determinants.

to the most medial portion of the mediodorsal globus pallidus interna and to the rostromedial substantia nigra pars reticulata.[25] The ventromedial caudate also sends an indirect loop through the dorsal globus pallidus externa to the lateral subthalamic nucleus, which then projects to the globus pallidus interna and substantia nigra pars reticulata.[11] Neurons are sent from the globus pallidus and substantia nigra to the medial section of the magnocellular division of the ventral anterior thalamus as well as an inferomedial sector of the magnocellular division of the mediodorsal thalamus.[9,13] The circuit then closes with projections from this thalamic region to the lateral orbitofrontal cortex.[13] This anatomical segregation is illustrated in Figure 3–3.

The lateral orbitofrontal circuit mediates empathic, civil, and socially appropriate behavior and takes part in object-affect associations; personality change is the hallmark of orbitofrontal dysfunction. Irritability, lability (rapid shifts from one mood to another), tactless-ness, and fatuous euphoria have been described in patients with lesions of this area.[26–28] Patients do not respond appropriately to social cues, show undue familiarity in interpersonal relationships, and are unable to empathize with the feelings of others. Irritability and lability are often prominent. A positron-emission tomography (PET) activation study supports the involvement of the lateral orbitofrontal cortex in processing visual social cues; expressions of anger, presented in increasing intensity, activated the right lateral orbitofrontal cortex in control subjects.[29] Utilization behavior (inappropriate automatic use of tools and utensils in the patient's environment) and automatic imitation of the gestures and actions of others may occur with large lesions.[30] Similar behavioral changes are evident in patients with dysfunction of the subcortical structures of the lateral orbitofrontal subcortical circuit, including patients with Huntington's disease (caudate abnormalities) and manganese intoxication (globus pallidus lesions).[22,31]

Obsessive-compulsive disorder, a condition characterized by increased behavioral control, overconcern about social behaviors and contamination, and excessive investment in social appropriateness, is characterized by increased metabolic activity in the orbitofrontal cortex and increased caudate metabolism.[32–34] Lesions of the globus pallidus (by virtue of the resulting thalamic disinhibition) also have been associated with obsessive-compulsive disorder.[35] An inverse functional balance between the orbitofrontal cortex and the amygdala is best demonstrated in functional imaging studies of depression with an increase in amygdalar activity and a decrease in orbitofrontal activity associated with depression severity that normalizes with treatment response.[36] A serotonergic imbalance in the orbitofrontal cortex also may subserve aggressive behavior. Impulsively aggressive patients have significantly blunted metabolic responses on [18F]fluorodeoxyglucose-PET to serotonergic stimulation in orbitofrontal and adjacent ventromedial cingulate cortices compared with control subjects without impulsive aggression.[37]

The medial division of the orbitofrontal cortex (Brodmann's area 14, and the medial portion of 11 and 13 in monkeys—all equivalent to the gyrus rectus and medial orbital gyrus of area 11 in humans) mediates mood and neurovegetative function.[38] Brain areas that have reciprocal connections with the medial orbitofrontal cortex influence visceral function when stimulated,[39] probably because of their shared amygdalar connections that convey the visceral state of the organism to the entire orbitofrontal and medial posterior frontal cortex. The severity of negative symptoms in schizophrenia is significantly correlated with orbitofrontal grey matter volume.[40]

The medial orbitofrontal cortex, along with the medial infracallosal anterior cingulate (Brodmann's area 25 and the inferior portion of 24 and 32), share similar subcortical circuit members as well as efferent and afferent connections with visceromotor centers and with the magnocellular basolateral amygdala.[24] Mania has been observed in patients with orbitofrontal lesions, caudate dysfunction in basal ganglia disorders, and lesions of the thalamus.[41–43] Hypofunctioning of the medial division of the orbitofrontal cortex is associated with depressive symptoms in patients with Parkinson's disease[44] that normalize when the mood disorder is treated successfully. In nonhuman primates, the orbitofrontal cortex processes the motivation associated with rewards resulting from voluntary action.[45] Table 3–2 summarizes the principal abnormalities asso-

TABLE 3–2. Summary of cognitive and behavioral abnormalities associated with disorders of the medial and lateral orbitofrontal cortex

Medial orbitofrontal cortex	Lateral orbitofrontal cortex
Personality change	**Personality change**
Anergy	Irritability
Anhedonia	Tactlessness
Neurovegetative changes	Fatuous euphoria
Hyper- or hypophagia	Impulsivity
Circadian dysfunction	Undue familiarity
Alimentary changes	**Environmental dependency**
Mood disorders	Utilization behavior
Depression	Imitation behavior
Dysphoria	**Mood disorders**
Obsessive-compulsive disorder	Lability
	Mania
	Obsessive-compulsive disorder

ciated with dysfunction of the lateral and medial orbitofrontal cortex.

Anterior Cingulate Circuit

From the supracallosal anterior cingulate, Brodmann's area 24 (Figure 3–2C), input is provided to the ventral striatum,[9] which includes the ventromedial caudate, ventral putamen, nucleus accumbens, and olfactory tubercle. This area is termed the *limbic striatum*.[46] Projections from the ventral striatum innervate the rostromedial globus pallidus interna and ventral pallidum (the region of the globus pallidus inferior to the anterior commissure) as well as the rostrodorsal substantia nigra.[47] An indirect loop also may project from the ventral striatum to the rostral pole of the globus pallidus externa.[47] The external pallidum in turn connects to the medial subthalamic nucleus, which returns projections to the ventral pallidum.[11] The ventral pallidum provides some input to the magnocellular mediodorsal thalamus.[48] The anterior cingulate circuit closes with projections from the dorsal portion of the magnocellular mediodorsal thalamus to the anterior cingulate.[15,49] The anatomy of this circuit is illustrated in Figure 3–3.

The anterior cingulate subcortical circuit mediates motivated behavior, and apathy is the marker behavior of dysfunction of structures of this circuit. Akinetic mutism occurs with bilateral lesions of the anterior cingulate. Patients are profoundly apathetic. They rarely move, are incontinent, and eat and drink only when fed; if speech occurs, it is limited to monosyllabic responses to others' questions. Displaying no emotions, even when in pain, patients show complete indifference to their circumstances.[50–52] Transient akinetic mutism with similar features occurs with unilateral lesions.[53] Transcortical motor aphasia is also the result of left anterior cingulate or anterior dorsolateral prefrontal lesions.[54,55] The classic syndrome of transcortical motor aphasia is initial mutism that resolves in days to weeks, yielding delayed initiation of brief phrases without impaired articulation, excellent repetition, inappropriate word selection, agrammatism, and poor comprehension of complex syntax.[56,57] Direct damage to the anterior cingulate, its outflow to other cortical areas (9, 10, and 46) or to the caudate—via the subcallosal fasciculus,[58] just inferior to the frontal horn of the lateral ventricle—will disrupt the frontal subcortical circuits involved in motivation and executive cognitive functions.[59] Failure of response inhibition on go/no-go tests is the major neuropsychological deficit in patients with medial frontal damage.[60,61] Apathy is also prominent in patients with disorders affecting the subcortical links of the anterior cingulate circuit, including Parkinson's disease, Huntington's disease, progressive supranuclear palsy,[62] and thalamic lesions.[63–65] Table 3–3 summarizes the principal abnormalities associated with dysfunction of the anterior cingulate cortex.

CIRCUIT CONNECTIONS

The activity within each frontal subcortical circuit constitutes a closed loop of neural processing dedicated to the specific functions subserved by that circuit. Neuronal activity in brain areas outside the member structures of a particular circuit may provide functionally relevant input to a circuit via efferent connections to the prefrontal cortex, striatum, globus pallidus, substantia nigra, or thalamus. The circuits also send efferents outside the loop to functionally related brain areas. These noncircuit connections constitute the open aspects of circuits.

An examination of the open aspects of each circuit facilitates understanding of how information processed in different brain regions can be integrated and synthesized in the processing cascade of the closed loop. Open aspects of the circuits serve to unify di-

TABLE 3–3. Summary of cognitive and behavioral abnormalities associated with disorders of the anterior cingulate prefrontal cortex

Impaired motivation
    Akinetic mutism
    Marked apathy
    Psychic emptiness/reduced creativity
    Transcortical motor aphasia
    Poverty of spontaneous speech

Indifference to pain

Poor response inhibition
    Impaired go/no-go test performance

verse brain regions into functional systems relevant to specific behaviors. The frontal subcortical circuits provide the anatomical framework for the final effector mechanisms of these distributed systems. Open elements of the circuits relate systematically to other brain regions that both mediate related functions and have similar phylogenetic origins. Review of the evolutionary development of cortical and subcortical structures makes these functional and phylogenetic alliances apparent.

At the subcortical level, two cytoarchitectonic divisions are evident. These are most apparent in the thalamus, where one is termed *magnocellular* because of the larger cell bodies of the neurons compared with the smaller sized cells of the *parvocellular* regions.[66] The larger magnocellular neurons predominate in phylogenetically older regions of the thalamus and participate in more primitive functions mediated by the limbic system, whereas the parvocellular regions have appeared more recently in phylogenetic development and participate in more recently acquired cognitive functions.

The cerebral cortex also has two regions with distinct evolutionary origins that are reflected in their different architectural organization and contrasting functions. Cortical development across mammals occurred in two waves originating from two primordial regions within the limbic ring (Figure 3–4). One developmental wave began in the orbitofrontal region of the olfactory *paleocortex* in primitive monotremes such as the duck-billed platypus, whose cortex is almost entirely olfactory in function. This paleocortical progression spread ventrolaterally up through the insula, temporal pole, and anterior parahippocampal area. The inte-

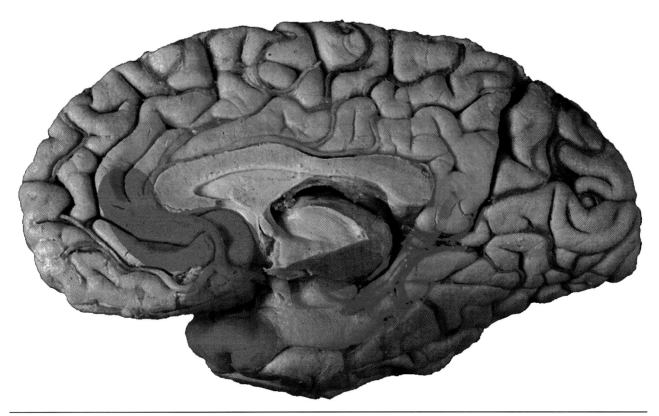

FIGURE 3–4. Paralimbic trends of evolutionary cortical development.
The paleocortical orbitofrontal-centered belt (red) extends into the subcallosal cingulate, temporal polar region, and the anterior insula (not shown). The archicortical hippocampal-centered trend (blue) extends its wave of cortical development dorsally through the posterior and anterior cingulate.

gration of appetitive drives with aversion or attraction to stimuli dominated paleocortical function. A second nidus of cortical development was centered in the *archicortex* of the hippocampus and spread posteriorly through the entorhinal, posterior parahippocampal regions, and through the cingulate. The archicortex was largely concerned with the integration of information from different sensory modalities—the first step away from thalamic control, as seen in reptiles, toward cortical dominance. By virtue of their connections and the parallel development of other brain regions linked to these two limbic divisions, the behavioral evolution of mammals mirrored the progressive trend toward cytoarchitectural complexity emanating from both the olfactory and the hippocampal centers.[67] Mesulam[68] described these two allocortical divisions as *paralimbic belts*.

The olfactory orbitofrontal belt is closely associated with the amygdala. Through mammalian evolution, the paleocortical division paralleled phylogenetic development of the amygdala. Two basic divisions of the amygdala in higher primates include the anterior cor-

ticobasolateral group, which supports cortical association connections, and the centromedian nuclear group, which is related to the olfactory bulb, diencephalon, and brain stem. The archicortical division has the hippocampus as its center, emphasizes pyramidal cells, and gives rise to the medial supplementary sensory and motor areas. The dorsal visual system, which processes the *location* of objects,[69] also is associated with the hippocampal archicortical paralimbic belt. The paleocortical division emphasizes granular cells as it differentiates into secondary somatosensory, auditory, and visual cortices; it is more directly coupled with the ventral visual system involved in object *feature* analysis.[67]

The highly differentiated dorsolateral prefrontal region mediates executive function, the medial prefrontal cortex provides motivation, and the orbitofrontal regions mediate mood and object-affect associations. The parvocellular and magnocellular regions of the dorsomedial thalamus project to the most differentiated and least differentiated prefrontal cortical areas, respectively. These prefrontal areas connect with other cortical areas that serve as open inputs to the circuits. In each case, the circuit connections share phylogenetic, cytoarchitectonic, and functional features. We emphasize the cortical regions related to the cortical source of the three frontal subcortical circuits.

Dorsolateral Prefrontal Circuit: Reciprocal Connections and Open Afferents and Efferents

In addition to Brodmann's areas 9 and 10, which serve as the frontal origin of the closed loop for the circuit, Brodmann's prefrontal area 46,[9] area 8, and area 7a of the caudal superior parietal lobe[70] are reciprocally connected to the cortical source of the dorsolateral prefrontal subcortical circuit (Figure 3–5A). Open afferents, which terminate in the dorsolateral caudate (not shown in Figure 3–5), are listed in Table 3–4. These include the dorsal parafascicular thalamus, the medial pars compacta of the substantia nigra, the dorsal raphe, and the central midbrain tegmentum.[71,72] The efferent projections of the dorsolateral circuit, emanating from the parvocellular ventral anterior and mediodorsal thalamus, close the circuit by terminating in areas 9 and 10 of the dorsolateral frontal lobe. A major open target is the anterior supplementary motor cortex of area 6.[15]

Parietal area 7a subserves visuospatial attention, visually guided reaching, and planning of visuospatial strategies. There are rich interconnections between area 7a and frontal areas 9, 10, and 46.[70] The minor open aspects of the executive circuit provide ascending thalamic, nigral, and brain stem input to the dorsolateral caudate. The parafascicular thalamus receives input primarily from the supplementary frontal eye fields, superior colliculus, and prefrontal cortex.[71] The entire substantia nigra pars compacta receives significant input from the ventral pallidum, which allows limbic influence to reach the striatum via dopaminergic projections from the substantia nigra pars compacta.[48] Serotonergic and noradrenergic modulatory influences reach the dorsolateral circuit from the dorsal raphé and central midbrain tegmentum. Open output to the supplementary motor area assists in the integration of executive and motor function. These reciprocal and open cortical regions are within the same dorsal architectonic derivation as the source (areas 9 and 10) of the circuit. The phylogenetically similar regions also connect with parvocellular regions of the thalamus dedicated to the dorsolateral prefrontal circuit.

TABLE 3–4. Reciprocal connections and open afferents and efferents of the dorsolateral circuit

Reciprocal connections
  Dorsofrontal area 46
  Frontal eye fields area 8
  Dorsofrontal area 7a

Open afferents
  Dorsal parafascicular thalamus
  Medial pars compacta of substantia nigra
  Dorsal raphé
  Central midbrain tegmentum

Open efferents
  Anterior frontal area 6

Orbitofrontal Circuit: Reciprocal Connections and Open Afferents and Efferents

The major reciprocal connections with the source of the lateral orbitofrontal circuit are with the dorsal and caudal portions of the basal and the accessory basal (magnocellular division) amygdala,[23,73–76] supracallosal cingulate areas 24 and 32,[75,77,78] dorsolateral temporal pole area 38,[23,75,79] inferior temporal cortex TE area 20,[23] and the supplementary eye field in the dorsal portion of area 6.[24] Open afferent inputs to the lateral orbitofrontal cortex originate in the rostromedial parafascicular thalamus,[71] medial substantia nigra pars compacta, dorsal raphe, and central midbrain tegmentum.[72] Open efferent targets of the orbitofrontal circuit receiving projections from the medial division of magnocellular ventral anterior and mediodorsal thalamus are areas 33 and 25 in the infracallosal cingulate, area 32 in the inferorostral cingulate gyrus, and the anterior agranular insular cortex.[15,49] The major cortical regions connected with the lateral division of the orbitofrontal subcortical circuit are shown in Table 3–5 and Figure 3–5B.

The lateral orbital cortex is a gateway for highly processed sensory information into the orbitofrontal paralimbic center. The dorsal portion of the basal amygdala is the source of projections to the ventral visual processing system in the inferior temporal cortex. The supracallosal anterior cingulate assists in the dorsolateral attentional system and effects cognitive engagement. The rostral auditory association cortex in the superior temporal area provides auditory information to the lateral orbitofrontal cortex; and the inferior

Frontal Subcortical Circuits 25

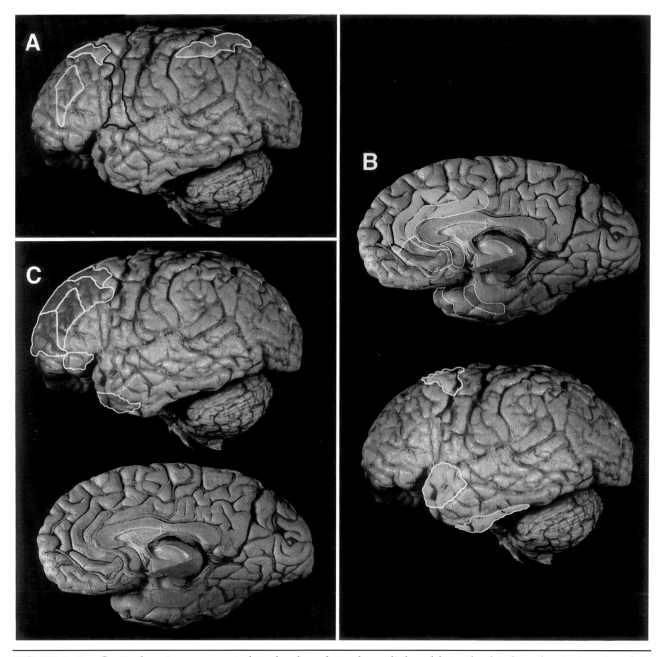

FIGURE 3–5. Cortical regions connected to the dorsolateral, medial and lateral orbital, and anterior cingulate frontal subcortical circuits.

A: The cortical regions that have major reciprocal connections (outlined in yellow) with the cortical origin of the dorsolateral frontal subcortical circuit include dorsolateral prefrontal areas 46 and 8 and caudal superior parietal area 7a. The major open efferent target (outlined in black) of the dorsolateral circuit arising from the parvocellular anterior and mediodorsal thalamus is the anterior supplementary motor cortex of area 6.   **B:** The cortical regions that have major reciprocal connections (outlined in yellow) with the cortical origin of the medial portion (red) of the orbitofrontal subcortical circuit include infracallosal areas 25, 24, and 32; ventromedial temporal area 38; and anterior entorhinal area 36 (amygdala and insular regions are not shown). The cortical regions that have major reciprocal connections with the lateral portion (green) of the orbitofrontal subcortical circuit include supracallosal areas 24 and 32, dorsolateral temporal pole area 38, inferior temporal area 20, and the dorsal supplementary eye fields of area 6 (amygdala regions are not shown).   **C:** The cortical regions that have major reciprocal connections (outlined in yellow) with the cortical origin of the anterior cingulate circuit include dorsolateral prefrontal areas 8, 9, 10, and 46; anterior parahippocampal areas 35 and 36; caudal lateral orbitofrontal area 47; and anterior inferior temporal pole area 38 (amygdala, insula, and claustrum are not shown). The major cortical open afferent inputs (outlined in blue) to the anterior cingulate circuit project from entorhinal area 28 and perirhinal area 35.

TABLE 3–5. Reciprocal connections and open afferents and efferents of the medial and lateral orbitofrontal circuits

Medial orbitofrontal division	Lateral orbitofrontal division
Reciprocal connections	
Medial portion of the basal amygdala	Dorsal and caudal portions of the basal amygdala
Accessory basal magnocellular amygdala	Accessory basal magnocellular amygdala
Infracallosal areas 25, 24, and 32	Supracallosal areas 24 and 32
Rostral (agranular) insula	Dorsolateral temporal pole area 38
Ventromedial temporal pole area 38	Inferior temporal cortex TE area 20
Anterior entorhinal cortex area 36	Supplementary eye field dorsal portion of area 6
Open afferents	
Anterior subiculum of hippocampus	Rostromedial parafascicular thalamus
Medial pars compacta of substantia nigra	Medial pars compacta of substantia nigra
Dorsal raphé	Dorsal raphé
Central midbrain tegmentum	Central midbrain tegmentum
Open efferents	
Area 33 in the infracallosal cingulate	Areas 33 and 25 in the infracallosal cingulate
Anterior agranular insular cortex	Area 32 in the infracallosal cingulate gyrus
	Anterior agranular insular cortex

temporal region TE is the last processing step for the ventral visual system devoted to object feature analysis. The reciprocal connections with the supplementary eye field in the dorsal portion of area 6 highlight the control over sensory information acquisition within lateral orbitofrontal cortex. The open afferents supply ascending reticular and modulatory innervation from the brain stem. Most of the open efferents of the orbitofrontal circuit correspond to the olfactory-centered paralimbic belt.[68]

The medial division of the orbitofrontal cortex has reciprocal connections with the medial portion of the basal and the accessory basal (magnocellular division) amygdala[23,73–76]; medial infracallosal cingulate areas 25, 24, and 32[75,77,78]; the rostral (agranular) insula[75,76,80]; ventromedial temporal pole area 38[23,75,79]; and anterior entorhinal area 36.[23,81] Brain areas that have reciprocal connections with the medial orbitofrontal cortex also influence visceral function when stimulated,[39] probably because of their shared amygdalar connections that convey the visceral state of the organism to the orbitofrontal region. The visceral effector region of the infracallosal cingulate adds motivational input to gustatory, olfactory, and alimentary information from anterior insular regions connected to the medial orbitofrontal cortex. The rostromedial entorhinal cortex is a paleocortical extension providing hippocampal interaction. No visual information has direct access to the medial division of the orbitofrontal center, which

serves as an integrator of visceral drives while modulating the organism's internal milieu. Open afferents and efferents to the medial orbitofrontal cortex are similar to those of the lateral division except for anterior subicular input from the hippocampal region.[23] The major cortical regions connected to the medial division of the orbitofrontal paralimbic center are shown in Table 3–5 and Figure 3–5B.

Anterior Cingulate Circuit: Reciprocal Connections and Open Afferents and Efferents

Reciprocal connections to area 24, the source of the anterior cingulate circuit, are with prefrontal areas 8, 9, 10, and 46,[75,82] the basal amygdala (magno- and parvocellular divisions),[73–76] anterior parahippocampal areas 35 and 36,[75,78,83] caudal lateral orbitofrontal area 12 in monkeys (equivalent to area 47 in humans),[75,77,78] anterior inferior temporal pole area 38,[75,79] the rostral (agranular) insula,[75,76,80] and the anterior medial claustrum.[83,84] Areas reciprocally connected to the anterior cingulate frontal subcortical circuit are more phylogenetically recent neocortical regions of dorsolateral prefrontal areas 8, 9, 10, and 46 devoted to cognitive executive function. The amygdala provides internal affective input to area 24. The distribution of amygdala efferents delineates the dorsal boundary of the cingulate as a functional system. Reciprocal connections with the orbitofrontal, insular, and temporal polar areas also convey affect and visceral information. Rostral insular cortex is a transitional paralimbic region that integrates visceral alimentary input with olfactory and gustatory afferents.[85] Auditory input arises from the anterior medial claustrum, as well as a minor link with the auditory association area of the superior temporal gyrus.[75] Connections with the anterior parahippocampal areas 35 and 36 allow the anterior cingulate circuit to influence multimodal sensory afferents entering the hippocampus. Open afferent sources projecting to area 24 include the hippocampus, entorhinal and perirhinal areas 28 and 35, the subparafascicular thalamus, the dorsal raphe, and the central midbrain tegmentum.[71,72]

The projections from the dorsal portion of the magnocellular mediodorsal thalamus close the anterior cingulate circuit by terminating in area 24 of the anterior cingulate.[15,49] Major open targets of the anterior cingulate circuit from the ventral pallidum are the entire mediolateral range of the substantia nigra pars compacta, the medial subthalamic nucleus, and its extension into the lateral hypothalamus.[48] Other minor open ventropallidal efferent targets include the midline nuclei of the thalamus, which have a major projection to the anterior cingulate,[86] the dorsal portion of both the globus pallidus interna and the globus pallidus externa, the lateral habenula, the central gray regions of the midbrain, and the pedunculopontine nucleus of the midbrain tegmentum.[48] The major cortical regions connected to the anterior cingulate frontal subcortical circuit are shown in Table 3–6 and Figure 3–5C.

The major afferent input to the anterior cingulate circuit represents the dorsal archicortical region originating in the hippocampus.[68] This hippocampal-centered system contains the cingulate and parahippocampal components of the paralimbic cortex. The anterior cingulate also has strong paleocortical input; it represents a convergence zone between the two limbic divisions. Each reflects different phylogenetic organizations within the limbic system. The orbitofrontal-centered belt is involved with the internal state of the organism. The hippocampal-centered belt is the externally directed division of the limbic system. The two divisions work in concert. Processing in the anterior cingulate circuit provides motivation for the intentional selection of environmental stimuli based on the internal relevance of those stimuli for the organism. Input about that internal relevance is provided by the orbitofrontal circuit. Damage to this circuit would disrupt the integration of emotional information with motivational mechanisms and produce unmotivated, apathetic behavior.

TABLE 3–6. Reciprocal connections and open afferents and efferents of the anterior cingulate circuit

Reciprocal connections
Prefrontal areas 8, 9, 10, and 46
Basal amygdala (magno- and parvocellular)
Anterior parahippocampal areas 35 and 36
Caudal lateral orbitofrontal cortex area 47
Anterior inferior temporal pole area 38
Rostral insula
Anterior medial claustrum

Open afferents
Hippocampus
Entorhinal area 28
Perirhinal area 35
Subparafascicular thalamus
Dorsal raphé
Central midbrain tegmentum

Open efferent targets
Pars compacta of substantia nigra
Medial subthalamic nucleus
Lateral hypothalamus
Midline thalamic nuclei
Dorsal globus pallidus interna/externa
Lateral habenula
Central gray region
Pedunculopontine nucleus

NEUROCHEMICAL ORGANIZATION

The striatum has two distinct organizational systems, the striosomes and the matrix. These two components are differentiated by their chemical, ontological, and connectional properties.[87] The acetylcholine-poor neurons of the striosomes mature earlier than the acetylcholine-rich cells of the matrix. Striosomes also have lower concentrations of dopamine and serotonin than do the matrix cells.[88] Striosomes have a high concentration of limbic-associated membrane protein[89] and receive dense orbitofrontal and insular input. In contrast, input to the matrix originates predominantly from the sensorimotor cortex. Dopaminergic input to striosomes is derived from the ventral tier of the substantia nigra pars compacta, in contrast to the more dorsal tier nigral input to the matrix.[90] GABAergic output from the striosomes is to the medial portion of the pars compacta of the substantia nigra, dedicated to the orbitofrontal circuit and other limbic sites, whereas GABAergic output from the matrix targets the external and internal globus pallidus and pars reticulata portion of the substantia nigra.

The effect of transmitter dysfunction within the circuits has been extensively studied in Parkinson's disease. The loss of striatal dopamine decreases thalamocortical activation by decreasing the inhibitory outflow of the direct loop (Figure 3–1) and increasing activity in the indirect loop.[91] The direct loop's D_1 receptors, which stimulate the second messenger adenylyl cyclase, are excitatory and thus release more GABA to inhibit the globus pallidus interna/substantia nigra pars reticulata. The D_2 receptors of the indirect loop inhibit adenylyl cyclase, causing decreased GABAergic inhibition of the globus pallidus externa. This results in an increased GABAergic inhibition of the excitatory outflow from the subthalamic nucleus to the globus pallidus interna/substantia nigra pars reticulata. The direct loop's inhibition and indirect loop's excitation imposed on the outflow of the basal ganglia are normally balanced by the differential effect nigral dopamine has on the striatum. Pallidal outflow inhibits thalamocortical excitation. Parkinson's disease, by decreasing direct loop inhibition, leads to an unchecked increase in indirect loop excitation on pallidal outflow, resulting in an attenuation of normal thalamocortical activation. Reduced cortical activation correlates with the clinical phenomenology of parkisonism.

The subcortical dopaminergic deficit in each circuit may differ in degenerative disease. The ventral tegmental area and medial portion of the ventral tier of the substantia nigra pars compacta provide dopaminergic innervation to the cortical and subcortical limbic forebrain.[92–94] The severity of dementia in Parkinson's disease is related to decreased cortical dopamine[95,96] and ventral tegmental area cell loss.[97] For these patients with dementia and Parkinson's disease, more thalamocortical deactivation occurs in the anterior cingulate circuit than occurs in the nondemented patients, an effect that may contribute to apathy and anhedonia. Dopaminergic projections from the pars compacta of the substantia nigra innervate the entire striatum and thus may influence all frontal subcortical circuits. The pars compacta of the substantia nigra receives diffuse input from the anterior cingulate circuit and thus provides a means for limbic *motivational* input to influence both motor activity and cognition. This anatomical arrangement provides an important convergence of limbic activation within the otherwise segregated frontal subcortical circuits.

The distribution of the D_3 receptor subtype localizes to limbic regions similar to the D_4 receptor, which may have a greater concentration in the amygdala and frontal cortex. The D_5 receptor is found in the hippocampus and hypothalamus, whereas the D_2 subtype is found in sensorimotor striatal regions. Regional difference in dopamine receptor subtypes has promoted the development of dopamine receptor antagonists specific to limbic regions, such as the D_4 antagonist clozapine, with fewer motor side effects than typical neuroleptics for the treatment of psychosis. Dopaminergic innervation of the anterior cingulate may be disrupted with subcortical lesions of the medial forebrain bundle[98] or the ventral pallidum, resulting in profound apathy or even akinetic mutism that responds to agents such as bromocriptine. Dopaminergic modulation of all the prefrontal subcortical circuits provides an anatomical basis for the multifaceted effects of dopaminergic agents, including improved motor function in Parkinson's disease, enhanced motivation in akinetic mutism, elevated mood, and hallucinations and delusions.[98,99]

The cholinergic system also has a differential input to the frontal subcortical circuits. Acetylcholine facilitates thalamic activation of the cortex. Most thalamic cholinergic input originates in the pedunculopontine and laterodorsal tegmentum; however, portions of the mediodorsal, ventroanterior, and reticular nuclei that participate in the cognitive and behavioral prefrontal subcortical circuits receive input from the nucleus basalis of Meynert in the basal forebrain.[100] The brain stem cholinergic nuclei are affected in progressive supranuclear palsy but not in Alzheimer's disease, which preferentially affects the nucleus basalis.[101] Thus, the cognitive differences between these two degenerative disorders may, in part, have a basis in the specific disruption each has in restricted portions of the frontal subcortical circuits and related cholinergic systems.

Serotonin (5-hydroxytryptamine; 5-HT) receptors are differentially distributed in the frontal subcortical circuits. The 5-HT_1 receptor is the most abundant serotonin receptor in the basal ganglia. The ventral striatum, the principal striatal structure of the anterior cingulate subcortical circuit, is the exception in that the 5-HT_3 receptor predominates there.[88] This finding mirrors the distribution of 5-HT_3 receptors in other areas functionally related to the anterior cingulate circuit: hippocampus, septum, and amygdala.

Immunohistochemical markers of the second messenger systems (phosphoinositide, adenylyl cyclase) in nonhuman primates appear to reflect the segregated anatomy of the frontal subcortical circuits. The phosphoinositide system is selectively concentrated in striosomes of the medial and ventral striatum, whereas the matrix selectively stains for adenylyl cyclase.[102] The phosphoinositide system has been hypothesized to play a prominent role in the mechanism of action of lithium's mood-stabilizing effect.[103] The association of this second messenger system with the limbic striatum may provide insight into how lithium exerts its effects on mood and suggests that frontal subcortical circuits may provide an anatomical basis for these effects.

The complexity created by the multiple neurotransmitter systems, the specific distribution of their receptor subtypes, the presence of several neuromodulators, and the actions of second messengers within the frontal subcortical circuits are daunting. This complexity makes predicting drug effects difficult and offers exciting possibilities for understanding the pharmacoanatomy of drug interventions as they relate to frontal subcortical circuits.

CONCLUSIONS

Frontal subcortical circuits are effector mechanisms that allow the organism to act on the environment. The dorsolateral prefrontal subcortical circuit mediates the organization of information to facilitate a response, the anterior cingulate subcortical circuit is required for motivated behavior, and the lateral orbitofrontal circuit allows the integration of limbic and emotional information into contextually appropriate behavioral responses. Neuropsychiatric syndromes observed with dysfunction of the frontal subcortical circuits are disorders of action rather than of perception or of stimulus integration. Thus, impaired executive functions, apathy, and impulsivity are hallmarks of frontal subcortical circuit dysfunction. Obsessive-compulsive behavior occurs when orbitofrontal structures are hyperactive. The mood disorders associated with frontal subcortical circuit dysfunction include mania, depression, and lability. Mania has many effector elements (hyperactivity, pressured speech, increased sexual drive, exaggerated appetite), and depression also has effector aspects (anhedonia, psychomotor retardation, anorexia).

Circuit-specific behaviors reveal an underlying organizational principle of neuropsychiatric disorders.

Neurobehavioral disorders such as aphasia arise from lesions of the cortex and have signature syndromes, such as Wernicke's aphasia or Broca's aphasia, that indicate a specific anatomical lesion. By contrast, neuropsychiatric disorders reflect circuit dysfunction, and the same syndrome can be seen with involvement of several structures of the circuit.

Neurobehavioral disorders associated with signature syndromes have proved to be treatment resistant, whereas circuit-mediated behaviors such as reduced motivation and mood abnormalities are more amenable to pharmacotherapy. The circuits involve a number of transmitters, receptor subtypes, and second messengers that can be manipulated pharmacologically. As the chemoarchitecture of the circuits is revealed, there will be an increased opportunity to construct a pharmacoanatomy that will guide circuit-specific and syndrome-specific interventions.

REFERENCES

1. Alexander GE, DeLong MR, Strick PL: Parallel organization of functionally segregated circuits linking basal ganglia and cortex. Annu Rev Neurosci 9:357–381, 1986
2. Cummings JL: Frontal-subcortical circuits and human behavior. Arch Neurol 50:873–880, 1993
3. Albin RL, Young AB, Penney JB: The functional anatomy of basal ganglia disorders. Trends Neurosci 12:366–375, 1989
4. Alexander GE, Crutcher MD: Functional architecture of basal ganglia circuits: neural substrates of parallel processing. Trends Neurosci 13:266–271, 1990
5. Groenewegen HJ, Roeling TAP, Voorn P, et al: The parallel arrangement of basal ganglia-thalamocortical circuits: a neuronal substrate for the role of dopamine in motor and cognitive functions?, in Mental Dysfunction in Parkinson Disease. Edited by Wolters EC, Scheltens P. Amsterdam, The Netherlands, Vrije Universiteit, 1993, pp 3–18
6. Brodmann K: Vergleichende Lokalisationslehre der Grosshirnrinde in ihren Prinzipien dargestellt auf Grund des Zellenbaues. Leipzig, Germany, Barth, 1909
7. Carmichael ST, Price JL: Architectonic subdivisions of the orbital and medial prefrontal cortex in the macaque monkey. J Comp Neurol 346:366–402, 1994
8. Zald DH, Kim SW: Anatomy and function of the orbital frontal cortex, I: anatomy, neurocircuitry, and obsessive-compulsive disorder. J Neuropsychiatry Clin Neurosci 8:125–138, 1996
9. Selemon LD, Goldman-Rakic PS: Longitudinal topography and interdigitation of corticostriatal projections in the rhesus monkey. J Neurosci 5:776–794, 1985

10. Parent A, Bouchard C, Smith Y: The striatopallidal and striatonigral projections: two distinct fiber systems in primate. Brain Res 303:385–390, 1984

11. Smith Y, Hazrati L-N, Parent A: Efferent projections of the subthalamic nucleus in the squirrel monkey as studied by the PHA-L anterograde tracing method. J Comp Neurol 294:306–323, 1990

12. Kim R, Nakano K, Jayaraman A, et al: Projections of the globus pallidus and adjacent structures: an autoradiographic study in the monkey. J Comp Neurol 169:263–290, 1976

13. Ilinsky IA, Jouandet ML, Goldman-Rakic PS: Organization of the nigrothalamocortical system in the rhesus monkey. J Comp Neurol 236:315–330, 1985

14. Kievit J, Kuypers HGJM: Organization of the thalamocortical connections to the frontal lobe in the rhesus monkey. Exp Brain Res 29:299–322, 1977

15. Giguere M, Goldman-Rakic PS: Mediodorsal nucleus: areal, laminar, and tangential distribution of afferents and efferents in the frontal lobe of rhesus monkey. J Comp Neurol 277:195–213, 1988

16. Milner B: Effects of different brain lesions on card sorting. Arch Neurol 9:90–100, 1963

17. Benton AL: Differential behavioral effects in frontal lobe disease. Neuropsychologia 6:53–60, 1968

18. Jones-Gotman M, Milner B: Design fluency: the invention of nonsense drawings after focal cortical lesions. Neuropsychologia 15:653–674, 1977

19. Cummings JL: Clinical Neuropsychiatry. New York, Grune & Stratton, 1985

20. Robinson RG, Starkstein SE: Current research in affective disorders following stroke. J Neuropsychiatry Clin Neurosci 2:1–14, 1990

21. Starkstein SE, Cohen BS, Federoff P, et al: Relationship between anxiety disorders and depressive disorders in patients with cerebrovascular injury. Arch Gen Psychiatry 47:246–251, 1990

22. Folstein SE: Huntington's Disease: A Disorder of Families. Baltimore, MD, Johns Hopkins University Press, 1989

23. Carmichael ST, Price JL: Limbic connections of the orbital and medial prefrontal cortex in Macaque monkeys. J Comp Neurol 363:615–641, 1995

24. Mega MS, Cummings JL: The cingulate and cingulate syndromes, in Contemporary Behavioral Neurology. Edited by Trimble MR, Cummings JL. Boston, MA, Butterworth-Heinemann, 1997, pp 189–214

25. Johnson TN, Rosvold HE: Topographic projections on the globus pallidus and substantia nigra of selectively placed lesions in the precommissural caudate nucleus and putamen in the monkey. Exp Neurol 33:584–596, 1971

26. Logue V, Durward M, Pratt RTC, et al: The quality of survival after an anterior cerebral aneurysm. Br J Psychiatry 114:137–160, 1968

27. Hunter R, Blackwood W, Bull J. Three cases of frontal meningiomas presenting psychiatrically. BMJ 3:9–16, 1968

28. Bogousslavsky J, Regli F: Anterior cerebral artery territory infarction in the Lausanne stroke registry. Arch Neurol 47:144–150, 1990

29. Blair RJR, Morris JS, Frith CD, et al: Dissociable neural responses to facial expressions of sadness and anger. Brain 122:883–893, 1999

30. Lhermitte F, Pillon B, Serdaru M: Human autonomy and the frontal lobes, part I: imitation and utilization behavior: a neuropsychological study of 75 patients. Ann Neurol 19:326–334, 1986

31. Mena I, Marin O, Fuenzalida S, et al: Chronic manganese poisoning. Neurology 17:128–136, 1967

32. Baxter LR, Phelps ME, Mazziotta JC, et al: Local cerebral glucose metabolic rates in obsessive-compulsive disorder. Arch Gen Psychiatry 44:211–218, 1987

33. Rauch SL, Jenike MA, Alpert NM, et al: Regional cerebral blood flow measured during symptom provocation in obsessive-compulsive disorder using oxygen 15-labeled carbon dioxide and positron emission tomography. Arch Gen Psychiatry 51:62–70, 1994

34. McGuire PK, Bench CJ, Firth CD, et al: Functional anatomy of obsessive-compulsive phenomena. Br J Psychiatry 164:459–468, 1994

35. Cummings JL, Cunningham K: Obsessive-compulsive disorder in Huntington's disease. Biol Psychiatry 31:263–270, 1992

36. Drevets WC: Prefrontal cortical-amygdalar metabolism in major depression. Ann N Y Acad Sci 877:614–637, 1999

37. Siever LJ, Buchsbaum MS, New AS, et al: d,l-Fenfluramine response in impulsive personality disorder assessed with [^{18}F]fluorodeoxyglucose positron emission tomography. Neuropsychopharmacology 20:413–423, 1999

38. Price JL: Prefrontal cortical networks related to visceral function and mood. Ann N Y Acad Sci 877:383–396, 1999

39. Kaada BR, Pribram KH, Epstein JA: Respiratory and vascular responses in monkeys from temporal pole, insula, orbital surface and cingulate gyrus. J Neurophysiol 12:347–356, 1949

40. Baare WF, Hulshoff Pol HE, Hijman R, et al: Volumetric analysis of frontal lobe regions in schizophrenia: relation to cognitive function and symptomatology. Biol Psychiatry 45:1597–1605, 1999

41. Bogousslavsky J, Ferrazzini M, Regli F, et al: Manic delirium and frontal-like syndrome with paramedian infarction of the right thalamus. J Neurol Neurosurg Psychiatry 51:116–119, 1988

42. Jorge RE, Robinson RG, Starkstein SE, et al: Secondary mania following traumatic brain injury. Am J Psychiatry 150:916–921, 1993

43. Starkstein SE, Pearlson GD, Boston J, et al: Mania after brain injury: a controlled study of causative factors. Arch Neurol 44:1069–1073, 1987

44. Mayberg H, Mahurin RK, Brannan SK, et al: Parkinson's depression: discrimination of mood-sensitive and mood-insensitive cognitive deficits using fluoxetine and FDG PET. Neurology 45 (suppl 4):A166, 1995

45. Tremblay L, Schultz W: Relative reward preference in primate orbitofrontal cortex. Nature 398:704–708, 1999

46. Heimer L: The olfactory cortex and the ventral striatum, in Limbic Mechanisms. Edited by Livingston KE, Hornykiewisz O. New York, Plenum, 1978, pp 95–187

47. Haber SN, Lynd E, Klein C, et al: Topographic organization of the ventral striatal efferent projections in the rhesus monkey: an anterograde tracing study. J Comp Neurol 293:282–298, 1990

48. Haber SN, Lynd-Balta E, Mitchell SJ: The organization of the descending ventral pallidal projections in the monkey. J Comp Neurol 329:111–128, 1993

49. Goldman-Rakic PS, Porrino LJ: The primate mediodorsal (MD) nucleus and its projection to the frontal lobe. J Comp Neurol 242:535–560, 1985

50. Barris RW, Schuman HR: Bilateral anterior cingulate gyrus lesions. Neurology 3:44–52, 1953

51. Fesenmeier JT, Kuzniecky R, Garcia JH: Akinetic mutism caused by bilateral anterior cerebral tuberculous obliterative arteritis. Neurology 30:1005–1006, 1990

52. Nielsen JM, Jacobs LL: Bilateral lesions of the anterior cingulate gyri. Bulletin of the Los Angeles Neurological Society 16:231–234, 1951

53. Damasio H, Damasio AR: Lesion Analysis in Neuropsychology. New York, Oxford University Press, 1989

54. Freedman M, Alexander MP, Naeser MA: Anatomic basis of transcortical motor aphasia. Neurology 34:409–417, 1984

55. Masdeu JC, Schoene WC, Funkenstein HH: Aphasia following infarction of the left supplementary motor area: a clinicopathologic study. Neurology 28:1220–1223, 1978

56. Goodglass H, Menn L: Is agrammatism a unitary phenomenon?, in Agrammatism. Edited by Kean ML. London, Academic Press, 1985, pp 1–26

57. Nadeau SE: Impaired grammar with normal fluency and phonology: implications for Broca's aphasia. Brain 111:1111–1137, 1988

58. Yakovlev PI, Locke S: Limbic nuclei of thalamus and connections of limbic cortex. Arch Neurol 5:364–400, 1961

59. Mega MS, Alexander MP: Subcortical aphasia: the core profile of capsulostriatal infarction. Neurology 44:1824–1829, 1994

60. Drewe EA: Go-no go learning after frontal lobe lesions in humans. Cortex 11:8–16, 1975

61. Leimkuhler ME, Mesulam M-M: Reversible go-no go deficits in a case of frontal lobe tumor. Ann Neurol 18:617–619, 1985

62. Litvan I, Mega MS, Cummings JL, et al: Neuropsychiatric aspects of progressive supranuclear palsy. Neurology 47:1184–1189, 1996

63. Burns A, Folstein S, Brandt J, et al: Clinical assessment of irritability, aggression, and apathy in Huntington and Alzheimer disease. J Nerv Ment Dis 178:20–26, 1990

64. Starkstein SE, Mayberg HS, Preziosi TJ, et al: Reliability, validity, and clinical correlates of apathy in Parkinson's disease. J Neuropsychiatry Clin Neurosci 4:134–139, 1992

65. Stuss DT, Guberman A, Nelson R, et al: The neuropsychology of paramedian thalamic infarction. Brain Cogn 8:348–378, 1988

66. Yakovlev PI: Development of the nuclei of the dorsal thalamus and the cerebral cortex: morphogenetic and tectogenetic correlation, in Modern Neurology. Edited by Locke S. Boston, MA, Little Brown, 1969, pp 15–53

67. Pandya DN, Yeterian EH: Architecture and connections of cortical association areas, in Cerebral Cortex, Vol 4. Edited by Peters A, Jones EG. New York, Plenum, 1985, pp 3–55

68. Mesulam M-M: Patterns in behavioral neuroanatomy: association areas, the limbic system, and hemispheric specialization, in Behavioral Neurology. Edited by Mesulam M-M. Philadelphia, PA, FA Davis, 1985, pp 1–70

69. Posner MI, Walker JA, Friedrich FA, et al: How do the parietal lobes direct covert attention? Neuropsychologia 25:135–145, 1987

70. Yeterian EH, Pandya DN: Striatal connections of the parietal association cortices in rhesus monkeys. J Comp Neurol 332:175–197, 1993

71. Sadikot AF, Parent A, Francois C: Efferent connections of the centromedian and parafascicular thalamic nuclei in the squirrel monkey: a PHA-L study of subcortical projections. J Comp Neurol 315:137–159, 1992

72. Parent A, Mackey A, DeBellefeuille L: The subcortical afferents to caudate nucleus and putamen in primate: a fluorescence retrograde double labeling study. Neuroscience 10:1137–1150, 1983

73. Amaral DG, Price JL, Pitkänen A, et al: Anatomical organization of the primate amygdaloid complex, in The Amygdala. Edited by Aggleton JP. New York, Wiley-Liss, 1992, pp 1–66

74. Amaral DG, Price JL: Amygdalo-cortical projections in the monkey (Macaca fascicularis). J Comp Neurol 230:465–496, 1984

75. Vogt BA, Pandya DN: Cingulate cortex of the rhesus monkey, II: cortical afferents. J Comp Neurol 262:271–289, 1987

76. Müller-Preuss P, Jürgens U: Projections from the "cingular" vocalization area in the squirrel monkey. Brain Res 103:29–43, 1976

77. Morecraft RJ, Geula C, Mesulam M-M: Cytoarchitecture and neural afferents of orbitofrontal cortex in the brain of the monkey. J Comp Neurol 323:341–358, 1992

78. Pandya DN, Van Hoesen GW, Mesulam M-M: Efferent connections of the cingulate gyrus in the rhesus monkey. Exp Brain Res 42:319–330, 1981

79. Moran MA, Mufson EJ, Mesulam M-M: Neural inputs to the temporopolar cortex of the rhesus monkey. J Comp Neurol 256:88–103, 1987

80. Mufson EJ, Mesulam M-M: Insula of the old world monkey, II: afferent cortical input and comments on the claustrum. J Comp Neurol 212:23–37, 1982

81. Insausti R, Amaral DG, Cowan WM: The entorhinal cortex of the monkey, II: cortical afferents. J Comp Neurol 264:356–395, 1987

82. Morecraft RJ, Van Hoesen GW: A comparison of frontal lobe afferents to the primary, supplementary and cingulate cortices in the rhesus monkey. Society of Neuroscience Abstracts 17:1019, 1991

83. Baleydier C, Mauguière F: The duality of the cingulate gyrus in monkey: neuroanatomical study and functional hypothesis. Brain 103:525–554, 1980

84. Van Hoesen GW, Morecraft RJ, Vogt BA: Connections of the monkey cingulate cortex, in Neurobiology of Cingulate Cortex and Limbic Thalamus: A Comprehensive Handbook. Edited by Vogt BA, Gabriel M. Boston, MA, Birkhäuser, 1993, pp 249–284

85. Mesulam M-M, Mufson EJ: The insula of Reil in man and monkey: architectonics, connectivity, and function, in Cerebral Cortex. Edited by Jones EG, Peters AA. New York, Plenum, 1985, pp 179–226

86. Vogt BA, Pandya DN: Cingulate cortex of the rhesus monkey, I: cytoarchitecture and thalamic afferents. J Comp Neurol 262:256–270, 1987

87. Graybiel AM: Neurotransmitters and neuromodulators in the basal ganglia. Trends Neurosci 13:244–254, 1990

88. Lavoie B, Parent A: Immunohistochemical study of the serotoninergic innervation of the basal ganglia in the squirrel monkey. J Comp Neurol 299:1–16, 1990

89. Chesselet M-F, Gonzales C, Levitt P: Heterogeneous distribution of the limbic system–associated membrane protein in the caudate nucleus and substantia nigra of the cat. Neuroscience 40:725–733, 1991

90. Gibb WRG: Melanin, tyrosine hydroxylase, calbindin and substance P in the human midbrain and substantia nigra in relation to nigrostriatal projections and differential neuronal susceptibility in Parkinson's disease. Brain Res 581:283–291, 1992

91. Stoof JC, Drukarch B, Vermeulen RJ: Dopamine and glutamate receptor subtypes as (potential) targets for the pharmacotherapy of Parkinson's disease, in Mental Dysfunction in Parkinson Disease. Edited by Wolters EC, Scheltens P. Amsterdam, The Netherlands, Vrije Universiteit, 1993, pp 19–34

92. Thierry AM, Tassin JP, Blanc G, et al: Studies on mesocortical dopamine systems. Adv Biochem Psychopharmacol 19:205–216, 1978

93. Moore RY, Bloom FE: Central catecholamine neuron systems: anatomy and physiology of the dopamine system. Annu Rev Neurosci 1:129–169, 1978

94. Oades RD, Halliday GM: Ventral tegmental (A10) system: neurobiology, 1: anatomy and connectivity. Brain Res Rev 12:117–165, 1987

95. Scatton B, Javoy-Agid F, Rouquier L, et al: Reduction of cortical dopamine, noradrenaline, serotonin and other metabolites in Parkinson's disease. Brain Res 275:321–328, 1983

96. Agid Y, Rugerg M, Dubois B, et al: Biochemical substrates of mental disturbances in Parkinson's disease, in Advances in Neurology, Vol 40. Edited by Hassler RG, Christ JF. New York, Raven, 1984, pp 211–218

97. Rinne JO, Rummukainen J, Paljärvi L, et al: Dementia in Parkinson's disease is related to neuronal loss in the medial substantia nigra. Ann Neurol 26:47–50, 1989

98. Ross ED, Stewart RM: Akinetic mutism from hypothalamic damage: successful treatment with dopamine agonists. Neurology 31:1435–1439, 1981

99. Cummings JL: Behavioral complications of drug treatment of Parkinson's disease. J Am Geriatr Soc 39:708–716, 1991

100. Parent A, Pare D, Smith Y, et al: Basal forebrain cholinergic and noncholinergic projections to the thalamus and brainstem in cats and monkeys. J Comp Neurol 277:281–301, 1988

101. Brandel JP, Hirsch EC, Malessa S, et al: Differential vulnerability of cholinergic projections to the mediodorsal nucleus of the thalamus in senile dementia of Alzheimer type and progressive supranuclear palsy. Neuroscience 41:25–31, 1991

102. Fotuhi M, Dawson TM, Sharp AH, et al: Phosphoinositide second messenger system is enriched in striosomes: immunohistochemical demonstration of inositol 1,4,5-triphosphate receptors and phospholipase C β and gamma in primate basal ganglia. J Neurosci 13:3300–3308, 1993

103. Snyder SH: Second messengers and affective illness. Focus on the phosphoinositide cycle. Pharmacopsychiatry 25:25–28, 1992

4

The Orbitofrontal Cortex

David H. Zald, Ph.D., Suck Won Kim, M.D.

Since the famous case of Phineas Gage,[1] investigators have speculated that dysfunction of the orbitofrontal cortex (OFC) plays an important role in neuropsychiatric illnesses. Recent neuroimaging and neurophysiological studies increasingly support this speculation and implicate the OFC in several neuropsychiatric conditions. This chapter reviews the current state of knowledge on the neurocircuitry and function of the OFC with the aim of providing a framework for understanding how dysfunction of this region contributes to psychophathological conditions.

ANATOMY OF THE ORBITOFRONTAL CORTEX

The OFC comprises the ventralmost regions of the prefrontal cortex. Several gyri constitute the OFC of humans, including 1) the *gyrus rectus,* which forms the boundary between the ventral and medial surface of the prefrontal cortex; 2) the *medial orbital gyrus,* which runs lateral to the olfactory sulcus; 3) a *central region,* which is disrupted by the arcuate or transverse orbital sulcus (the regions anterior and posterior to the transverse orbital sulcus are often labeled the *anterior orbital gyrus* and *posterior orbital gyrus,* respectively, but some

anatomists refer to this area more generally as the *middle orbital gyrus*); 4) a *lateral orbital gyrus;* and 5) the orbital portion of the *inferior frontal gyrus* on the lateral boundary of the ventral prefrontal surface (in some cases, there is no clear division between the lateral orbital gyrus and the inferior frontal gyrus pars orbitalis). The specific shapes of the orbital gyri and sulci vary substantially across individuals.[2] Indeed, although prominent medial and lateral sulci usually can be identified in human brain samples, the common presence of additional or free-standing sulci, and the variability in the degree to which the gyri connect with the transverse orbital sulcus, often leads to confusion in labeling this region. Because of this, some neuroanatomical atlases generically label everything between the olfactory sulcus and inferior frontal gyrus as *orbital gyri* and label all of the sulci by the generic term *orbital sulci.*

Several different parcellation schemes exist for designating the different regions within the OFC. The most widely used parcellation scheme is that of Brodmann,[3] who divided the OFC into two major regions (area 47 and 11) (see Figure 4–1). Unfortunately, Brodmann's system treats regions with substantially different cyto- and chemoarchitecture as if they were homogeneous. Other researchers who used classical histologi-

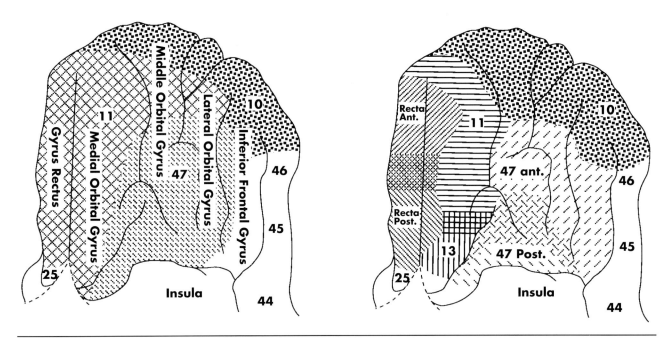

FIGURE 4–1.   Left: Ventral view of the human orbitofrontal cortex (OFC) according to Brodmann.[3]   **Right:** The parcellation of Beck,[8] in which area 11 is restricted to the anterior portion of the medial orbital gyrus and area 13 is defined in the posterior portion of the gyrus.
Note the wide area of the OFC that Brodmann treats as homogeneous. Additionally, Brodmann's area 47 has been subdivided into anterior and posterior regions based on the transition posterior-anterior gradient of granulization. Beck's system was never widely accepted but shows greater similarity to Walker's system in the macaque and shows a rough correspondence to Hof's chemoarchitectural parcellation.

cal techniques defined far more regions within the OFC.[4,5] The precedence of Brodmann's system, combined with the significant individual differences in the specific topography of the OFC and the transitional nature of OFC architectural features, limited widespread acceptance of more detailed parcellation schemes in humans. However, the human OFC has several clearly definable features that allow reliable parcellation with greater precision than with Brodmann's system. At the most general level, the area consists of three broad zones, with a posterior agranular region, middle dysgranular region, and anterior granular region (see Figure 4–2).[6–9] Using modern cyto- and chemoarchitectural techniques, Hof and colleagues[9] recently provided a general parcellation scheme based on reliable and statistically definable divisions between OFC subregions. This system divides the OFC into anteromedial, posteromedial, medial-orbital (central), anterolateral, and posterolateral segments. As can be seen in Figure 4–2, the chemoarchitectural boundaries defined by Hof et al. do not map exactly to the agranular-dysgranular and dysgranular-granular boundaries. Parcellation systems that take into account additional chemoarchitec-

tural subdivisions that have been defined in the monkey OFC are currently under development.[10]

The nonhuman primate OFC shares many features in common with the human OFC, and much of what is known about the neurocircuitry of the OFC derives from studies in nonhuman primates. Walker[11] divided the OFC into five separate areas in the macaque, which he numbered 10, 11, 12, 13, and 14 (Figure 4–3). Walker's system appears to correspond well with many of the features of Hof's parcellation of the human OFC. Table 4–1 lists the human OFC regions with their corresponding regions in the macaque. The cytoarchitectural features of the medial OFC regions appear extremely similar across primate species. Over the years, there has been greater disagreement on the extent to which the more lateral sections of the OFC reflect architecturally homologous regions across species, but the lateral segments of the OFC in human and nonhuman primates clearly share many features in common. Specifically, Walker's area 12 in the macaque shares homologous features with the inferior frontal gyrus and lateral orbital gyrus in humans.[10,12] Some neuroanatomists now refer to this inferior frontal gyrus/lateral orbital gyrus area as 47/12 to highlight this commonality across primate species.[12]

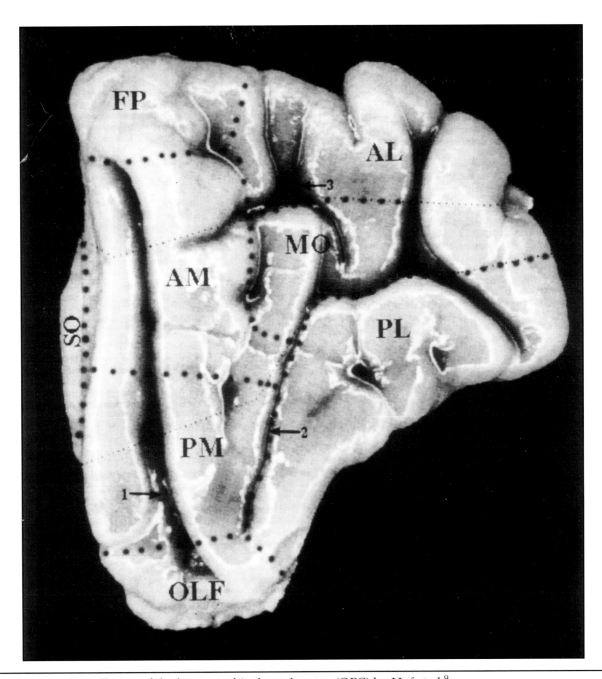

FIGURE 4–2. Parcellation of the human orbitofrontal cortex (OFC) by Hof et al.[9]

Large dots represent divisions between major chemoarchitectural areas. Thin dashed lines represent the transition points between agranular (posterior), dysgranular (middle), and granular cortex (anterior). Note that the chemoarchitectural divisions defined by Hof et al. do not match the architectonic transitions between the dysgranular and granular zones, and in some cases, transitions cannot be defined precisely but represent prototypical transition points. AL=anterior lateral; AM=anterior medial; FP=frontal pole; MO=medial orbital (central); PL=posterior lateral; PM=posterior medial; SO=sus orbital; OLF=olfactory tubercle. Arrow 1=olfactory sulcus. Arrow 2=MO sulcus. In this brain, the MO sulcus merges with the transverse orbital sulcus, which runs horizontally between the PM and MO sections (some anatomists refer to the sulcus labeled by arrow 2 as a PM branch of the transverse orbital sulcus because of its continuity with the transverse orbital sulcus). As is frequently the case, the lateral end of the transverse orbital sulcus joins with a perpendicular running sulcus, which is typically labeled as the lateral orbital sulcus. The labeling of the sulci in the AM and MO regions is less clear in this brain sample and displays some of the idiosyncratic features that can be observed in this region (arrow 3).

Source. Adapted from Hof PR, Mufson EJ, Morrison JH: "Human Orbitofrontal Cortex: Cytoarchitecture and Quantitative Immunohistochemical Parcellation." *Journal of Comparative Neurology* 359:48–68, 1995. Copyright 1995 John Wiley and Sons, Inc. Reprinted by permission of Wiley-Liss, Inc., a subsidiary of John Wiley and Sons, Inc.

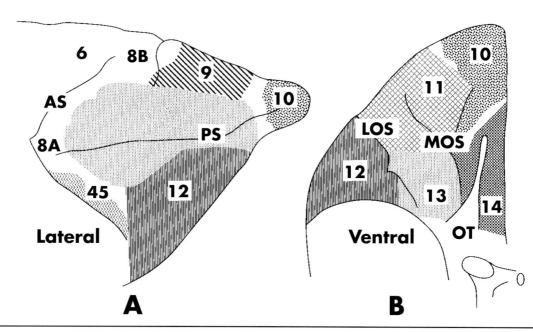

FIGURE 4–3. Lateral **(A)** and ventral **(B)** views of the macaque prefrontal cortex based on the parcellation system of Walker.[11]

AS=arcuate sulcus; LOS=lateral orbital sulcus; MOS=medial orbital sulcus; OT=olfactory tuberule; PS=principal sulcus.

Based on detailed investigations of the cyto- and chemoarchitectural features of the OFC, Carmichael and Price[13] divided Walker's areas into a series of subregions (Figure 4–4). This system labels the posterior agranular portion of the medial wall of the olfactory sulcus as area 13a. Just anterior to this lies a dysgranular region labeled 13b. The posterior third of the area between the medial and lateral orbital sulci forms area 13 proper. Carmichael and Price further subdivided this region into a lateral (13l) and a medial (13m) segment. Walker's area 12 is also subdivided into several separate subregions. The posterior orbital portion of area 12, which has only a thin, light, granular layer, forms area 12o. The more anterior regions of area 12 are composed of a rostral granular region (12r) and lateral and medial granular regions labeled 12l and 12m. Carmichael and Price also subdivided the band of agranular cortex at the posterior boundary of the OFC into five separate subregions, including a medial (Iam), intermediate (Iai), lateral (Ial), posterior-lateral (Iapl), and posterior-medial (Iapm) segments. This region lies continuous with the insula, and they refer to it as an insular subregion. In this chapter, we use the term *posterior agranular OFC* to refer to this band of cortex. However, in referring to the specific subregions, we retain the nomenclature of Carmichael and Price.

Each of the subregions defined by Carmichael and Price in the macaque has a corresponding homolo-

TABLE 4–1. Correspondence between human and macaque parcellation systems

Hof et al. (human)	Walker (macaque)	Brodmann (human)
Frontopolar	10	10, 11
Anteromedial	11	11
Anterolateral	12	11
Medial-orbital	12, 13	11
Posteromedial	13, 14	11
Posterolateral	13	11, 47
Sus-orbital sulcus	10, 11	12

gous subregion in the human brain.[10] Although the exact boundaries of these subregions remain under study in humans, they show a relatively similar layout to that seen in the monkey. Human areas 13a, 13b, 13m, and 13l occur within the posterior-medial sector defined by Hof (refer to Figure 4–2), with areas 13m and 13l falling between the olfactory and the medial orbital sulci. Areas 11m and 11l lie anterior to this, with the division between 11m and 11l falling about halfway between the olfactory and the medial orbital sulci. Area 47/12m occupies much of the area between the medial and the lateral orbital sulci (Hof's posterolateral and central areas), with 12r falling anterior to this in part of Hof's anterolateral area). Area 47/12l

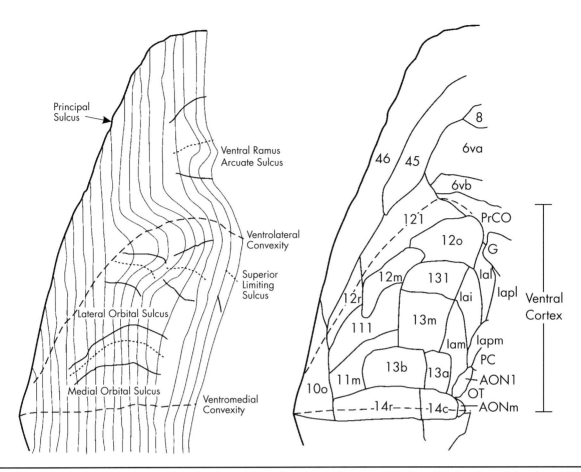

FIGURE 4–4.   Left: The unfolded topography of the orbitofrontal cortex (OFC).   **Right:** Carmichael and Price's parcellation of the OFC.

Note in this system the agranular band in the posterior of the OFC is labeled as part of the insula. This differs from the system of labeling used by Mesulam and Mufson[6] and Morecraft et al.,[7] who labeled these regions as orbital frontal agranular zones. AON=anterior olfactory nucleus; G=gustatory cortex; i=intermediate; Ia=agranular insula; l=lateral; m=medial; o=orbital; OT=olfactory tubercle; p=posterior; PC=pyriform (primary olfactory) cortex; PrCO=precentral opercular area; r=rostral; v=ventral.

Source.   Adapted from Carmichael ST, Price JL: "Architectonic Subdivision of the Orbital and Medial Prefrontal Cortex in the Macaque Monkey." *Journal of Comparative Neurology* 346:366–402, 1994. Copyright 1994 John Wiley and Sons, Inc. Reprinted by permission of Wiley-Liss, Inc., a subsidiary of John Wiley and Sons, Inc.

appears mostly lateral to the lateral orbital sulcus. The homologue to the macaque 12o in monkeys falls posterior to this and appears buried in the rostral extension of the superior limiting sulcus, where it extends into the frontal lobe.

Unfortunately, the vast majority of studies reviewed in this chapter predate Carmichael and Price's parcellation system in monkeys and its recent extension to the human OFC. Wherever possible, we use Carmichael and Price's terminology because of its exquisite detail, but in situations in which such precision is lacking, we use Walker's more general parcellation scheme. Many studies actually encompass more than one of Walker's regions. The lack of specificity frequently results because the transition points between different cytoarchitectural regions in the OFC are often gradual, and substantial intra- and interspecies differences exist in the location of these transition points. Investigations often involve either a broad medial or a broad lateral segment of the OFC. Studies of the medial OFC generally encompass Walker's area 13 and, to a greater or lesser extent, also may include part of area 14 and/or the medial part of area 11. Such investigations often focus on the posterior agranular-dysgranular portion of this area. The lateral OFC is generally viewed as consisting of the lateral portion of Walker's area 11 and most or all of area 12. Although there exist marked differences in some of the innervation characteristics of areas 11 and 12, functional studies rarely distinguish between the two areas. Instead, lesion studies often involve a strip of cortex known as the *inferior convexity*. The inferior convexity includes the lateral part of area 11 and most or all of area 12 and, depending on the species and the cytoarchitectural system used, often intrudes on the ventral segment of area 46 along the inferior boundary of the principal sulcus. Unfortunately, the involvement of multiple regions in inferior convexity lesions frequently makes it difficult to determine the extent to which area 11, area 12, and ventral area 46 individually relate to many functions.

SENSORY INNERVATION OF THE ORBITOFRONTAL CORTEX

The development of all prefrontal cortex areas in mammalian species derives from two prime moieties: a paleocortical moiety that evolved from a primitive olfactory core and an archicortical moiety that developed from hippocampal archicortex.[14,15] These two moieties are distinguishable on both cytoarchitectural and functional grounds throughout the cerebral cortex. At a broad level, structures within the archicortical trend support functions related to the localization of stimuli in space, whereas structures within the paleocortical trend support stimulus recognition functions.[15] Walker's areas 11, 12, and 13 derive exclusively from the paleocortical moiety. The primary source of sensory input into the OFC derives from cortical regions that also evolved from the paleocortical core. These connections provide the OFC with substantial sensory input from cortical regions involved in the recognition of stimuli. In contrast, the gyrus rectus forms a transition to portions of the medial prefrontal cortex that derive from hippocampal archicortex.

The OFC receives well-processed unimodal and polymodal, exteroceptive and interoceptive sensory information from every sensory modality (see Table 4–2). These afferents tend to follow a general pattern: more highly differentiated sensory association cortices project to the more differentiated regions of the OFC, whereas the more cytoarchitecturally primitive sensory association regions direct their projections to the agranular or dysgranular cortices in the more posterior OFC.[5,6,16–19] This pattern provides the OFC with multiple parallel sensory projections originating from association cortices of different phylogenetic age.

TABLE 4–2. Overview of primary and major secondary targets of sensory input to the orbitofrontal cortex

Modality	Principal recipient regions
Olfactory	Iam, Iapm, 13a, 13m
Gustatory	Ial, Iapm, 13l
Visual	12l, 11
Auditory	12r, 12m, 11l
Somatosensory	12m, 13l
Visceral	Iapm, Ial, 13a

Note.   See text for details.

Olfactory

The primary (pyriform) olfactory cortex and the anterior olfactory nucleus project extensively to the posterior agranular portions of the OFC. Areas Iam and Iapm receive the heaviest input from primary olfactory regions, but significant direct afferents also reach areas 13a, Iai, and Ial, and lighter projections directly reach areas 13m and Iapl.[19,20] Although area 13m receives only a light direct projection from the primary olfactory cortex, it receives heavy indirect olfactory projections via the mediodorsal nucleus of the thalamus, pars magnocellularis (MDmc),[21–24] and projections from areas Iam and Iapm.[25] Together, these OFC regions act as a cortical association area for the olfactory system. Neurophysiological studies indicate that cells in olfactory recipient regions of the OFC show robust and often highly selective responses to olfactory stimuli.[26–29] In fact, many if not most of the olfactory responsive cells in the OFC show far greater stimulus selectivity than is observed in the pyriform cortex and olfactory bulb. Lesions to the OFC in humans damage olfactory discrimination, identification, and recognition memory without altering olfactory detection thresholds.[30–32] Olfactory identification abilities show relatively equal levels of deterioration following left and right OFC lesions. In contrast, olfactory recognition memory and discrimination appear specifically sensitive to right OFC lesions. Recent positron-emission tomography (PET) studies in humans also indicated that the OFC shows significant increases in activity during exposure to odorants.[33–35] The right OFC is more consistently involved in olfactory processing, although the left OFC shows a substantial involvement in some olfactory tasks. For instance, the left OFC has activated during exposure to odorants with strong appetitive or aversive properties.

Gustatory

Rolls and colleagues[36,37] identified a secondary taste association area within a caudally located dysgranular portion of the OFC, which appears to most closely correspond to area 13l. This region receives projections from both the frontal opercular taste cortex and the insular taste cortex.[38] The agranular posterior regions Iapm and Ial receive substantial gustatory information and project this information to dysgranular areas 13l and 13m.[18,25,38] Area 13 differs dramatically from other gustatory cortical areas in that it lacks direct innervation from the thalamic taste region (ventral posterior medial nucleus). Instead, its thalamic input derives from the MDmc.[24] The OFC taste region has both unimodal (gustatory) and polymodal (gustatory/olfactory and gustatory/visual) responsive cells.[36,39,40] The convergence of olfactory and gustatory modalities in these regions distinguishes the OFC from primary taste areas that lack significant olfactory input. This suggests that the OFC provides an interface zone through which olfactory and gustatory information interact to determine the perception of flavor. As in the olfactory modality, gustatory responsive cells in the OFC show a high level of stimulus specificity. Many of the OFC gustatory cells respond to only one or two tastes.[37] This differs dramatically from the responsivity to multiple gustatory stimuli that occurs in earlier gustatory processing stages. Functional neuroimaging studies have repeatedly confirmed the presence of a gustatory responsive area in the human OFC. However, the location of these responses often appears more anterior than the secondary gustatory area defined in the monkey.[41]

Visual

Visual input reaches multiple subregions of the OFC through projections from inferior temporal visual association areas.[17,18,42] These association areas represent the last stages of the ventral visual processing pathway dedicated to object recognition.[43,44] The most prominent of these projections derives from area TE (VA2) in the inferior temporal lobe, which projects to area 12l and the adjacent ventral portion of area 46 (Figure 4–5).[18] In contrast, more medial orbital areas (11 and 13) receive input from VA3, which occupies a more anterior portion of the inferior temporal cortex. VA3 represents a later stage in the ventral visual pathway than the area projecting to lateral area 12. Only a few studies have examined the visual properties of OFC cells. Cells in area 12l and ventral area 46 (which

also reciprocally connects with area 12l) appear to have response properties similar to those of the inferior temporal cortices that project to them. These cells respond best to foveal stimulation with complex stimuli such as objects or patterns.[45,46] The medial OFC also possesses many visually responsive cells.[47] As in the olfactory and gustatory domains, visually responsive cells appear in close proximity to cells responsive to other sensory modalities, and many of these cells show bimodal responses.[40,47] To the extent to which they have been studied, visually responsive cells in the OFC also show a high level of stimulus specificity.

Auditory

Well-processed auditory information arrives via the rostral superior temporal gyrus and the neighboring rostral auditory parabelt.[42,48–50] This input principally innervates rostral-lateral (Walker's area 12) sectors of the OFC, but auditory responses have been observed in both the lateral and the medial OFC. As is typical of OFC sensory processing, auditory-responsive cells in this region appear to have a high level of stimulus specificity, but information on this subject remains scarce. Specifically, the cells show a high degree of frequency selectivity.[45] These cells occur close to cells responsive to other modalities, and many of the cells show bimodal responses.[40,45] The nature of auditory processing in the areas projecting to the OFC suggests that the OFC may receive information about certain types of vocalizations. PET studies have found a clear involvement of the OFC in music perception.[51,52]

Somatosensory

Somatosensory projections innervate the OFC from the parietal operculum (including both SII and areas 1 and 2), the inferior parietal lobule (area 7b), and the posterior granular insula.[13,15,24,53] These projections focus most strongly on area 12m, with additional projections reaching areas 13m and 13l. These projections convey somatosensory information for the orofacial area and the digits of the hand. Little is known about the nature of somatosensory coding in the OFC. Interestingly, the information about the orofacial area converges with gustatory information in area 13l and appears to convey information about the texture of food.[54]

Visceral

The OFC has long been known to receive interoceptive (somatovisceral) sensory information. As early as

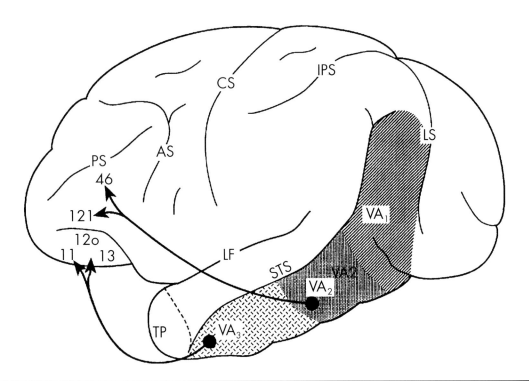

FIGURE 4–5.   Projections from temporal lobe visual association areas to the orbitofrontal cortex (OFC).
AS=arcuate sulcus; CS=central sulcus; IPS=inferior parietal sulcus; LF=longitudinal fissure; LS=lunate sulcus; PS=principal sulcus; STS=superior temporal sulcus; TP=temporal pole; VA=visual association areas 1–3.

1938, stimulation of the vagus nerve was reported to produce alterations in electrical potentials in the OFC of cats.[55] The OFC probably receives visceral information through multiple sources. The most substantial source involves projections from the ventral posterior medial nucleus of the thalamus (parvocellular division) to posterior agranular regions, specifically areas Iapm and Ial.[17] These regions in turn project to agranular and dysgranular regions of the OFC, including all subdivisions of areas 13 and 12m.[24] A second source of information involves a projection through the submedial nucleus of the thalamus. This projection relays information from the spinal cord and appears to provide the primary route through which visceral nociceptive information reaches the OFC.[56] In lower mammals, the areas of the OFC receiving submedial inputs respond to visceral nociceptive information.[57] To date, nociceptive responses in primates have not been examined. However, the projection of the submedial nucleus to the OFC is retained in primates and focuses on area 13a. Intralaminar and midline nuclei of the thalamus may additionally augment the visceral and autonomic information reaching the OFC. The submedial nucleus also appears to relay information from the trigeminal nerve.[56] The function of this projection has received little attention, but it may relate to the burn-

ing sensation of trigeminal irritants and could provide a source for integrating olfactory and trigeminal coding of airborne chemicals. A final potential source of information on visceral states derives from connections with area 25, which is situated just above area 14c on the posterior medial wall. This area appears to represent a cortical center for the visceral motor system and possesses afferents and efferents directly associated with autonomic functions.[58,59] The gyrus rectus (especially area 14c) and, to a lesser extent, areas Iai and 13a, connect with this region.[25]

Polymodal

The OFC's innervation by multiple sensory modalities implicates it as a critical convergence zone capable of integrating diverse sources of information. In general, each modality projects to specific subregions of the OFC. However, the pattern of interconnections between OFC subregions allows for substantial multimodal sensory integration.[25] Cells in much of areas 13 and 12 have access to different combinations of olfactory, visceral, gustatory, somatosensory, visual, and auditory information depending on their specific connections. Additionally, the OFC receives polymodal information via projections from heteromodal areas of the temporal pole and insula.[60–62] Areas 13a, Iai, and 12o also receive prominent projections from polymodal regions of the superior temporal gyrus.[17] As already noted, the OFC possesses many bimodal and polymodal cells. The stimulus specificity of bimodal cells in the OFC has not been thoroughly examined. However, at least some of these cells show a high degree of stimulus selectivity across sensory domains. For instance, Thorpe et al.[47] observed a cell that responded to both the sight and the taste of a banana but did not respond to either the sight or the taste of other foods.

ASSOCIATIONS

Medial Frontal Lobe and Cingulate Cortex

Because of its position at the boundary between the orbital and medial surface of the frontal lobe, investigators have often disagreed on whether to consider the gyrus rectus as part of the orbital or medial frontal cortex. In terms of its connections, the gyrus rectus has far more intimate connections with other medial frontal areas than with the OFC, indicating that if a categorization has to be made, then the gyrus rectus should be considered as part of a medial frontal network.[17] However, the gyrus rectus has significant connections with the immediately neighboring medial OFC regions (13a and 13b). Areas 13a and 12o (which are themselves heavily interconnected) provide a critical interface between the medial and the orbital prefrontal cortex. These two areas have substantial, often bidirectional connections with both medial and orbital regions, indicating that they integrate or coordinate both medial and orbital activity. Three other areas on the orbital surface (11m, 10o, Iai) connect primarily with the medial prefrontal cortex rather than with other OFC structures. Each of these three regions has strong connections with area 12o and/or 13a, further highlighting the importance of 12o and 13a in medial and orbital prefrontal cortex integration. Interestingly, areas 12o and 13a, along with area Iai, show substantially different patterns of connections than other orbital regions. These differences include an exclusive input from polymodal regions of the superior temporal gyrus, as well as unique amygdala and thalamic projections.

Multiple portions of the cingulate cortex reciprocally connect with the OFC.[7,17,63–66] The most prominent connections with the anterior cingulate (Walker's area 24) involve areas 12o laterally, area Iai posteriorly, and areas 13a, 13b, and especially area 11m in the medial OFC. The posterior cingulate area also projects to the more granulated area 11m.

Dorsolateral Prefrontal Cortex and Posterior Parietal Cortex

The OFC has reciprocal connections with both the dorsolateral prefrontal cortex and the frontal eye fields.[7,67–70] Dorsolateral prefrontal cortex connections derive primarily from the lower bank of the principal sulcus and the region ventral to the principal sulcus and are heavily associated with the more rostral and lateral granular areas of the OFC. The heaviest connections focus on area 12l. In the medial OFC, area 13a also receives a significant dorsolateral prefrontal cortex projection. Associations between the frontal eye fields and the OFC appear limited to the more granular portions of area 12. The spatial processing functions of the dorsolateral prefrontal cortex closely reflect its intimate reciprocal connections with the posterior parietal lobe.[71] Similarly, the attention-related functions of the frontal eye fields appear highly dependent on the frontal eye field's connections with an adjacent area of the posterior parietal lobe.[72] It is interesting to note that the parietal lobe has restricted connections with the lateral granular OFC and that these connections lie directly adjacent to dorsolateral prefrontal cortex– and frontal eye field–labeled bands of the lateral OFC.

Orbitofrontal Cortex, Temporal Pole, and Insula

Mesulam and colleagues[6,7,61] use the term *paralimbic* to describe the OFC, temporal pole, and insula. These three regions evolved as a series of concentric rings deriving from olfactory paleocortex (Figure 4–6). The rings consist of agranular cortex surrounding the olfactory core, granular cortex farthest from the core, and dysgranular cortex in between. Each ring within the OFC continues uninterrupted into the insula and temporal pole. Given this shared evolution, it is not surprising that the three regions have tight reciprocal connections.[7,60–62] Specifically, the agranular-dysgranular portions of the posterior OFC show their strongest associations with the agranular and dysgranular sections of the temporal pole and insula, whereas more anterior granular portions of the OFC are primarily associated with granular regions of the temporal pole and insula. The three areas also show similar patterns of connections with other structures in the paleo-

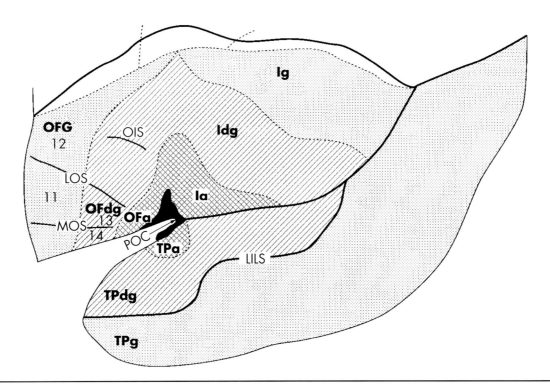

FIGURE 4–6.   Orbital-insular-temporal bands of cortical differentiation.

a=agranular; dg=dysgranular; g=granular; I=Insula; LILS=lateral inferior limiting sulcus; LOS=lateral orbital sulcus; MOS=medial orbital sulcus; OF=orbital frontal; OIS=orbital-insula sulcus; POC=primary olfactory cortex; TP=temporal pole.

Source.   Adapted from Mesulam MM, Mufson EJ: "Insula of the Old World Monkey, I: Architectonics in the Insulo-Orbito-Temporal Component of the Paralimbic Brain." *Journal of Comparative Neurology* 212:1–22, 1982; and Morecraft RJ, Geula C, Mesulam MM: "Cytoarchitecture and Neural Afferents of Orbitofrontal Cortex in the Brain of the Monkey." *Journal of Comparative Neurology* 323:341–358, 1992.

cortical moiety. Specifically, the agranular-dysgranular regions in the OFC, temporal pole, and insula have a closer relation to limbic structures such as the amygdala, whereas granular regions show greater associations with structures that act as higher-order association cortices.

Based on commonalties in the connections and the effects of stimulation and lesions in these three regions, Mesulam and Mufson[61] argued that these regions evolved as an integrated functional network engaged in integrating sensory information with inner motivational states.

Amygdala-Orbitofrontal Interconnections

The functions of the OFC are critically intertwined with the functions of the amygdala. A substantial literature implicates the amygdala in the process of evaluating the affective or behavioral significance of stimuli.[73–75] The OFC and medial wall of the prefrontal cortex are the only regions of the prefrontal cortex that have strong connections with the amygdala. Amygdalar projections to the OFC focus on the agranular band in the posterior OFC; areas 13a, 13b, and 12o; and the gyrus rectus.[7,66,76–79] Few amygdalar fibers reach area 13 proper or area 11, and only light projections reach the more anterior and lateral portions of area 12. Amygdalar fibers reaching the OFC derive largely from the basolateral nucleus of the amygdala, with additional projections arriving from the basal accessory nucleus and to a lesser extent the dorsomedial part of the lateral nucleus (Figure 4–7). Retrograde tracing data further indicate that different sections of the basolateral nucleus project to different subregions of the OFC based on the subregion's level of connection with the medial prefrontal cortex.[66]

Studies of the afferent, efferent, and intrinsic connections of the amygdala have identified a critical pathway through which information proceeds through the amygdala. The lateral nucleus acts as a crucial zone of sensory input, whereas the central nucleus is the major source of efferents to brain stem and hypo-

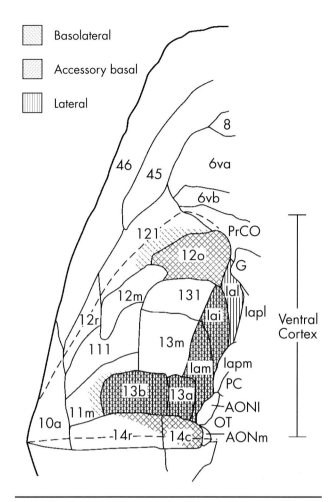

FIGURE 4–7. Amygdala input to the orbitofrontal cortex (OFC).

AON=anterior olfactory nucleus; G=gustatory cortex; i=intermediate; Ia=agranular insula; l=lateral; m=medial; o=orbital; OT=olfactory tubercle; p=posterior; PC=pyriform (primary olfactory) cortex; PrCO=precentral opercular area; r=rostral; v=ventral.

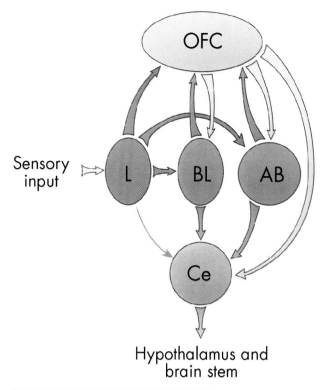

FIGURE 4–8. Interaction of the amygdala and orbitofrontal cortex (OFC).

AB= accessory basal; BL=basolateral; Ce= central; L= lateral.

thalamic structures controlling a spectrum of endocrine, autonomic, and involuntary behavioral responses.[74,75,80] The vast majority of information flow from the lateral nucleus travels through the basolateral and basal accessory nucleus before reaching the central nucleus (Figure 4–8). As a recipient of lateral, basolateral, and accessory basal innervation, the OFC receives information from the critical input and sensory/response interface zones of the amygdala. In return, the OFC sends prominent projections back to the basolateral and basal accessory nuclei of the amygdala.[77,80] The majority of the OFC-amygdala interaction involves this sensory/response interface zone. However, the caudal OFC also projects directly to the central nucleus of the amygdala, providing a route

through which the OFC may exert a direct influence on the amygdala's output.[81]

A less substantial amygdala projection derives from the medial and anterior cortical nuclei of the amygdala. These nuclei represent the "olfactory amygdala" because they retain afferents from the primary olfactory cortex and/or the lateral olfactory tract.[22] They primarily project to the agranular areas in the posterior OFC (Ial and Iapm), with sparse projections reaching areas 13a, 13b, and 14c from the anterior cortical nucleus.[66] A secondary pathway through the MDmc provides an indirect, but substantial, route through which the amygdala directs information toward the OFC.[21,23,79] All regions receiving direct amygdalar input receive indirect input via the MDmc. In addition, areas 11 and 13 proper, which receive only sparse and patchy direct amygdalar input, receive input from regions of the MDmc that are innervated by the amygdala.[23]

Medial Temporal Lobe

The OFC was once thought to lack prominent connections with the hippocampus. However, a region near the border of the subiculum and the CA1/CA3 region of the hippocampus send a projection to the medial OFC (particularly areas 13a, 13b, and 14c, with lighter projections to 14r and 11m).[7,66,82,83] There is some controversy over whether the area sending this projection should be defined as CA1/CA1′ or the subiculum, although its staining features appear more consistent with CA1/CA1′ than subiculum. The OFC does not directly reciprocate these projections but instead sends fibers to the entorhinal, perirhinal, and parahippocampal regions, which in turn project to the hippocampus (Figure 4–9). The OFC's reciprocal connections with the entorhinal cortex appear particularly important in this regard and largely focus on the agranular regions in the posterior OFC and medial areas 13a, 13b, 14c, and 11m.[7,66,84] The reciprocal parahippocampal connections largely overlap with the medial regions receiving direct hippocampal projections.[66,85] In contrast, the reciprocal perirhinal projection to the OFC primarily involves the posterior agranular OFC and areas 13m and 13l.[66,84]

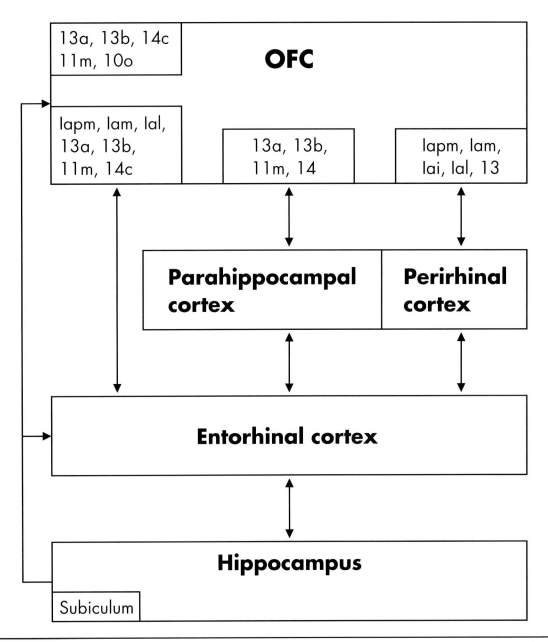

FIGURE 4–9.   Schematic of the orbitofrontal cortex's (OFC's) interconnections with the hippocampal complex.
Iai = intermediate; Ial = lateral; Iam = medial; Iapm = posterior-medial.

Hypothalamus and Brain Stem

In addition to its connections to the amygdala, the OFC projects to several areas critically involved in the coordination of autonomic and behavioral responses to emotional stimuli. The lateral hypothalamus represents a major output channel for the limbic system.[75] The lateral hypothalamus, and to a lesser extent the medial hypothalamus, send nonselective projections to much of the OFC.[7,86] In contrast, posterior and medial areas of the OFC selectively innervate the lateral hypothalamus.[86–88] The densest frontal lobe projections to the hypothalamus derive from structures along the ventromedial wall (especially area 25). Areas on the orbital surface that are heavily connected with the ventromedial wall, such as the gyrus rectus and areas 13a and Iai, provide a dense projection to the hypothalamus. Lighter projections also reach the hypothalamus from other sectors of the OFC, including 12o and the other subregions of area 13. This pattern of connections indicates that the OFC (particularly the posterior and medial OFC) can directly influence hypothalamic output channels.

The OFC subregions that send strong projections to the lateral hypothalamus also innervate the ventrolateral column of the periaqueductal gray.[89] Taken together with its hypothalamic projections, these connections indicate that the OFC influences two of the most critical structures involved in activating visceral responses to emotionally salient stimuli. Interestingly, the same areas of the lateral hypothalamus and periaqueductal gray that receive OFC projections also receive projections from the central nucleus of the amygdala. Thus, the OFC not only interacts with the amygdala but also appears capable of directly manipulating some of the same output pathways as the amygdala. The caudal section of the OFC additionally sends a projection to the septal region.[90,91] This may allow the OFC to influence processing within the septum, which has long been known to play a role in modulating certain types of aggression. Taken together with its lateral hypothalamic and periaqueductal gray connections, the OFC is thus well positioned to exert an influence over multiple areas involved in responses to emotionally salient stimuli.

Orbitofrontal Cortex and the Thalamus

The mediodorsal nucleus is the primary source of thalamic input to the OFC.[21,23,92–94] These projections derive primarily from the MDmc, which projects to the OFC in a topographically organized manner. Projec-

tions from the MDmc to areas 11, 12o, 12 proper, 13a, 13b, and 13 proper are reciprocated by significant projections from the OFC to the MDmc. Similar to their distinction in amygdala connections, areas 13a, 12o, and Iai connect with portions of the MDmc that primarily connect with the medial prefrontal cortex rather than with the rest of the OFC.[23,24] Area 13a also receives projections from the submedial nucleus, which lies ventral to the mediodorsal nucleus. On the other hand, area 12l receives projections from the most medial edge of the parvocellular division of the mediodorsal nucleus, which is consistent with its close involvement with the dorsolateral prefrontal cortex.

Multiple structures project indirectly to the OFC via the MDmc. These structures include the amygdala; temporal pole; primary olfactory, entorhinal, and perirhinal cortices; substantia innominata (including the ventral pallidum); and lighter projections from the superior and inferior temporal gyri and the insula.[22,79,93] It is unlikely that the MDmc acts as a simple relay station for these structures because all of these areas (with the exception of the substantia innominata) also project directly to the OFC (Figure 4–10). Although projections to the OFC and the MDmc appear to arise from similar cortical and subcortical regions, there appears to be a difference in the nature of the cells projecting to the MDmc and OFC, respectively. Direct projections to the OFC arise from numerous small cells, whereas projections to the MDmc derive from a few sparsely labeled large neurons with long, radiating dendrites.[21,23] This suggests that the direct projections to the OFC may be more suited for carrying detailed information, whereas projections to the MDmc may carry more integrated information.

In contrast to the combination of direct and indirect projections that characterizes most input into the OFC, the substantia innominata (including the ventral pallidum) only influences the OFC via projections to the thalamus.[21] Lacking direct projections to the OFC, this transthalamic projection appears to be the primary route through which basal ganglia functions influence the OFC.

The medial structures of the OFC, which receive projections from the subiculum, also receive a projection from the anteromedial nucleus of the thalamus.[64] The same portion of the anteromedial nucleus that projects to the OFC also receives a projection from the subiculum. The triangular arrangement of the hippocampus, anteromedial thalamus, and OFC thus parallels the triangular arrangement of the amygdala, MDmc, and OFC. Some less significant projections

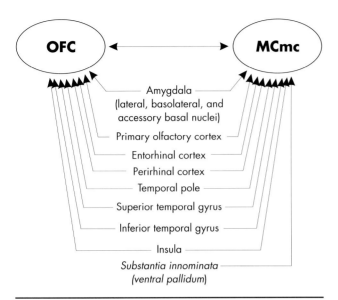

FIGURE 4–10. Triangular organization of afferent input into the orbitofrontal cortex (OFC) and pars magnocellularis (MDmc).

also reach the OFC from the pulvinar, midline, and intralaminar nuclei.[7,92,95,96] The association with the pulvinar appears relatively limited to granular (visual recipient) OFC regions. In contrast, midline and intralaminar nuclei only project to the poorly granulated medial areas.[15] These midline and intralaminar nuclei appear to transfer information related to nociceptive, autonomic, and visceral functions and likely provide a transthalamic pathway through which the medial OFC receives interoceptive information.[97,98]

Orbitofrontal Cortex–Basal Ganglia Loops

Both the lateral OFC and the medial OFC direct significant projections toward the basal ganglia. These projections contribute to a pair of segregated loops connecting the OFC, striatum, globus pallidus, and thalamus.[99–101] In both cases, the flow of information follows a unidirectional course from the OFC to the striatum to the globus pallidus and then returns to the OFC via projections through the MDmc and, to a lesser extent, the ventral anterior thalamic nucleus. The lateral OFC loop originates with a projection from the lateral OFC to a ventral and central strip of the head and body of the caudate nucleus and a medial portion of the putamen (Figure 4–11). The same region of the striatum also receives projections from the superior and inferior temporal (auditory and visual) association cortices. In contrast, the medial OFC loop projects to a more extreme ventromedial segment of the caudate extending

into adjacent portions of the putamen and other aspects of the ventral striatum (Figure 4–12). The ventral striatum consists of the nucleus accumbens, part of the olfactory tubercle, and the extreme edge of the ventral caudate. It primarily receives projections from limbic and paralimbic regions, including the basolateral nucleus of the amygdala; the anterior cingulate; and entorhinal, perirhinal, and temporal lobe structures.[102,103] Thus, many of the key structures that interact with the lateral OFC project to the same region of the striatum that is innervated by the lateral OFC, whereas the key structures that interact with the medial OFC project to the same region of the caudate and ventral striatum that is innervated by the medial OFC.

The medial OFC targeting of the ventral striatum likely plays a critical role in its ability to influence motivation-related functions. A wealth of evidence implicates the ventral striatum, specifically the nucleus accumbens, in brain-reward mechanisms activated by habit-forming drugs, other reinforcers, and the initiation of behaviors aimed at gaining these reinforcers.[104] The posterior agranular OFC (area 13/anterior insula) also sends a highly selective projection to the "striosomes" of the striatum.[105] Along with the agranular medial prelimbic regions, these form the only prefrontal projections to the striosomes. This projection is of interest because the striosomes appear to project directly to the dopamine-containing cells of the substantia nigra or its immediate vicinity, allowing the posterior OFC to selectively modulate the firing of dopamine projections to the basal ganglia. This may allow the OFC to play a selective role in controlling the initiation of basal ganglia–controlled processes. These projections, along with the other OFC projections to the "matrix" compartments of the basal ganglia, also may allow the OFC to influence the initiation of routinized, sequential, or habit-based processes typically attributed to striatal functioning.[106]

FUNCTIONAL CHARACTERISTICS OF THE ORBITOFRONTAL CORTEX

The anatomical characteristics of the OFC provide the basis for the OFC's involvement in normal functioning and psychopathology. The area forms a critical convergence zone for exteroceptive sensory association cortices, interoceptive information, limbic regions involved in emotional processing and memory, and subcortical regions involved in the control of auto-

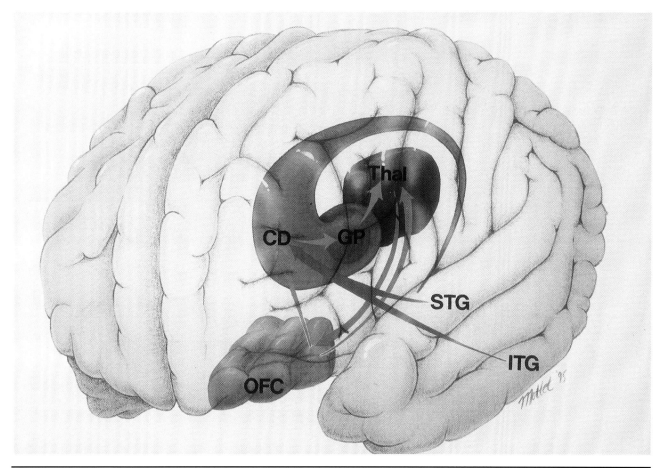

FIGURE 4–11. Lateral orbitofrontal cortex (OFC)–basal ganglia loop.

CD=caudate nucleus; GP=globus pallidum; ITG=inferior temporal gyrus; STG=superior temporal gyrus; Thal=thalamus.

nomic and motor effector pathways. Sensory information is already well processed by the time it reaches this region, and the OFC codes this information with an exquisite level of stimulus specificity. Yet, it is clear that with the exception of the olfactory modality, the region is less involved in perception per se. Rather, the region is involved in the recognition of biologically significant stimuli and their associates and modulating responses to these stimuli based on the current motivational state of the organism.

RECOGNITION OF REINFORCING STIMULI

Cellular and Behavioral
Responses to Appetitive Reinforcers

Food is a powerful reinforcer. The gustatory projections to the OFC provide specific information about the physical properties of food, whereas projections from other sensory areas provide information about stimuli associated with food. This convergence of information provides the ability to make cross-modal associations related to food reward. OFC cells that fire in response to visual presentation of reinforcing foods provide a clear demonstration of this capacity.[47] These cells often show bimodal responses to both the taste and the sight of food. Cells that respond to the visual presentation of appetitive stimuli also exist in the lateral hypothalamus, the substantia innominata, and the amygdala.[107–110] However, the cells in the OFC show a far greater level of stimulus specificity than do cells in these other regions. Cells with responses to visually presented food or aversive stimuli in the substantia innominata, lateral hypothalamus, and amygdala generally respond to multiple aversive or hedonic stimuli, whereas OFC cells have been observed to respond to as few as one appetitive stimulus.

A similar process of association occurs between olfactory and gustatory information in the OFC.[28] The robust ability to associate odors with foods likely reflects the anatomical proximity of secondary taste

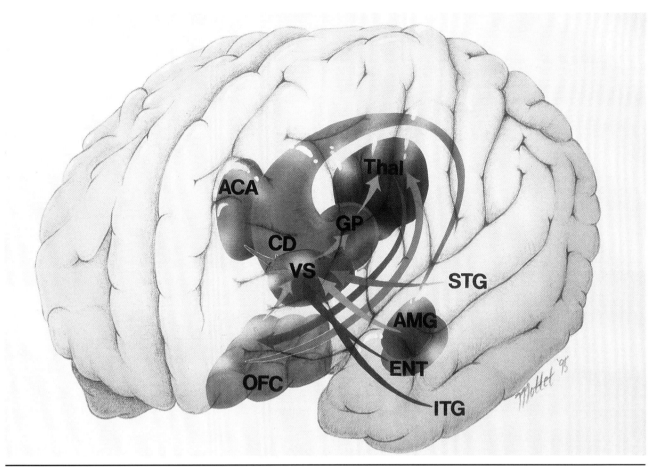

FIGURE 4–12.   The medial orbitofrontal cortex (OFC)–basal ganglia loop.

ACA=anterior cingulate area; AMG=amygdala; CD=caudate nucleus; ENT=entorhinal cortex; ITG=inferior temporal gyrus; STG=superior temporal gyrus; Thal=thalamus; VS=ventral striatum.

cortex and olfactory-dedicated areas of the OFC. Lesions of the OFC cause marked alterations in food preferences and impair the discrimination of food from nonfood objects.[111–113] For instance, OFC-lesioned monkeys will eat foods such as raw meats that nonlesioned monkeys treat as unpalatable.[111,113] These animals also show a hyperorality in which they both place nonfood objects in their mouths and show a readiness to eat nonfood items.[112,114] This hyperorality resembles aspects of the Klüver-Bucy syndrome arising from bilateral temporal lobectomy (amygdalectomy).[115] OFC-lesioned animals appear to treat these nonfood objects as if they had the same reinforcement value as food, and they will even perform operant responses at high levels in order to eat them.

By far, the most commonly used appetitive reinforcer in behavioral and neurophysiological studies is food. During the course of studies that use food reward, cells in the OFC frequently respond to the presentation of food reward or stimuli that signal upcoming food reward.[47,116–118] This reinforcement-related activity occurs in both the lateral and the medial OFC.

The OFC's responsiveness to appetitive stimuli is not limited to food reward. Intracerebral self-stimulation has been widely used to map the neural network involved in reward.[119] The only region of the neocortex in primates that reliably supports intracerebral self-stimulation is the OFC. Self-stimulation sites are primarily found in the posterior-medial OFC (area 13).[119] These intracerebral self-stimulation sites are closely connected to intracerebral self-stimulation sites in the amygdala, lateral hypothalamus, and nucleus accumbens. Indeed, intracerebral self-stimulation of area 13 activates lateral hypothalamic cells, and intracerebral self-stimulation within the lateral hypothalamus or nucleus accumbens activates cells within the posterior OFC.[119] Dopamine antagonists injected into the OFC dose-dependently attenuate the operant responding for intracerebral self-stimulation in the OFC.[120] These OFC injections also significantly decrease operant responding for intracerebral self-stimulation in the amygdala and the lateral hypothalamus. Thus, the OFC is intimately connected to other regions in the brain's reward network and appears to directly influence the ability of these regions to support intracerebral self-stimulation.

An important aspect of the OFC's cellular responses to food reinforcers and intracerebral self-stimulation lies in the reduction or cessation of these neurophysiological responses when the motivational or affective value of these stimuli decreases. For instance, many OFC cells that show activity in response to specific foods when an animal is hungry become unresponsive or show substantially reduced responsiveness after the animal has been satiated on that specific food.[121] Similarly, OFC cells that respond when a thirsty animal receives fluids show decreased firing when the animal is no longer thirsty. The gustatory processing that occurs in the OFC differs dramatically from what is seen in the earlier stages of the gustatory system, where activity occurs independent of motivational state.[122–124]

Sensory-specific satiety also extends into the visual and olfactory domains. OFC cells that respond to the sight or taste of a specific food decrease or cease firing when the animal sees or smells the food after being fed to satiety.[125] These findings indicate that the activity of these cells does not just reflect a process of cross-modal sensory integration but rather reflects the current motivational or reinforcement value of the gustatory stimuli.

In nonlesioned animals, the readiness to perform operant responses for food reward inversely relates to the animal's level of satiety. Animals without lesions significantly reduce their operant responding for food when satiated. In contrast, animals with lesions that include the OFC do not show as great a decrement in operant responses when satiated.[126] These animals sometimes have seemingly insatiable appetites.[126,127] Similarly, several case reports have noted the presence of voracious appetites in humans following OFC lesions.[128–132] The exact focus within the OFC necessary to produce this effect is not clear, although some reports suggested that damage to the more anterior regions of the OFC or the frontal poles forms the critical focus in these cases.[132]

Satiety not only decreases operant responses for food but also attenuates operant responses for intracerebral self-stimulation in the OFC and the lateral hypothalamus.[133] This highlights the close linkage between reward and gustatory processing at the level of the OFC. Furthermore, it suggests that the OFC's modulation of the primary reinforcement value of food reward reflects a more general role in processing the reward value of appetitive reinforcers. Indeed, the OFC appears to process information about positively valenced stimuli in every sensory modality. Even in the somatosensory modality, greater OFC activity emerges during exposure to pleasant stimuli than during neutral stimulation.[134] Thus, while responses to food-related stimuli provide one of the easiest to observe manifestations of OFC processing, it probably represents a more general process that affects all classes of appetitive reinforcers.

Cellular Responses to Aversive Stimuli

Some OFC cells respond to olfactory, gustatory, and visual stimuli that act as unconditioned or conditioned aversive reinforcers.[28,47] The lateral hypothalamus, amygdala, and substantia innominata also have cells that respond to the visual presentation of aversive stimuli.[107,108,110,135] As is the case in the processing of appetitive reinforcers, the cells in the OFC process aversive stimuli with greater specificity than do the cells in these other areas. Whereas cells in these other regions respond to multiple aversive stimuli, OFC cells respond to as few as one aversive stimulus. Studies examining aversive responses in the primate OFC have primarily focused on aversive gustatory stimuli (e.g., an aversive saline solution). However, data in lower mammals further indicate that OFC cells respond to somatovisceral nociception.[57] Thus, both interoceptive and exteroceptive stimuli with aversive properties activate OFC cells.

Olfactory stimuli may possess unconditional aversive properties. Some cells in the primate OFC respond to aversive odorants.[28] In a PET study of olfactory hedonics in humans, aversive odorants produced significant increases in left posterior-lateral OFC activity, and the magnitude of the increase correlated significantly with ratings of aversiveness.[33] Interestingly, this increase also correlated with activity in the left amygdala, indicating that humans retain the close functional relationship between the OFC and the amygdala seen in nonhuman primates. Aversive gustatory stimuli also have been observed to activate the OFC in humans.[136] Surprisingly, this activation occurs far more anteriorly than the caudolateral OFC and thus appears to represent activity within a section of the OFC other than that described as secondary gustatory cortex by Rolls and colleagues.[36–38]

STIMULUS-REINFORCER LEARNING

Amygdala–Orbitofrontal Cortex Interactions in Creating Stimulus-Reward Associations

In many cases, OFC neurons only respond to a sensory stimulus after it has become associated with an appetitive or aversive reinforcer. For instance, Thorpe et al.[47] observed an OFC cell that responded to the visual presentation of a syringe only after the syringe had become associated with an unpleasant-tasting fluid. Many olfactory-responsive cells in the OFC have activity patterns that reflect stimulus-reinforcer learning. A recent neurophysiological study reported that approximately 35% of the olfactory-responsive neurons in the OFC depend on the association of odorants with a rewarding or aversive gustatory stimulus.[137] Such neurons also may code for incidental associations, such as the place where the rewarded odorants occur.[138]

Lesions of the OFC impair the ability to directly associate visual stimuli with food reward (without relying on a secondary reinforcer).[139–141] Lesions of the amygdala produce impairments of similar severity to those produced by lesions of the OFC.[142] Similar impairments also arise following lesions of the MDmc.[140] Thus, lesions at any point in the triangular circuit connecting the amygdala, OFC, and MDmc disrupt the ability to make direct stimulus-reinforcer associations.

Despite its involvement in directly associating visual stimuli with food reward, the OFC is not essential for the acquisition of numerous tasks involving reinforcement. Conditioning of operant responses[126] and fear conditioning to contextual cues[143] are both acquired at normal levels in the face of OFC damage. Similarly, OFC-lesioned animals perform tasks such as the positional response task[144–146] and temporal reinforcement schedules[147] at normal levels. Medial OFC lesions also leave many visual and auditory discrimination tasks unimpaired.[148] Thus, despite the OFC's critical participation in directly associating stimuli with reward, many tasks and conditioning paradigms can proceed without OFC involvement. This parallels findings from nonhuman primates with amygdala lesions, which showed intact learning of tasks that allow secondary or indirect associations with reward, despite impairments in direct stimulus-reinforcer learning.[140,141]

Coding Changes in Reinforcement Contingencies

Many OFC cells show alterations in their firing pattern that coincide with alterations in reinforcement contin-

gencies. For instance, on a go/no-go visual discrimination task, in which visual stimuli were associated with food reward and aversive saline, respectively, 71% of the cells (mainly lateral OFC cells) that selectively responded to the visual stimuli reversed their firing pattern when the visual-gustatory pairings were reversed.[137] These changes occurred extremely rapidly (sometimes after only one trial) and usually coincided with or preceded behavioral reversal. Another 23.5% of the visually responsive cells showed extinction of differential responses after the reversal. In a similar paradigm involving the olfactory-responsive cells of the OFC (primarily medial OFC), 25% of the odor-responsive cells showed full reversal of their firing after reversal of the stimulus association, whereas 43% showed extinction of selective responding to the stimuli. These physiological and behavioral reversals and extinctions in the olfactory domain take substantially longer than the rapid reversals and extinctions in the visual domain.

In addition to possessing cells that show reversals and extinctions, the OFC has cells that fire when there is a discrepancy between the expected reward and the actual consequences of a behavior. For instance, Rosenkilde et al.[118] observed "error detection" cells in the OFC that did not fire when a response was rewarded but fired vigorously after responses if the expected reward was withheld. After a few extinction trials, the firing decreased, suggesting that the cells were primarily involved in registering the absence of an expected reinforcer. A similar pattern of activity occurs in response to the removal of food or preferred objects.[133] Most "error detection" or "reinforcer withdrawal" cells localize to the medial OFC, although a few error detection cells have been found in other prefrontal regions.[149,150] The only other area where error detection cells of this sort have been reported is the anterior cingulate.[149] A subpopulation of reinforcement-sensitive cells in ventral area 46/lateral area 12 also appear sensitive to changes in reinforcement contingencies. These cells have been observed to respond to unreinforced trials with changes in firing activity opposite to their firing on reinforced trials.[118]

Orbitofrontal Cortex Involvement in Extinction and Reversal

Error detection cells and cells that extinguish selective responding following changes in reinforcement contingencies likely play a critical role in the OFC's ability to modify behavior when reinforcement contingencies change. Lesions encompassing or focused on the medial OFC (especially Walker's area 13) result in a marked tendency toward continued (perseverative) responding in extinction paradigms.[114,126,143,151]

The medial OFC's role in reversal learning is more complicated. Medial OFC–lesioned animals are not impaired in learning an initial reversal.[148,151] However, these animals often have difficulty acquiring subsequent reversals.[148,152] This deficit arises only after both stimuli have been associated with reward and nonreward. In such situations, a simple associative process alone cannot be used for determining which stimulus is the correct one to respond to because both stimuli have been associated with reward and nonreward. Rather, some mechanism for retaining or using information about the most recently reinforced object is required. The reliability and focus of this multiple reversal deficit remain in question. Restricted lesioning of the posterior medial OFC or more anterior OFC areas produce no impairment or only mild impairment on reversal tasks.[151] The lesions that produce multiple reversal deficits appear more widespread than those that do not and may involve a more laterally placed area of the OFC. However, the perseverative pattern of errors typically observed following lateral OFC lesions was not observed in these animals.

In contrast, inferior convexity lesions produce severe impairments in the acquisition of spatial and object reversals and alternations.[148,151,153–155] A major cause of this impairment has been traced to the strong tendency for inferior convexity–lesioned animals to perseveratively respond to stimuli.[148,155] This perseverative behavior occurs on such a wide variety of tasks that it is often viewed as a defining characteristic of intracerebral lesions.[156] Originally, this behavior was described in terms of a "drive disinhibition" syndrome because the response occurred in the context of perseverative go responses in go/no-go paradigms.[132,157] However, the drive disinhibition hypothesis fails to explain why inferior convexity–lesioned animals respond perseveratively on two choice alternation tasks[148,153,154] or why these animals engage in perseverative nonresponding following reversals of go and no-go stimuli.[158,159] A simple inability to inhibit motor responses cannot explain these impairments. A consistent component of tasks on which inferior convexity–lesioned animals perseverate is the requirement that the animal alter its behavior away from a predominant or previously reinforced response style.[156,160] In order to do this, an animal must recognize that the previously rewarded or predominant response is not

generating the expected reward and then use this information to select a different response. The presence in the lateral OFC of cells responsive to the withholding of reward (or showing rapid reversal for reward and punishment) could provide a basis through which response failures get coded.[117,118] The inferior convexity region also has cells that show activity correlated to both go and no-go responses.[117,161] The region is thus in a position to act as an interface between error detection and response selection. Inferior convexity–lesioned animals who lack this interface would be unable to modulate their behavior appropriately in the face of changing reinforcement contingencies.

In contrast to the effects of medial OFC lesions, lesions of the lateral OFC do not impair extinction learning.[151] The lateral OFC and medial OFC thus appear to play complementary and dissociable roles in situations in which rewards are withheld. The medial OFC appears necessary for normal extinction, whereas the lateral OFC is required for modulating behavior in situations in which more than one choice (including no response) is reinforced over time. Interestingly, error detection cells in the medial OFC show different neurophysiological features than do lateral OFC error detection cells.[118] Medial OFC error detection cells frequently fail to respond except when reward is withheld. In contrast, the error detection cells in the lateral OFC alter their firing in response to both reward and nonreward.[118] This difference between lateral and medial OFC cells may relate to differences in the ease of extinction and reversal in the olfactory and visual domains. Although reversal and extinction cells are observable in both the medial and the lateral OFC, the medial region is more involved in olfaction, and more olfactory-responsive cells extinguish rather than reverse their firing following a reversal in olfactory-gustatory reward reinforcement contingencies.[137] In contrast, visually responsive cells, which are more prominent in the lateral OFC, more frequently reverse rather than extinguish their firing.

The OFC's ability to reverse and extinguish firing to reinforcers, especially its ability to rapidly reverse firing to visual stimuli, critically distinguishes it from other areas involved in stimulus-reinforcer associations. For instance, the amygdala, which is clearly involved in forming stimulus-reinforcer associations, does not show equivalently rapid reversal abilities.[162] Because of this, normal OFC processing becomes paramount in situations in which reinforcement changes occur too rapidly for the amygdala to alter its less fluid stimulus-reinforcer associations. The OFC's involvement in fluidly coding changes in stimulus-response-reinforcer contingencies appears to relate directly to many of the deficits observed in humans with OFC lesions. Humans with OFC lesions show both reversal and extinction deficits similar to those seen in nonhuman primates.[163] Moreover, the degree of impairment on these tasks is associated with the social and emotional dysfunction that characterizes OFC-lesioned patients.

Coding of Expectancies and Relative Reward Value

As already noted, the OFC has cells that code when expected reinforcers are withheld. This indicates that the OFC processes information about not only reinforcers that are currently present but also expected (future) reinforcers. Single-cell studies have directly observed cells in the OFC that fire in anticipation of appetitive or aversive reinforcers.[164–166] During instrumental learning, these cells appear to modify their firing even before the animal has learned to reliably perform the reinforced behavior. Thus, the cells are not merely firing as a consequence of learned behavior. Rather, they appear to provide information about reinforcers that helps guide the learning of the behavior.

Schultz and colleagues[165] have conducted some of the most thorough investigations of expectancy representations in the OFC. They used a delayed go/no-go task with monkeys and observed OFC cells that fire during the period preceding a reward and terminate soon after the receipt of the reward. These cells fire after the animal has already performed the necessary movement or nonmovement and thus do not reflect what the animal did. Strikingly, these cells show prolonged activity if the reward is delayed and abbreviated activity if the reward arrives early. Thus, these cells appear specifically linked to the anticipation of the reward, with their offset occurring once the reward is received.

To date, the neural bases of expectancies have received little attention in the cognitive neuroscience literature. However, a recent PET study suggests that the human OFC becomes active during breaches in expectancies.[167] This converges with the primate literature indicating the presence of OFC cells that specifically fire when expected outcomes fail to materialize. In many cases, the OFC's processing of rewarding stimuli does not consist of a simple representation of the reinforcer. Instead, many reward-related cells in the OFC appear to code for the relative reward value

of stimuli.[166] Thus, the OFC not only participates in determining whether a rewarding stimulus (or its associated conditioned stimulus) is present but also codes for the reinforcer's relative reward value. Not surprisingly, animals with OFC lesions are unable to modify their behavior during reinforcer devaluations.[168]

EMOTIONAL AND SOCIAL BEHAVIOR

Effects of Lesions on Emotional Behavior in Animals

OFC lesions produce robust alterations in emotional behaviors in animals. In cats, prefrontal lesions that impinge on the OFC produce a general lowering of thresholds for emotional reactions, especially rage reactions.[169] OFC lesions in vervet monkeys produce increases in aggressive responses in certain settings,[170] but lesions in rhesus monkeys produce robust long-term and stable decrements in aggressive responses and increases in fearful withdrawal.[114,171] In rhesus monkeys, the posterior portion of Walker's area 13 appears to represent the critical lesion site for producing these behavioral alterations. In both species, the animals show increased social withdrawal. This has most closely been observed with vervet monkeys who show dramatic decreases in social grooming and other affiliative behaviors as well as substantial declines in social rank.[172] In summary, OFC lesions produce robust changes in affiliative and other emotional behaviors in animals. The specific changes differ depending on the species and probably the size and location of the lesion focus, but the lesions consistently reduce the ability to function within a social environment.

Effects of Lesions on Affect in Humans

OFC lesions in humans produce alterations in a wide range of affective behavior.[173–180] Approximately half of the patients with bilateral or right OFC lesions in one study required psychiatric treatment.[174] In contrast, unilateral left OFC lesions appear to produce less dramatic psychiatric problems than do right lesions. Patients with right OFC lesions appear particularly susceptible to increases in negative emotions, reporting heightened incidences of depression, anger, irritability, and anxiety. OFC lesions also appear to lead to increased overt hostility and verbal aggressiveness, although subjects with these lesions sometimes show little awareness of their increased aggessiveness.[181]

In contrast to the increased negative emotionality associated with OFC lesions, euphoria, exuberance, and hyperactivity sometimes increase as a consequence of reduced OFC functioning.[176,177,180] These intense affective responses may reach maniclike levels. Alternatively, patients may show a global heightening of emotional responsivity to socially relevant stimuli. Intense (pseudobulbar-like) emotional expressions disconnected from relevant social stimuli also may occur in such individuals. For instance, Damasio and Anderson[182] described a patient who would frequently laugh or cry in social situations despite the absence of humorous or sorrowful stimuli. When questioned while laughing or crying, the patient denied feeling particularly happy or sad. Paradoxically, a blunting of affect sometimes occurs following these lesions.

The Pseudopsychopathic Personality

The alterations in emotional responsivity that occur in humans with OFC lesions are frequently accompanied by a characteristic pattern of social disinhibition.[1,173,182–184] OFC-lesioned patients often are described as coarse, tactless, and generally lacking in empathy and social restraints. Reports of excessive involvement in pleasure-seeking behaviors, especially sexual behaviors, are common with such individuals. This excessive involvement in pleasurable activities is compounded by an apparent reduction in sensitivity to negative risks. Reports of patients making risky business decisions with disastrous consequences, despite the advice of others, repeatedly appear in the literature. In addition, these patients show impulsive and antisocial behavior. However, despite an apparent disregard for social rules, they usually lack the intentional viciousness or organization of a true antisocial personality disorder.[182] Blumer and Benson[173] aptly referred to these lesion-induced personality traits as "pseudopsychopathic."

The functional basis of the pseudopsychopathic personality is unclear. But several clear deficits emerge with regularity in OFC-lesioned patients that may explain some of these behaviors. First, patients with OFC lesions show a marked loss of empathy.[185] Second, humans with OFC lesions show impairments in emotional facial and vocal identification.[186] Thus, these patients not only lack empathy for others but also have substantial difficulties identifying the emotional experience that others are experiencing based on emotional cues. Saver and Damasio[193] examined a

"pseudopsychopathic" patient with ventromedial lesions on a series of probes of social reasoning. Compared with control subjects, this patient showed no deficits in moral or social reasoning, and the patient's ability to consider response options and predict the consequences of these responses was normal.

The inability of OFC-lesioned patients to appropriately identify facial emotion converges with neuroimaging studies implicating the OFC in the learning and recognition of faces and the identification of facial expressions of emotion.[187–193] These abilities appear critical to the maintenance of appropriate social functioning in a complex society. The emotional reactions of other people that occur in response to one's own behavior often act as primary or secondary reinforcers and provide important information about when one needs to modify one's behavior. It is not difficult to see how the lack of such abilities could lead to socially inappropriate behavior, especially in someone with diminished inhibitory control.

Saver and Damasio concluded that the patient's disregard for social rules and his disastrous decision making could not be attributed to a lack of social knowledge or moral reasoning, inability to generate appropriate response options, or inability to consider the consequences or risks associated with responses or social configurations.

Recent investigations using gambling simulations also have started to delineate the basis of the risk-taking behavior of these patients.[194,195] PET data indicate that when persons without lesions make choices between high reward/high risk and low reward/low risk options, they activate portions of the right OFC and ventral frontal pole.[196] Not surprisingly, patients with ventral frontal lesions perform poorly on gambling simulations. In particular, when given gambling tasks in which subjects have to balance future risks or punishment with immediate rewards or punishments, patients with ventromedial frontal (i.e., medial orbital gyrus, gyrus rectus, and subgenual cingulate) lesions show a relative insensitivity to the future consequences of behavior. These subjects do not appear to be simply hypersensitive to immediate reward or hyposensitive to immediate punishment. Rather, they appear to be largely uninfluenced by the potential for future reward or punishment compared with immediate reward or punishment. These studies suggest that the risky and often disastrous business decisions of OFC-lesioned individuals arise from a reduction of potential future consequences to influence decisions.

Autonomic Responses

Electrical stimulation of the OFC, particularly the posterior medial OFC, produces phasic changes in autonomic and endocrinological functions. Stimulation of this region produces both sympathetic and parasympathetic effects, including alterations in respiration, blood pressure, pupillary dilation, salivation, stomach tone, plasma cortisol levels, and inhibition of pyloric peristalsis.[197–202] Lesions of the OFC in both human and nonhuman primates do not produce changes in the tonic regulation of visceral systems.[202,203] Rather, they alter autonomic responses to stimuli that are behaviorally meaningful.[203–206] For instance, humans with ventromedial prefrontal cortex lesions show significantly blunted autonomic responses to socially meaningful stimuli. They also show blunted responses to conditioned stimuli that have been associated with a startling loud sound, despite having normal responses to unconditioned stimuli. In humans, these deficits particularly arise from posterior but not anterior ventromedial lesions, which is consistent with the visceral-related afferents and efferents in the posterior medial region of the OFC. In some cases, lesions causing these effects may have encroached on area 25 in the subgenual cingulate, but this does not appear to have been the central focus in many of these cases. It is unclear whether these blunted autonomic responses reflect a cause, a consequence, or an integral part of the deficient (affective) decision making of these patients. Regardless of its specific role, abnormal autonomic functioning appears intimately tied to the emotional and social dysfunction in these patients.

Positron-Emission Tomography Studies of Emotions

PET studies that use anxiety-provoking paradigms frequently report alterations in regional cerebral blood flow (rCBF) within the OFC. Increases in rCBF in the left posterior OFC and medial OFC have been reported in psychiatrically healthy individuals anxiously anticipating an electric shock and infusion of cholecystokinin tetrapeptide (CCK), respectively.[207,208] Furthermore, the amount of rCBF change in the left OFC appears to correlate with the level of induced anxiety.[209] Pardo et al.[210] observed significant rCBF increases in the inferior frontal gyrus, extending into the lateral OFC, in control subjects undergoing self-induced recall or imagining of dysphoric events.

Posterior lateral OFC activations also have been observed during script-induced anger.[211] In an important series of PET studies, Rauch and colleagues[212–214] and Shin and colleagues[215] exposed patients with anxiety disorders to anxiety-provoking stimuli. Patients with social phobia, obsessive-compulsive disorder (OCD), and posttraumatic stress disorder all had increased activity within posterior portions of the OFC compared with those who had neutral exposures. Other studies also have reported increased OFC activity in patients with anxiety disorders undergoing anxiety inductions.[216,217] Of particular note, patients with OCD exposed to stimuli that provoke obsessions show increased OFC blood flow.[213,217,218] Some data also suggest that psychiatrically healthy subjects exposed to auditory stimuli that provoke obsessive ruminations show increased OFC activity.[218]

In contrast to the increased OFC activity observed in many anxiety-induction studies, Fredrikson and colleagues[219–221] reported decreased OFC activity in two separate groups of patients with simple phobia undergoing exposure to a videotape presentation of phobogenic visual stimuli as compared with neutral stimuli. The Fredrikson studies differ from the other anxiety-induction studies in that in all of the other studies, subjects were not viewing a fear-inducing object at the time of the scans but instead were contemplating or anticipating an aversive event or object that was either not present or not visible at the time of imaging.

Taken together, these studies suggest that OFC activity increases when subjects contemplate or imagine phobic or traumatic stimuli, whereas OFC activity decreases when subjects actually view phobogenic stimuli. This hypothesis received its most direct testing in a PET study by Shin et al.,[222] who contrasted visual imagery of combat-related pictures with viewing of combat-related pictures in patients with posttraumatic stress disorder and healthy control subjects. Although no significant differences were observed in OFC activity between the two conditions in the patients with posttraumatic stress disorder, greater left OFC activity occurred when healthy subjects performed visual imagery of the combat scenes than when they perceived them. We hope that future studies will clarify this issue.

PET studies also implicate the OFC in processes related to drug craving and/or the effects of drugs. In one study, human subjects with a history of cocaine abuse showed increased regional brain metabolism in the OFC during the first week of cocaine withdrawal, and this activity correlated significantly with the level of craving for cocaine.[223] Cocaine abusers exposed to drug-related cues similarly showed increased metabolism in the OFC.[224]

MNEMONIC AND HIGHER COGNITIVE FUNCTIONS

Memory in Nonhuman Primates With Orbitofrontal Cortex Lesions

The connections of the medial OFC/gyrus rectus region with the hippocampus, entorhinal cortex, and thalamus suggest a role for medial OFC regions in processes related to mnemonic functions. OFC lesions that encompass areas 13 and 14 produce significant impairments on a visual delayed nonmatching-to-sample task (an object recognition task sensitive to hippocampal damage).[225] The extent of this impairment increases significantly with delay, indicating that the deficit arises from mnemonic dysfunction rather than other task demands. Electrophysiological data also support the hypothesis that the OFC participates in some aspect of mnemonic coding. The cortex surrounding the medial and middle orbital sulci contains cells that alter their firing patterns during the delay periods of visual delayed matching-to-sample tasks.[118] Some of these delay-period changes appear to occur only if the response made after the delay is correct.

Lesions elsewhere in the OFC of nonhuman primates frequently produce deficits on other memory tasks, but these deficits often reflect task-related problems that are not specific to mnemonic functions. For instance, ablations that include area 11 or 12 interfere with performance on tasks that require the retention of information about object or stimulus characteristics (such as color or pattern features) over brief delays.[153,154,226] However, several features call into question whether these deficits relate to the mnemonic components of these tasks. Many of the lesioned animals show a high rate of perseverative responding. In one experiment, the animals showed impairment even when there was no delay,[139] and in another experiment, increasing the delay time failed to increase the error rate.[226] Taken together, these factors suggest that the performance deficit is not related to the mnemonic aspects of the tasks. More clearly mnemonic-related deficits result from inferior convexity lesions. Reversible lesions of the prefrontal cortex that impinge on ventral area 46 and area 12l produce delay-sensitive deficits on nonspatial memory tasks.[227] However, the separate contributions of area 12l and ventral area 46 remain unclear. More evidence implicates ventral area 46 in these functions than area 12l.[46] Nevertheless, because of the close connections between area 12l and ventral area 46 and the similarity in many of the efferent connections of these structures, 12l's contribution to visual working memory remains unresolved.

Learning in Nonhuman Primates

In most tasks that are impaired by OFC lesions in nonhuman primates, the lesions disproportionately impair the acquisition component of the task. For instance, the deficit in acquiring the delayed nonmatching-to-sample task that arises from combined lesions of areas 13 and 14 is greater than that observed following medial temporal lobe (combined hippocampal-amygdala-entorhinal) lesions.[225,228] However, once the behavior is acquired, the impairment is less severe than that caused by medial temporal lobe lesions. A similar pattern characterizes the OFC's involvement in visual discrimination learning. Lesions of the OFC frequently impair the learning of object or pattern discriminations.[139,152,229–231] This deficit arises following large lesions to the OFC or inferior convexity, although selective medial OFC and inferior convexity lesions sometimes do not produce this deficit. To investigate the source of this visual discrimination deficit, Voytko[152] examined the ability of animals to perform already-learned discriminations under OFC cooling and found no deficit, despite the inability of these animals to learn new discrimination during OFC cooling. This suggests that the deficit arising from OFC lesions relates to the acquisition component of the task rather than reflecting an inability to perceptually discriminate objects or patterns. The learning deficits associated with the OFC lesions reflect a multimodal problem. Lesions of the inferior convexity produce impairments in learning auditory discriminations without impairing auditory sensory thresholds.[148] Inferior convexity lesions even impair performance of tactile discrimination tasks, which clearly does not arise from a basic perceptual deficit.[232]

The OFC performs several functions that could potentially interfere with task acquisition. First, the ability to establish new stimulus-reinforcer associations is critical to learning discrimination, unless other strategies such as verbalization are available. Both visual and auditory discrimination tasks require the establishment of stimulus-reinforcer associations. A second component of learning these tasks involves altering responses based on changing contingencies. Learning a new task often requires that prepotent stimulus-response bonds be suppressed or extinguished based on the new reinforcement contingency. The fact that OFC cells respond to alterations in reinforcement contingencies faster than do cells in other regions may allow the OFC to rapidly influence learning and unlearning. Finally, the presence of error detection cells may allow the OFC to help correct wrong or previously rewarded responses. In the absence of such reward- and error-related information, lesioned animals rely on prepotent and often perseverative response styles.

Memory in Humans With Orbitofrontal Cortex Lesions

Lesions of the OFC in humans produce no consistent deficits on traditional neuropsychological tests of memory.[182,183,233,234] However, memory impairments do arise on some less traditional mnemonic tasks. Prefrontal lesions involving an orbital focus have been reported to impair delayed-response and delayed-alternation tasks, even in the absence of impairment on the Wechsler Memory Scale.[235] These deficits were not observed following prefrontal cortex lesions that excluded the OFC. Consistent with this finding, robust bilateral OFC activity (measured with PET) has been reported during the acquisition of a delayed-response alternation task.[236] The greatest focus of activation on this task involved the anterior and lateral portions of the right OFC (Brodmann's areas 11 and 47). Several PET studies have reported OFC activations during the recall of different types of verbal information.[237–239] These activations have appeared in multiple areas of the OFC, with the right anterior extreme of the OFC (Brodmann's area 10) showing the greatest consistency across studies.

In a series of studies comparing OFC-leukotomized schizophrenic patients with nonleukotomized schizophrenic patients, Stuss and colleagues[234,240,241] found that leukotomized patients performed significantly worse than nonleukotomized patients when asked to recall consonant trigrams after an intervening interference task. All other memory tasks and attentional tasks were performed at an equivalent level to that attained by the nonleukotomized patients. These data suggest that the OFC plays a role in guiding memory during tasks with divided attentional demands. However, the generalizability of this result to nonschizophrenic individuals is questionable. Studies of nonpsychotic patients with ventromedial frontal lesions have not found a similar interference effect.[184] In sum-

mary, although several studies suggest a role for the OFC in some aspect of mnemonic functions, the specific role remains poorly defined.

Higher Cognitive Functions in Humans

In general, OFC lesions in humans produce only minimal effects on IQ.[184,234,241] These patients perform most neuropsychological functions, including language, visuospatial, attention, and executive functions, at normal levels. However, data from leukotomized schizophrenic patients suggest that some more subtle deficits may exist in OFC-lesioned patients. Leukotomized patients show difficulty making some conceptual shifts.[241] Nevertheless, these patients usually show little perseveration on the Wisconsin Card Sorting Test, and when problems do develop on the Wisconsin Card Sorting Test, they tend to relate to failures to maintain set rather than perseveration.[241] This is consistent with the heightened distractibility that occurs sometimes in such patients. In summary, patients with OFC lesions frequently have relatively normal neuropsychological abilities, and to the extent that neuropsychological deficits arise from these lesions, they appear far subtler than those arising from either the dorsolateral prefrontal or more posterior lesions. The subtlety of these deficits contrasts with the deficits in empathy, recognizing the emotions of others, and affiliative behavior, as well as the disastrous real-life decision making that characterizes these patients.

THE ORBITOFRONTAL CORTEX IN NEUROPSYCHIATRIC ILLNESS

In most cases, the link between OFC functioning and specific forms of psychopathology remains speculative. However, the OFC's involvement in a wide range of functions related to emotional processing suggests a likely role for the OFC in a variety of neuropsychiatric conditions. Many of the functions subserved by the OFC directly relate to abnormal psychological processes that characterize neuropsychiatric illness. For instance, the OFC's involvement in modulating the motivational value of appetitive reinforcers implicates it in processes directly pertinent to substance abuse and other addictive behaviors.

In considering the OFC's potential role in substance abuse, it is important to recall that the OFC sends direct projections to the ventral striatum, including the nucleus accumbens. A wealth of evidence implicates the nucleus accumbens in the substrates of brain reward, especially those related to habit-forming drugs.[119,242] Dopaminergic modulation of this region critically mediates initiation of a range of incentive-motivated behavior for naturally occurring rewards (e.g., sex, food).[104,243] The OFC's direct input into the ventral striatum allows it to modulate and provide current reward-related information to this pivotal brain-reward structure. Phylogenetically, the OFC is a more recently developed structure than the ventral striatum, and, as such, it appears to critically modulate the more primitive functions of the ventral striatum. The OFC processes reward-related activity with far greater flexibility than does the ventral striatum. For instance, satiety does not appear to reduce self-stimulation in the nucleus accumbens in the manner that it does in the OFC.[133] The coding of satiety essentially involves a reduction in the motivational value of stimuli with prolonged exposure. Failure or weakness of this process leads to prolonged exposure to reinforcers and the continued high evaluation of their reinforcement value. In the case of habit-forming drugs, such prolonged exposure increases the vulnerability to the physiological effects of reinforcers such as tolerance and withdrawal. Thus, a failure of the OFC coding of satiety may lead to prolonged desire and exposure to drugs as well as increasing the risk of developing symptoms of dependency. Another potential source of OFC involvement in substance abuse relates to its high level of stimulus specificity in recognizing cues associated with reinforcers. Recognition of such associations triggers approach and other incentive-motivated behaviors aimed at obtaining the primary reinforcer. Studies of cocaine abusers highlight the importance of this role, indicating OFC activation during exposure to drug-related cues and suggesting a possible involvement of the OFC in craving.[223,224]

The OFC's role in gustatory reward and satiety suggests similar links to binge-eating behavior. As already noted, OFC lesions sometimes produce a failure to satiate in both human and nonhuman primates.[126–131] Alternatively, the recognition of the associates of specific foods could influence the incentive craving for these foods. Although studies of reward-related functions in the OFC usually focus on intracerebral self-stimulation and gustatory reward, the OFC's reward-related processes likely reflect a general process in modulating reward-related behaviors. This suggests that the OFC's coding of satiety and reinforcer associations may play an active role in other impulse-control

and compulsive behaviors in which individuals fail to stop behaviors once started or experience impulses when exposed to cues related to these rewarding actions.

On the surface, reducing the reinforcer value of stimuli based on satiety and recognizing reinforcer associates may appear to reflect contradictory processes. However, these both reflect variations of a general role in modulating behavior based on a comparison of potential reinforcers in the environment and the current needs of the organism. The rapid coding and integration of changes in external stimuli, internal states, and stimulus-reinforcer contingencies are necessary for the flexible adaptation of behavior in rapidly changing environments. In these situations, the OFC appears to perform essential operations. The OFC's involvement in coding and modulating the motivational value of stimuli also suggests a potential role in affective disorders, in which the sensitivity to reward is either elevated (mania) or depressed (major depression). Whether primary or secondary to lesions, these affective episodes may be conceptualized in terms of abnormal coding of the motivational value of potential appetitive reinforcers. The frequency of depressive episodes and the occurrence of maniclike episodes following OFC lesions underscore the importance of the OFC in regulating these processes.[174–178,180] Indeed, decreased orbital rCBF has been observed in manic patients.[244]

Of course, OFC functions may be disrupted, or biased by far more subtle processes. Specifically, emerging data suggests that alterations in serotonergic functioning may powerfully modulate the OFC's processing of affective information. Powerful alterations in serotonergic functioning may modulate the OFC's processing of affective information. For instance, depressive relapses caused by tryptophan depletions are specifically associated with reductions in OFC metabolism.[245]

OFC involvement in processes related to empathy and recognition of affect provides another area through which OFC dysfunction might relate to psychopathology. In particular, disorders such as psychopathy (antisocial personality disorder), in which individuals show a lack of empathy, excessive aggression, and a reduced sensitivity to risks, show direct parallels to the effects of OFC lesions in humans. The effects of OFC lesions in nonhuman primates also provide parallels to the emotional and affiliative dysfunction seen in Asperger's disorder or even in the schizophrenic spectrum.

The OFC also processes aversive stimuli. Of particular interest, OFC cells can associate previously neutral stimuli with aversive stimuli.[28,47] This involvement in recognizing aversive stimuli provides a strong theoretical link to the anxiety disorders. Learning the associates of aversive stimuli and recognizing conditioned and unconditioned stimuli with aversive properties lie at the core of behavioral conceptualizations of anxiety disorders. Many investigators have emphasized the amygdala's role in these processes.[75,80] The differential roles of the OFC and amygdala are unclear. The OFC has not received as close scrutiny as the amygdala in this regard. This partly reflects the fact that rodents do not provide a good model for studying OFC functions, whereas more substantial similarities exist between the amygdala in the rodent and the primate. However, lesions of the ventral portions of the medial prefrontal cortex in rodents (which shows similarities to the medial OFC in primates) do not affect the acquisition of aversive conditioning.[143] They do, however, disrupt the extinction of aversive conditioning. Thus, at least in rodents, the critical role of the OFC appears to be in altering already-established aversive reinforcement contingencies. This corresponds to studies in nonhuman primates, which indicate that the OFC has greater flexibility and speed than the amygdala in processing changes in aversive reinforcement contingencies. For instance, when a visual stimulus that was previously rewarded starts being punished, OFC cells rapidly alter their firing.[137] A similarly rapid process of learning appears in OFC cells when a previously punished response becomes rewarded. To our knowledge, alterations in responses of similar speed and flexibility have never been reported in studies examining the amygdala. Furthermore, the OFC shows greater stimulus specificity in its coding of aversive stimuli, possibly allowing detection of more subtle discrimination of specific stimulus-reinforcer contingencies. PET stimulation studies in patients with anxiety disorders and healthy control subjects further suggest the importance of activity in the OFC for anxiety disorders.[207–209,212–215] Of all the anxiety disorders, OCD shows the most robust and replicated link to OFC functioning. Therefore, in the remainder of this chapter, we focus on the potential role of the OFC in the expression of obsessive-compulsive symptoms.

Obsessive-Compulsive Disorder

PET studies frequently report OFC hypermetabolism in OCD patients at rest.[246–249] OCD patients also show robust increases in OFC activity immediately after or during exposure to triggering stimuli.[213,217,250] Furthermore, successful pharmacological treatment of OCD with selective serotonin reuptake inhibitors is associated with significant reductions in OFC metabolism.[251,252] Both pharmacological and behavioral treatments of OCD alter the pattern of correlations between OFC, basal ganglia, and thalamic metabolism, consistent with previous evidence implicating the OFC–basal ganglia loops in OCD.[252–257]

The specific role that the OFC plays in OCD remains speculative. However, several possibilities arise based on the normal functions subserved by the OFC. We examine these possibilities in the following paragraphs. The focus on the OFC is not intended to imply that other areas such as the cingulate do not participate in OCD but to stimulate research on the specific contributions of the OFC to obsessive-compulsive symptoms.

The OFC's role in processing information about aversive stimuli and their associates provides a useful starting point. For instance, OFC hyperactivity might be theorized to relate to a hypervigilance or hypersensitivity to detecting conditioned and unconditioned aversive stimuli. Similarly, OFC hyperactivity might simply reflect heightened anxiety or anxiety sensitivity. However, these possibilities fail to capture the unique properties of OFC processing. To clarify the OFC's role, it is useful to return to what distinguishes OFC processing from amygdala processing. The distinguishing characteristics relate to the OFC's high degree of flexibility and stimulus specificity in coding reinforcement-related information. Patients with OCD are frequently inflexible in how they code the affective value of stimuli over time. For instance, many individuals without OCD experience discomfort associated with a desire to wash after touching a dirty bathroom stall. However, this discomfort and desire decrease rapidly following washing. In contrast, OCD patients do not appropriately modify their coding of the affective value of the situation following washing but continue to experience discomfort or desire. In essence, these patients show an inflexibility in modulating their coding of stimulus-reinforcer contingencies once they have been activated by exposure to a triggering stimulus. Thus, it may be speculated that dysfunction of the normal flexible coding of the OFC could result in the perseverative affective coding that occurs in OCD.

Behavioral researchers have often noted that the performance of compulsions is reinforced in that compulsions almost always lead to a temporary reduction in anxiety or distress.[258,259] Relief from anxiety represents a negative reinforcement. As such, the OFC may act to motivate operant responses (compulsive behaviors) to receive this type of reinforcement in the same manner as its acts for gustatory reward and intracerebral self-stimulation. Thus, although motivated by different types of reinforcers, similar processes and neural substrata may mediate the urge to perform compulsions and other addictive behaviors.

Sensory-specific satiety forms the basis of one of the OFC's most unique contributions to the brain-reward system. It may be hypothesized that a similar process of satiety acts during avoidance responding. Such a process would help limit continued avoidance responding when the aversive reinforcer is no longer pertinent. It is this very process that often seems to be lacking in OCD patients, who in essence fail to reach a point at which they feel "satiated" in their safety. The failure to reach this "satiety" for safety would directly explain why OCD patients with washing compulsions continue to feel compelled to wash long after a person without OCD would consider such behavior unnecessary. Although the OFC's mediation of such a process remains purely theoretical, it is consistent with its role in handling appetitive reinforcers.

Another distinguishing feature of the OFC is its apparent ability to engage internal representations of the current reinforcement value of stimuli that are not actually present at the current time. Many of the studies reporting increased OFC activity in humans involved paradigms in which subjects were not actually exposed to an aversive stimulus during the scan period itself. Rather, the subjects were asked to think about or contemplate a recently presented stimulus or told that they would receive a stimulus that they did not actually receive during the scan period. Several additional lines of evidence support the contention that the OFC generates or accesses internal representations of aversive events. First, cells that are engaged by unconditioned reinforcers (gustatory stimuli) are similarly engaged by the olfactory and visual associates of the reinforcer, and the extent of the engagement depends not on the reinforcer being present but on the motivational value of the reinforcer. Second, OFC activity increases when subjects specifically attempt to imagine or recall emotional events. Third, OFC lesions decrease the influence of future consequences of behavior. Fourth, some OFC cells show activity that appears to represent the expectancy of a reward in behavioral paradigms. Furthermore, the presence of error detec-

tion cells in the OFC implies the presence of an expectancy for reward. Such expectancies must exist for cells to fire specifically when a reward that would normally have occurred is withheld. If the OFC processes information about aversive expectancies, hyperactivity in this region could therefore lead to the excessive representations of future aversive events or stimuli.

Internal representations or expectancies of future aversive events or consequences of behavior dominate the clinical picture of OCD. Internal representations (repetitive thoughts and images) of dreaded events, such as getting ill, hurting someone, or causing some calamity, frequently lie at the core of the obsessive-compulsive symptom picture. Therefore, OFC hyperactivity may reflect or cause overengagement of aversive expectancies. Furthermore, because of the OFC's involvement in stimulus-reinforcer associations, these internal representations of aversive events may become associated with neutral stimuli that happen to be present at the same time as the internal representation. In other words, the OFC could potentially provide a substrate for the behavioral conditioning of external stimuli with internally generated reinforcer representations.

Goldman-Rakic[71] suggested that the OFC is involved in maintaining internal representations of the reinforcement value of stimuli in working memory. Although speculative, the presence of OFC cells that maintain their firing during delay tasks supports this possibility. Viewed from this working memory perspective, the inability of OCD patients to inhibit intrusive thoughts and images could reflect a hyperactive working memory process in which internally generated representations (expectancies) are maintained indefinitely in a state of moment-to-moment awareness. In the extreme case, this information might become locked "on-line," despite repeated attempts to eliminate the representation. In such cases, the individual may repeatedly perform behaviors aimed at reducing the anxiety associated with the representation. However, because the representation continues to be maintained on-line, the individual feels compelled to repeat the behaviors to avert the dreaded event.

Another potential source of obsessive-compulsive behaviors arises from the activity of error detection cells in the OFC. OCD patients frequently perceive that they performed previous responses inadequately. If the error coding of OFC cells were hypersensitive, such that responses consistently were coded as errors, individuals might repeatedly experience their responses as inadequate. In extreme cases, this could lead to repetitive attempts to perform acts "just right." To date, our understanding of such error detection cells is limited to animal paradigms, but with the increased temporal resolution of functional magnetic resonance imaging, it might be possible to design paradigms for studying the neural substrates of error detection in healthy control subjects.

Finally, OFC hyperactivity may relate to the very processes that appear so deficient in the pseudopsychopathic condition. For instance, whereas the pseudopsychopathic individual participates in risky behavior despite knowledge of the risks, OCD patients appear excessively concerned with such risks. The pseudopsychopathic individual shows a lack of concern and an irresponsibility toward others, but OCD patients often show excessive concern with how their actions will affect others.[260,261] Similarly, feelings of guilt, shame, anxiety, and concern for social norms, which seem so lacking in pseudopsychopathic persons, appear accentuated in OCD patients.

The source of OFC hyperactivity in OCD remains unclear. Given the responsivity of OCD to serotonin reuptake inhibitors,[262] and the abnormal serotonergic functioning observed in some neuroendocrine challenge studies,[263] the possibility that a specific serotonergic abnormality leads to OFC hyperactivity must be considered. Consistent with this possibility, cerebrospinal fluid levels of the serotonin metabolite 5-hydroxyindoleacetic acid negatively correlate with OFC metabolic levels in nonhuman primates.[264]

An important source of OFC regulation arises within the OFC–basal ganglia loops. Heightened caudate nucleus metabolism has been observed in OCD patients at rest, and these levels decline following successful behavioral and pharmacological therapy.[249,251,252] Moreover, these declines are associated with a reduction in the effective connectivity (correlation of metabolism) between the caudate and OFC. These changes in OFC–basal ganglia–thalamic correlations have led to the hypothesis that abnormal functioning within the basal ganglia loops represents the core pathological process in OCD. Based on the neurochemical properties of the connections within the OFC–basal ganglia loops, three hypotheses have been proposed.

First, hyperactivity within the caudate is proposed to lead to a disinhibition of the MDmc. The thalamus acts as a gate or filter, which if disinhibited releases information to its efferent targets. Disinhibition thus would allow information that is normally gated in the MDmc to be passed through to the OFC.[254,256,265] This adventitiously released information would be experienced as intrusive because of its inappropriate release into moment-to-moment awareness. Because intrusive information reaching the OFC likely reflects information related to aversive reinforcers or expectancies (i.e., the normal information processed in these loops), these stimuli would not be experienced as neutral because of the aversive nature of information processed in this circuit. Of course, appetitive reinforcer information also might be adventitiously released, but such information might not be experienced as ego-dystonic or intrusive.

A second effect of overactivity within these loops arises from the reciprocal connections between the OFC and the MDmc. Both projections use the excitatory neurotransmitter glutamate as their primary neurotransmitter. Because of this, a disinhibition of the thalamus could lead to the establishment of a positive feedback loop.[256] Once activated, information transmitted between the two regions would be trapped in a perseverative feedback loop. In this manner, stimulus-reinforcer information, and other information related to OFC/MDmc processing, would get trapped on-line by feedback in the OFC/MDmc axis. Once such a feedback loop is established, even performance of activities such as compulsions aimed at responding to this information would likely fail to halt the feedback. Finally, disinhibition at core points within the OFC–basal ganglia circuit might lead to a feedback loop involving the entire OFC-striatal-pallidal-MDmc loop.[266] Such feedback again would lead to perseveration of the normal processing within these connected structures.

Given the projections from the OFC to the caudate nucleus, OFC hyperactivity may cause caudate hyperactivity rather than the reverse. The specific functions of the portions of the caudate that receive OFC projections are not well known. Investigators sometimes label this as part of the "cognitive" striatum, but beyond indicating that this part of the striatum does not directly affect motor execution, this label has limited utility. In primates, cells in the OFC-recipient regions of the caudate show responses that suggest that they are directly influenced by OFC processing. Specifically, cells in this area respond to gustatory reward, and in at least one case, a caudate cell was reported to reduce its responsivity following satiety.[267] Other portions of the caudate show activity in relation to routinized, habit-based behaviors, especially those involving sequentially chained actions. This has most clearly been demonstrated in terms of rat grooming behavior.[268,269] Whether OFC-recipient portions of the caudate participate in routinized or sequential processes remains to be determined. If this were the case, however, it might help to explain the sequential nature of many compulsive behaviors, including compulsions related to activities such as counting.

The ability of pharmacological treatment to normalize OFC metabolism raises the possibility that OFC hyperactivity reflects a state, as opposed to a trait, marker of OCD. Most discussions of the pathophysiology of OCD (including the preceding paragraphs) conceptualize the pathophysiology as causing obsessive-compulsive symptoms. However, the causal direction of the OFC hyperactivity in OCD is unknown. Cottraux et al.[218] recently reported that both non-OCD and OCD subjects showed increases in OFC rCBF when presented with sentences containing obsessive compared with neutral content. Because OFC activation occurred in both patients and control subjects, it could reflect a "normal" process activated by obsessive rumination. Andreasen and colleagues[270] recently argued that "resting" activity in the OFC reflects a process of silent mentation. If correct, this could suggest that the increased resting OFC metabolism in OCD simply reflects a greater engagement of obsessive ruminations in OCD patients than in control subjects without OCD.

CONCLUSIONS

In conclusion, the OFC forms a critical convergence zone between sensory and limbic regions. As such, it forms a pivotal substrate through which exteroceptive and interoceptive stimuli influence motivated behavior. Clearly, we have a long way to go in understanding how this region influences neuropsychiatric illness. However, our knowledge of the neurocircuitry and function of this region has increased dramatically in recent years. Future research aimed at unraveling the specific functions of the different OFC regions will likely produce a far greater understanding of the physiological basis of a broad spectrum of neuropsychiatric illness.

REFERENCES

1. Harlow JM: Recovery from the passage of an iron bar through the head. Publications of the Massachusetts Medical Society 2:327–347, 1868
2. Ono M, Kubik S, Abernathy CD: Atlas of the Cerebral Sulci. New York, Thieme Medical Publishers, 1990
3. Brodmann K: Physiologie des Gehrins. Neue Deutsche Chirugie 2:85–426, 1914
4. von Economo C, Koskinas GN: Die Cytoarchitektonik der Hirnrinde des erwachsenen Menschen. Berlin, Germany, Springer, 1925
5. von Bonin G, Bailey P: The neocortex of *Macaca mulatta*, in Illinois Monographs in the Medical Sciences. Urbana, IL, University of Illinois Press, 1947, pp 1–163
6. Mesulam MM, Mufson EJ: Insula of the old world monkey, I: architectonics in the insulo-orbito-temporal component of the paralimbic brain. J Comp Neurol 212:1–22, 1982
7. Morecraft RJ, Geula C, Mesulam MM: Cytoarchitecture and neural afferents of orbitofrontal cortex in the brain of the monkey. J Comp Neurol 323:341–358, 1992
8. Beck E: A cytoarchitectural investigation into the boundaries of cortical areas 13 and 14 in the human brain. J Anat 83:147–157, 1949
9. Hof PR, Mufson EJ, Morrison JH: Human orbitofrontal cortex: cytoarchitecture and quantitative immunohistochemical parcellation. J Comp Neurol 359:48–68, 1995
10. Öngür D, Price JL: Architectonic subdivisions of the human orbital and medial prefrontal cortex (abstract). Society for Neuroscience Abstracts 25:362, 1999
11. Walker AE: A cytoarchitectural study of the prefrontal area of the macaque monkey. J Comp Neurol 73:59–86, 1940
12. Petrides M, Pandya DN: Comparative architectonic analyses of the human and the macaque frontal cortex, in Handbook of Neuropsychology, Vol 9. Edited by Booler F, Grafman J. Amsterdam, The Netherlands, Elsevier, 1994, pp 17–58
13. Carmichael ST, Price JL: Architectonic subdivision of the orbital and medial prefrontal cortex in the macaque monkey. J Comp Neurol 346:366–402, 1994
14. Sanides F: Comparative architects of the neocortex of mammals and their evolutionary interpretation. Ann N Y Acad Sci 167:404–423, 1969
15. Sanides F: Representation in the cerebral cortex and its areal lamination patterns, in Structure and Function of Nervous Tissue. Edited by Bourne GF. New York, Academic Press, 1972, pp 329–453
16. Pandya DN, Yeterian EH: Prefrontal cortex in relation to other cortical areas in rhesus monkey: architecture and connections. Prog Brain Res 85:63–94, 1990
17. Barbas H: Anatomic organization of basoventral and mediodorsal visual recipient prefrontal regions in the rhesus monkey. J Comp Neurol 276:313–342, 1988
18. Carmichael ST, Price JL: Sensory and premotor connections of the orbital and medial prefrontal cortex. J Comp Neurol 363:642–664, 1995
19. Barbas H: Organization of cortical afferent input to orbitofrontal areas in the rhesus monkey. Neuroscience 56:841–864, 1993

20. Carmichael ST, Clugnet MC, Price JL: Central olfactory connections in the macaque monkey. J Comp Neurol 346:403–434, 1994

21. Yarita H, Iino M, Tanabe T, et al: A transthalamic olfactory pathway to orbitofrontal cortex in the monkey. J Neurophysiol 43:69–85, 1980

22. Russchen FT, Amaral DG, Price JL: The afferent input to the magnocellular division of the mediodorsal thalamic nucleus in the monkey, *Macaca fascicularis*. J Comp Neurol 256:175–210, 1987

23. Price JL: The central olfactory and accessory olfactory systems, in Neurobiology of Taste and Smell. Edited by Finger TE, Silver WL. Malabar, FL, Krieger, 1991, pp 179–203

24. Ray JP, Price JL: The organization of projections from the mediodorsal nucleus of the thalamus to orbital and medial prefrontal cortex in macaque monkeys. J Comp Neurol 337:1–31, 1993

25. Carmichael ST, Price JL: Connectional networks within the orbital and medial prefrontal cortex of macaque monkeys. J Comp Neurol 346:179–207, 1996

26. Tanabe T, Yarita H, Iino M, et al: An olfactory projection area in orbitofrontal cortex of the monkey. J Neurophysiol 38:1269–1283, 1975

27. Takagi SF: Studies on the olfactory nervous system of the Old World monkey. Prog Neurobiol 27:195–250, 1986

28. Tanabe T, Iino M, Takagi SF: Discrimination of odors in olfactory bulb, pyriform-amygdaloid areas, and orbitofrontal cortex of the monkey. J Neurophysiol 38:1284–1296, 1975

29. Critchley HD, Rolls ET: Olfactory neuronal responses in the primate orbitofrontal cortex: analysis in an olfactory discrimination task. J Neurophysiol 75:1659–1672, 1996

30. Zatorre RJ, Jones-Gotman M: Human olfactory discrimination after unilateral frontal or temporal lobectomy. Brain 114 (part A):71–84, 1991

31. Jones-Gotman M, Zatorre RJ: Odor recognition memory in humans: role of right temporal and orbitofrontal regions. Brain Cogn 22:182–198, 1993

32. Jones-Gotman M, Zatorre RJ: Olfactory identification deficits in patients with focal cerebral excision. Neuropschologia 26:387–400, 1988

33. Zatorre RJ, Jones-Gotman M, Evans AC, et al: Functional localization and lateralization of human olfactory cortex. Nature 360:339–340, 1992

34. Zald DH, Pardo JV: The amygdala and emotion: amygdala activation during aversive olfaction. Proc Natl Acad Sci U S A 94:4119–4124, 1997

35. Zald DH, Pardo JV: Functional neuroimaging of the olfactory system in humans. Int J Psychophysiol 36:165–181, 2000

36. Rolls ET: Information processing in the taste system of primates. J Exp Biol 146:141–164, 1989

37. Rolls ET, Yaxley S, Sienkiewicz ZJ: Gustatory responses of single neurons in the caudolateral orbitofrontal cortex of the macaque monkey. J Neurophysiol 64:1055–1066, 1990

38. Baylis LL, Rolls ET, Baylis GC: Afferent connections of the caudolateral orbitofrontal cortex taste area of the primate. Neuroscience 64:801–812, 1995

39. Rolls ET, Sienkiewicz ZJ, Yaxley S: Hunger modulates the responses to gustatory stimuli of single neurons in the caudolateral orbitofrontal cortex of the macaque monkey. Eur J Neurosci 1:53–60, 1989

40. Rolls ET, Baylis LL: Gustatory, olfactory, and visual convergence within the primate orbitofrontal cortex. J Neurosci 14:5437–5452, 1994

41. Small DM, Zald DH, Jones-Gotman M, et al: Human cortical gustatory areas: a review of functional neuroimaging data. Neuroreport 10:7–14, 1999

42. Barbas H: Architecture and cortical connections of the prefrontal cortex in the rhesus monkey. Adv Neurol 57:91–115, 1992

43. Jones EG, Powell TP: An anatomical study of converging sensory pathways within the cerebral cortex of the monkey. Brain 93:793–820, 1970

44. Mishkin M, Ungerleider LG, Macko KA: Object vision and spatial vision: two cortical pathways. Trends Neurosci 6:414–417, 1983

45. Benevento LA, Fallon J, Davis BJ, et al: Auditory-visual interaction in single cells in the cortex of the superior temporal sulcus and the orbital frontal cortex of the macaque monkey. Exp Neurol 57:849–872, 1977

46. Wilson FA, Scalaidhe SP, Goldman-Rakic PS: Dissociation of object and spatial processing domains in primate prefrontal cortex. Science 260:1955–1958, 1993

47. Thorpe SJ, Rolls ET, Maddison S: The orbitofrontal cortex: neuronal activity in the behaving monkey. Exp Brain Res 49:93–115, 1983

48. Chavis DA, Pandya DN: Further observations on corticofrontal connections in the rhesus monkey. Brain Res 117:369–386, 1976

49. Hackett TA, Stepniewska I, Kaas JH: Prefrontal connections of the parabelt auditory cortex in macaque monkeys. Brain Res 817:45–58, 1999

50. Romanski LM, Bates JF, Goldman-Rakic PS: Auditory belt and parabelt projections to the prefrontal cortex in the rhesus monkey. J Comp Neurol 403:141–157, 1999

51. Platel H, Price C, Baron JC, et al: The structural components of music perception. A functional anatomical study. Brain 120:229–243, 1997

52. Zatorre RJ, Perry DW, Beckett CA, et al: Functional anatomy of musical processing in listeners with absolute pitch and relative pitch. Proc Natl Acad Sci U S A 95:3172–3177, 1998

53. Preuss TM, Goldman-Rakic PS: Connections of the ventral granular frontal cortex of macaques with perisylvian premotor and somatosensory areas: anatomical evidence for somatic representation in primate frontal association cortex. J Comp Neurol 282:293–316, 1989

54. Rolls ET, Critchley HD, Browning AS, et al: Response to the sensory properties of fat of neurons in the primate orbitofrontal cortex. J Neurosci 19:1532–1540, 1999

55. Bailey P, Bremmer F: A sensory cortical representation of the vagus nerve. J Neurophysiol 1:405–412, 1938

56. Coffield JA, Bowen KK, Miletic V: Retrograde tracing of projections between the nucleus submedius, the ventrolateral orbital cortex, and the midbrain in the rat. J Comp Neurol 321:488–499, 1992

57. Snow PJ, Lumb BM, Cervero F: The representation of prolonged and intense, noxious somatic and visceral stimuli in the ventrolateral orbital cortex of the cat. Pain 48:88–89, 1992

58. Hurley KM, Herbert H, Moga MM, et al: Efferent projections of the infralimbic cortex of the rat. J Comp Neurol 308:249–276, 1991

59. Neafsey EJ: Prefrontal cortical control of the autonomic nervous system: anatomical and physiological observations. Prog Brain Res 85:147–166, 1990

60. Mufson EJ, Mesulam MM: Insula of the old world monkey, II: afferent cortical input and comments on the claustrum. J Comp Neurol 212:23–37, 1982

61. Mesulam MM, Mufson EJ: Insula of the old world monkey, III: efferent cortical output and comments on function. J Comp Neurol 212:38–52, 1982

62. Moran MA, Mufson EJ, Mesulam MM: Neural inputs into the temporopolar cortex of the rhesus monkey. J Comp Neurol 256:88–103, 1987

63. Vogt BA, Pandya DN: Cingulate cortex of the rhesus monkey, II: cortical afferents. J Comp Neurol 262:271–289, 1987

64. Pandya DN, Van Hoesen GW, Mesulam MM: Efferent connections of the cingulate gyrus in the rhesus monkey. Exp Brain Res 42:319–330, 1981

65. Van Hoesen GW, Morecraft RJ, Vogt BA: Connections of the monkey cingulate cortex, in Neurobiology of Cingulate Cortex and Limbic Thalamus: A Comprehensive Handbook. Edited by Vogt BA, Gabriel M. Boston, MA, Birkhauser, 1993, pp 249–284

66. Carmichael ST, Price JL: Limbic connections of the orbital and medial prefrontal cortex of macaque monkeys. J Comp Neurol 363:615–641, 1995

67. Barbas H, Mesulam MM: Organization of afferent input to subdivisions of area 8 in the rhesus monkey. J Comp Neurol 200:407–431, 1981

68. Pandya DN, Dye P, Butters N: Efferent cortico-cortical projections of the prefrontal cortex in the rhesus monkey. Brain Res 31:35–46, 1971

69. Selemon LD, Goldman-Rakic PS: Common cortical and subcortical targets of the dorsolateral prefrontal and posterior parietal cortices in the rhesus monkey: evidence for a distributed neural network subserving spatially guided behavior. J Neurosci 8:4049–4068, 1988

70. Morecraft RJ, Geula C, Mesulam MM: Architecture of connectivity within a cingulo-fronto-parietal neurocognitive network for directed attention. Arch Neurol 50:279–284, 1993

71. Goldman-Rakic PS: Circuitry of primate prefrontal cortex and regulation of behavior by representational memory, in Handbook of Physiology: The Nervous System. Edited by Plum F, Mountcastle V. Bethesda, MD, American Physiological Society, 1987, pp 373–417

72. Mesulam MM: A cortical network for directed attention and unilateral neglect. Ann Neurol 10:309–325, 1981

73. Aggleton JP (ed): The Amygdala: Neurobiological Aspects of Emotion, Memory, and Mental Dysfunction. New York, Wiley, 1992

74. Aggleton JP, Mishkin M: The amygdala: sensory gateway to the emotions, in Biological Foundations of Emotion. Edited by Plutchik E, Kellerman H. New York, Academic Press, 1986, pp 281–299

75. Ledoux JE: Emotion, in Handbook of Physiology: The Nervous System. Edited by Plum F, Mountcastle V. Bethesda, MD, American Physiological Society, 1987, pp 419–459

76. Amaral DG, Price JL: Amygdalo-cortical projections in the monkey (*Macaca fascicularis*). J Comp Neurol 230:465–496, 1984

77. Amaral DG, Price JL, Pitkänen A, et al: Anatomical organization of the primate amygdaloid complex, in The Amygdala: Neurobiological Aspects of Emotion, Memory, and Mental Dysfunction. Edited by Aggleton JP. New York, Wiley, 1992, pp 1–66

78. Barbas H, De Olmos J: Projections from the amygdala to basoventral and mediodorsal prefrontal regions in the rhesus monkey. J Comp Neurol 300:549–571, 1990

79. Porrino LJ, Crane AM, Goldman-Rakic PS: Direct and indirect pathways from the amygdala to the frontal lobe in rhesus monkeys. J Comp Neurol 198:121–136, 1981

80. Davis M: The role of the amygdala in fear and anxiety. Annu Rev Neurosci 15:353–375, 1992

81. Van Hoesen GW: The differential distribution, diversity and sprouting of cortical projections to the amygdala in the rhesus monkey, in The Amygdaloid Complex. Edited by Ben-Ari Y. Amsterdam, The Netherlands, Elsevier/North Holland, 1981, pp 77–90

82. Barbas H, Blatt GJ: Topographically specific hippocampal projections target functionally distinct prefrontal areas in the rhesus monkey. Hippocampus 5:511–533, 1995

83. Cavada C, Companý T, Tejodor J, et al: The anatomical connections of the macaque monkey orbitofrontal cortex: a review. Cereb Cortex 10:220–242, 2000

84. Van Hoesen G, Pandya DN, Butters N: Some connections of the entorhinal (area 28) and perirhinal (area 35) cortices of the rhesus monkey, II: frontal lobe afferents. Brain Res 95:25–38, 1975

85. Van Hoesen GW: The parahippocampal gyrus: new observations regarding its cortical connections in the monkey. Trends Neurosci 5:345–350, 1982

86. Rempel-Clower NL, Barbas H: Topographic organization of connections between the hypothalamus and prefrontal cortex in the rhesus monkey. J Comp Neurol 398:393–419, 1998

87. Johnson TN, Rosvold HE, Mishkin M: Projections from behaviorally defined sectors of the prefrontal cortex to the basal ganglia, septum, and diencephalon of the monkey. Exp Neurol 21:20–34, 1968

88. Ongur D, An X, Price JL: Prefrontal cortical projections to the hypothalamus in macaque monkeys. J Comp Neurol 401:480–505, 1998

89. An X, Bandler R, Ongur D, et al: Prefrontal cortical projections to longitudinal columns in the midbrain periaqeductal gray in macaque monkeys. J Comp Neurol 401:455–479, 1998

90. Nauta WJ: The problem of the frontal lobe: a reinterpretation. J Psychiatr Res 8:167–187, 1971

91. Nauta WJH: Connections of the frontal lobe with the limbic system, in Surgical Approaches in Psychiatry. Edited by Laitinen LV, Livingston KE. Baltimore, MD, University Park Press, 1973, pp 303–314

92. Barbas H, Henion TH, Dermon CR: Diverse thalamic projections to the prefrontal cortex in the rhesus monkey. J Comp Neurol 313:65–94, 1991

93. Giguere M, Goldman-Rakic PS: Mediodorsal nucleus: areal, laminar, and tangential distribution of afferents and efferents in the frontal lobe of rhesus monkeys. J Comp Neurol 277:195–213, 1988

94. Siwek DF, Pandya DN: Prefrontal projections to the mediodorsal nucleus of the thalamus in the rhesus monkey. J Comp Neurol 312:509–524, 1991

95. Ilinsky IA, Kultas-Ilinsky K: Sagittal cytoarchitectonic maps of the *Macaca mulatta* thalamus with a revised nomenclature of the motor-related nuclei validated by observations on their connectivity. J Comp Neurol 262:331–364, 1987

96. Nakano K, Tokushige A, Kohno M, et al: An autoradiographic study of cortical projections from motor thalamic nuclei in the macaque monkey. Neurosci Res 13:119–137, 1992

97. Peschanski M, Guilbaud G, Gautron M: Posterior intralaminar region in rat: neuronal responses to noxious and nonnoxious cutaneous stimuli. Exp Neurol 72:226–238, 1981

98. Buchanan SL, Thompson RH, Powell DA: Midline thalamic lesions enhance conditioned bradycardia and the cardiac orienting reflex in rabbits. Psychobiology 17:300–306, 1989

99. Alexander GE, DeLong MR, Strick PL: Parallel organization of functionally segregated circuits linking basal ganglia and cortex. Annu Rev Neurosci 9:357–381, 1986

100. Alexander GE, Crutcher MD, DeLong MR: Basal ganglia-thalamocortical circuits: parallel substrates for motor, oculomotor, "prefrontal" and "limbic" functions. Prog Brain Res 85:119–146, 1990

101. Yeterian EH, Pandya DN: Prefrontal connections in relation to cortical architectonic organization in rhesus monkeys. J Comp Neurol 312:43–67, 1991

102. Heimer L, Switzer RD, Van Hoesen GW: Ventral striatum and ventral pallidum: components of the motor system? Trends Neurosci 5:83–87, 1982

103. Nauta HJ: A proposed conceptual reorganization of the basal ganglia and telencephalon. Neuroscience 4:1875–1881, 1979

104. Collins PF, Depue RD: A neurobehavioral systems approach to developmental psychopathology, in Developmental Perspectives on Depression, Vol. 4. Edited by Ciccetti D, Toth S. Rochester, NY, University of Rochester Press, 1992, pp 29–101

105. Eblen F, Graybiel AM: Highly restricted origin of prefrontal cortical inputs to striosomes in the Macaque monkey. J Neurosci 15:5999–6013, 1995

106. MacLean PD: The Triune Brain. New York, Plenum, 1990

107. Ono T, Nishijo H: Neurophysiological basis of the Klüver-Bucy syndrome: responses of monkey amygdaloid neurons to biologically significant objects, in The Amygdala: Neurobiological Aspects of Emotion, Memory, and Mental Dysfunction. Edited by Aggleton JP. New York, Wiley, 1992, pp 167–190

108. Rolls ET: Neurophysiology and functions of the primate amygdala, in The Amygdala: Neurobiological Aspects of Emotion, Memory, and Mental Dysfunction. Edited by Aggleton JP. New York, Wiley, 1992, pp 143–166

109. Rolls ET, Burton MJ, Mora F: Hypothalamic neuronal responses associated with the sight of food. Brain Res 111:53–66, 1976

110. Rolls ET, Sanghera MK, Roper-Hall A: The latency of activation of neurones in the lateral hypothalamus and substantia innominata during feeding in the monkey. Brain Res 164:121–135, 1979

111. Baylis LL, Gaffan D: Amygdalectomy and ventromedial prefrontal ablation produce similar deficits in food choice and in simple object discrimination learning for an unseen reward. Exp Brain Res 86:617–622, 1991

112. Butter CM, McDonald JA, Snyder DR: Orality, preference behavior, and reinforcement value of nonfood object in monkeys with orbital frontal lesions. Science 164:1306–1307, 1969

113. Ursin H, Rosvold HE, Vest B: Food preference in brain lesioned monkeys. Physiol Behav 4:609–612, 1969

114. Butter CM, Snyder DR, McDonald JA: Effects of orbital frontal lesions on aversive and aggressive behaviors in rhesus monkeys. Journal of Comparative and Physiological Psychology 72:132–144, 1970

115. Klüver H, Bucy PC: "Psychic blindness" and other symptoms following bilateral temporal lobectomy in rhesus monkeys. Am J Physiol 119:352–353, 1937

116. Niki H, Sakai M, Kubota K: Delayed alternation performance and unit activity of the caudate head and medial orbitofrontal gyrus in the monkey. Brain Res 38:343–353, 1972

117. Kubota K, Komatsu H: Neuron activities of monkey prefrontal cortex during the learning of visual discrimination tasks with go/no-go performances. Neurosci Res 3:106–129, 1985

118. Rosenkilde CE, Bauer RH, Fuster JM: Single cell activity in ventral prefrontal cortex of behaving monkeys. Brain Res 209:375–394, 1981

119. Mora F, Avrith DB, Rolls ET: An electrophysiological and behavioural study of self-stimulation in the orbitofrontal cortex of the rhesus monkey. Brain Res Bull 5:111–115, 1980

120. Mora F, Rolls ET, Burton MJ, et al: Effects of dopamine-receptor blockade on self-stimulation in the monkey. Pharmacol Biochem Behav 4:211–216, 1976

121. Rolls ET, Sienkiewicz ZJ, Yaxley S: Hunger modulates the responses to gustatory stimuli of single neurons in the caudolateral orbitofrontal cortex of the macaque monkey. Eur J Neurosci 1:53–60, 1989

122. Rolls ET, Scott TR, Sienkiewicz ZJ, et al: The responsiveness of neurones in the frontal opercular gustatory cortex of the macaque monkey is independent of hunger. J Physiol 397:1–12, 1988

123. Scott TR, Yaxley S, Sienkiewicz ZJ, et al: Gustatory responses in the nucleus tractus solitarius of the alert cynomolgus monkey. J Neurophysiol 55:182–200, 1986

124. Scott TR, Yaxley S, Sienkiewicz ZJ, et al: Gustatory responses in the frontal opercular cortex of the alert cynomolgus monkey. J Neurophysiol 56:876–890, 1986

125. Critchley HD, Rolls ET: Hunger and satiety modify the responses of olfactory and visual neurons in the primate orbitofrontal cortex. J Neurophysiol 75:1673–1686, 1995

126. Butter CM, Mishkin M, Rosvold HE: Conditioning and extinction of a food-rewarded response after selective ablations of frontal cortex in rhesus monkeys. Exp Neurol 7:65–75, 1963

127. Bachevalier J, Mishkin M: Visual recognition impairment follows ventromedial but not dorsolateral prefrontal lesions in monkeys. Behav Brain Res 20:249–261, 1986

128. Erb JL, Gwirtsman HE, Fuster JM, et al: Bulimia associated with frontal lobe lesions. Int J Eat Disord 8:117–121, 1989

129. Hecaen H: Mental symptoms associated with tumors of the frontal lobe, in The Frontal Granular Cortex and Behavior. Edited by Warren JM, Akert K. New York, McGraw-Hill, 1964, pp 335–352

130. Hofstatter L, Smolik EA, Busch AK: Prefrontal lobotomy in treatment of chronic psychoses with special reference to section of the orbital areas only. Archives of Neurology and Psychiatry 53:125–130, 1945

131. Kirschbaum WR: Excessive hunger as a symptom of cerebral origin. J Nerv Ment Dis 113:95–114, 1951

132. Brutkowski S: Prefrontal cortex and drive inhibition, in The Frontal Granular Cortex and Behavior. Edited by Warren JM, Akert K. New York, McGraw-Hill, 1964, pp 242–294

133. Mora F, Avrith DB, Phillips AG, et al: Effects of satiety on self-stimulation of the orbitofrontal cortex in the rhesus monkey. Neurosci Lett 13:141–145, 1979

134. Francis S, Rolls ET, Bowtell R, et al: The representation of pleasant touch in the brain and its relationship with taste and olfactory area. Neuroreport 10:453–459, 1999

135. Sanghera MK, Rolls ET, Roper-Hall A: Visual responses of neurons in the dorsolateral amygdala of the alert monkey. Exp Neurol 63:610–626, 1979

136. Zald DH, Lee JT, Fluegel KW, et al: Aversive gustatory stimulation activates limbic circuits in humans. Brain 121:1143–1154, 1998

137. Rolls ET, Critchley HD, Mason R, et al: Orbitofrontal cortex neurons: role in olfactory and visual association learning. J Neurophysiol 75:1970–1981, 1996

138. Lipton PA, Alvarez P, Eichenbaum H: Crossmodal associative memory representations in rodent orbitofrontal cortex. Neuron 22:349–359, 1999

139. Baylis LL, Gaffan D: Amygdalectomy and ventromedial prefrontal ablation produce similar deficits in food choice and in simple object discrimination learning for an unseen reward. Exp Brain Res 86:617–622, 1991

140. Gaffan D, Murray EA: Amygdalar interaction with the mediodorsal nucleus of the thalamus and the ventromedial prefrontal cortex in stimulus-reward associative learning in the monkey. J Neurosci 10:3479–3493, 1990

141. Gaffan D, Murray EA, Fabre-Thorpe M: Interaction of the amygdala with the frontal lobe in reward memory. Eur J Neurosci 5:968–975, 1993

142. Gaffan D: Amygdala and the memory of reward, in The Amygdala: Neurobiological Aspects of Emotion, Memory, and Mental Dysfunction. Edited by Aggleton JP. New York, Wiley, 1992, pp 471–484

143. Morgan MA, LeDoux JE: Differential contribution of dorsal and ventral medial prefrontal cortex to the acquisition and extinction of conditioned fear in rats. Behav Neurosci 109:681–688, 1995

144. Lawicka W, Mishkin M, Rosvold HE: Dissociation of deficits on auditory tasks following partial prefrontal lesions in monkeys. Acta Neurobiol Exp (Warsz) 35:581–607, 1975

145. Stamm JS: Functional dissociation between the inferior and arcuate segments of dorsolateral prefrontal cortex in the monkey. Neuropsychologia 11:181–190, 1973

146. Goldman PS, Rosvold HE, Mishkin M: Selective sparing of function following prefrontal lobectomy in infant monkeys. Exp Neurol 29:221–226, 1970

147. Manning FJ: Performance under temporal schedules by monkeys with partial ablations of prefrontal cortex. Physiol Behav 11:563–569, 1973

148. Iversen SD, Mishkin M: Perseverative interference in monkeys following selective lesions of the inferior prefrontal convexity. Exp Brain Res 11:376–386, 1970

149. Niki H, Watanabe M: Prefrontal and cingulate unit activity during timing behavior in the monkey. Brain Res 171:213–224, 1979

150. Kubota K, Komatsu H: Prefrontal neuron activity related to task reversal (abstract). Society for Neuroscience Abstracts 7:359, 1981

151. Butter CM: Perseveration in extinction and in discrimination reversal tasks following selective frontal ablations in *Macaca mulatta*. Physiol Behav 4:163–171, 1969

152. Voytko ML: Cooling orbital frontal cortex disrupts matching-to-sample and visual discrimination learning in monkeys. Physiological Psychology 13:219–229, 1985

153. Mishkin M, Manning FJ: Non-spatial memory after selective prefrontal lesions in monkeys. Brain Res 143: 313–323, 1978

154. Passingham R: Delayed matching after selective prefrontal lesions in monkeys (*Macaca mulatta*). Brain Res 92:89–102, 1975

155. Butter N, Butter C, Rosen J, et al: Behavioral effects of sequential and one-stage ablations of orbital prefrontal cortex in the monkey. Exp Neurol 39:204–214, 1973

156. Rosenkilde CE: Functional heterogeneity of the prefrontal cortex in the monkey: a review. Behavioral and Neurol Biology 25:301–345, 1979

157. Konorski J: Some hypotheses concerning the functional organization of prefrontal cortex. Acta Neurobiol Exp (Warsz) 32:595–613, 1972

158. McEnaney KW, Butter CM: Perseveration of responding and nonresponding in monkeys with orbital frontal ablations. Journal of Comparative Physiological Psychology 68:558–561, 1969

159. Ward K, Butter CM: Perseveration of responding and nonresponding in monkeys with orbital frontal lesions (abstract). Proceedings of the 76th Annual Convention of the American Psychological Association. Washington, DC, American Psychological Association, 1968, pp 271–272

160. Mishkin M: Perseveration of central sets after frontal lesions in monkeys, in The Frontal Granular Cortex and Behavior. Edited by Warren JM, Akert K. New York, McGraw-Hill, 1964, pp 219–241

161. Watanabe M: Prefrontal unit activity during delayed conditional go/no-go discrimination in the monkey, II: relation to go and no-go responses. Brain Res 382:15–27, 1986

162. Rolls ET: The orbitofrontal cortex. Philos Trans R Soc Lond B Biol Sci 351:1433–1444, 1996

163. Rolls ET, Hornak J, Wade D, et al: Emotion related learning in patients with social and emotional changes associated with frontal lobe damage. J Neurol Neurosurg Psychiatry 57:1518–1524, 1994

164. Schoenbaum G, Chiba AA, Gallagher M: Orbitofrontal cortex and basolateral amygdala encode expected outcomes during learning. Nature Neuroscience 1:155–159, 1999

165. Schultz W, Tremblay L, Hollerman JR: Reward processing in primate orbitofrontal cortex and basal ganglia. Cereb Cortex 10:272–283, 2000

166. Tremblay L, Schultz W: Relative reward preference in primate orbitofrontal cortex. Nature 398:704–708, 1999

167. Nobre AC, Coull JT, Frith CD, et al: Orbitofrontal cortex is activated during breaches of expectation in tasks of visual attention. Nature Neuroscience 2:11–12, 1999

168. Gallagher M, McMahan RW, Schoenbaum G: Orbitofrontal cortex and representation of incentive value in associative learning. J Neurosci 19:6610–6614, 1999

169. Fuster JM: The Prefrontal Cortex: New York, Raven, 1989

170. Raleigh MJ, Steklis HD, Ervin FR, et al: The effects of orbitofrontal lesions on the aggressive behavior of vervet monkeys (cercopithecus aethiops sabaeous). Exp Neurol 73:378–389, 1981

171. Butter CM, Mishkin M, Mirsky AF: Emotional responses toward humans in monkeys with selective frontal lesions. Physiol Behav 3:213–215, 1968

172. Raleigh MJ, Steklis HD: Effects of orbitofrontal and temporal neocortical lesions on the affiliative behavior of vervet monkeys. Exp Neurol 66:158–168, 1979

173. Blumer D, Benson DF: Personality changes with frontal and temporal lobe lesions, in Psychiatric Aspects of Neurological Disease. Edited by Blumer D, Benson DF. New York, Grune & Stratton, 1975, pp 151–170

174. Grafman J, Vance SC, Weingartner H, et al: The effects of lateralized frontal lesions on mood regulation. Brain 109:1127–1148, 1986

175. Irle E, Peper M, Wowra B, et al: Mood changes after surgery for tumors of the cerebral cortex. Arch Neurol 51:164–174, 1994

176. Rylander G: Personality Changes After Operations on the Frontal Lobes. London, Oxford University Press, 1939

177. Starkstein SE, Boston JD, Robinson RG: Mechanisms of mania after brain injury: 12 case reports and review of the literature. J Nerv Ment Dis 176:87–100, 1988

178. Starkstein SE, Migliorelli R, Teson A, et al: Specificity of changes in cerebral blood flow in patients with frontal lobe dementia. J Neurol Neurosurg Psychiatry 57:790–796, 1994

179. Malloy P, Bihrle A, Duffy J, et al: The orbitomedial frontal syndrome. Archives of Clinical Neuropsychology 8:185–201, 1993

180. Bakchine S, Lacomblez L, Benoit N, et al: Manic-like state after bilateral orbitofrontal and right temporoparietal injury: efficacy of clonidine. Neurology 39:777–781, 1989

181. Grafman J, Schwab K, Warden D, et al: Frontal lobe injuries, violence, and aggression: a report of the Vietnam Head Injury Study. Neurology 46:1231–1238, 1996

182. Damasio A, Anderson S: The frontal lobes, in Clinical Neuropsychology. Edited by Heilman KM, Valenstein E. New York, Oxford University Press, 1993, pp 409–460

183. Stuss DT, Benson DF: The Frontal Lobes. New York, Raven, 1986

184. Eslinger PJ, Damasio AR: Severe disturbance of higher cognition after bilateral frontal lobe ablation: patient EVR. Neurology 35:1731–1741, 1985

185. Grattan LM, Bloomer RH, Archambault FX, et al: Cognitive flexibility and empathy after frontal lobe lesion. Neuropsychiatry Neuropsychol Behav Neurol 7:251–259, 1994

186. Hornak J, Rolls ET, Wade D: Face and voice expression identification in patients with emotional and behavioural changes following ventral frontal lesions. Neuropsychologia 34:247–261, 1996

187. Andreasen NC, O'Leary DS, Arndt SA, et al: Neural substrates of facial recognition. J Neuropsychiatry Clin Neurosci 8:139–146, 1996

188. Haxby JV, Ungerleider LG, Horwitz B, et al: Face encoding and recognition in the human brain. Proc Natl Acad Sci U S A 93:922–927, 1996

189. Sprengelmeyer R, Rausch M, Eysel UT, et al: Neural structures associated with recognition of facial expressions of basic emotions. Proc R Soc Lond B Biol Sci 265:1927–1931, 1998

190. Morris JS, Friston KJ, Buchel C, et al: A neuromodulatory role for the human amygdala in processing emotional facial expressions. Brain 121:47–57, 1998

191. Blair RR, Morris JS, Frith CD, et al: Dissociable neural responses to facial expressions of sadness and anger. Brain 122:883–893, 1999

192. Nakamura K, Kawashima R, Ito K, et al: Activation of the right inferior frontal cortex during assessment of facial emotion. J Neurophysiol 22:1610–1614, 1999

193. Saver JL, Damasio AR: Preserved access and processing of social knowledge in a patient with acquired sociopathy due to ventromedial frontal damage. Neuropsychologia 29:1241–1249, 1991

194. Anderson SW, Bechara A, Tranel D, et al: Characterization of the decision making defect of subjects with ventromedial frontal damage (abstract). Society for Neuroscience Abstracts 22:1108, 1996

195. Damasio A: The somatic marker hypothesis and the possible functions of the prefrontal cortex. Philos Trans R Soc Lond B Biol Sci 351:1413–1420, 1996

196. Rogers RD, Owen AM, Middleton HC, et al: Choosing between small, likely rewards and large, unlikely rewards activates inferior and orbital prefrontal cortex. J Neurosci 19:9029–9038, 1999

197. Bailey P, Sweet WH: Effects on respiration, blood pressure and gastric motility of stimulation of orbital surface of frontal lobe. J Neurophysiol 3:276–281, 1940

198. Delgado JMR, Livingston RB: Some respiratory, vascular and thermal responses to stimulation of orbital surface of frontal lobe. J Neurophysiol 11:39–55, 1948

199. Hall RE, Marr HB: Influence of electrical stimulation of posterior orbital cortex upon plasma cortisol levels in unanesthetized sub-human primate. Brain Res 93:367–371, 1975

200. Hall RE, Livingston RB, Bloor CM: Orbital cortical influences on cardiovascular dynamics and myocardial structures in conscious monkeys. J Neurosurg 46:638–647, 1977

201. Kaada BR: Somato-motor, autonomic and electrocorticographic responses to electrical stimulation of "rhinencephalic" and other structures in primates, cat and dog: a study of responses from the limbic, subcallosal, orbito-insular, piriform and temporal cortex, hippocampus-fornix and amygdala. Acta Physiol Scand 24 (suppl 83):1–285, 1951

202. Kaada BR: Cingulate, posterior orbital, anterior insular and temporal pole cortex, in Handbook of Physiology. Edited by Field F, Magoun HW, Hall VE. Baltimore, MD, Williams & Wilkins, 1960, pp 1345–1372

203. Damasio AR, Tranel D, Damasio H: Individuals with sociopathic behavior caused by frontal damage fail to respond autonomically to social stimuli. Behav Brain Res 41:81–94, 1990

204. Elithorn A, Piercy MF, Crosskey MA: Prefrontal leucotomy and the anticipation of pain. J Neurol Neurosurg Psychiatry 18:34–43, 1955

205. Grueninger WM, Kimble DP, Grueninger JP, et al: GSR and corticosteroid response in monkeys with frontal. Neuropsychologia 3:205–216, 1965

206. Tranel D, Bechara A, Damasio H, et al: Fear conditioning after ventromedial frontal damage in humans (abstract). Society for Neuroscience Abstracts 22:1108, 1996

207. Drevets WC, Videen TO, Snyder AZ, et al: Regional cerebral blood flow changes during anticipatory anxiety (abstract). Society for Neuroscience Abstracts 20:368, 1994

208. Benkelfat C, Bradwejn J, Meyer E, et al: Functional neuroanatomy of CCK_4-induced anxiety in normal healthy volunteers. Am J Psychiatry 152:1180–1184, 1995

209. Chua P, Krams M, Toni I, et al: A functional anatomy of anticipatory anxiety. Neuroimage 9:563–571, 1999

210. Pardo JV, Pardo PJ, Raichle ME: Neural correlates of self-induced dysphoria. Am J Psychiatry 150:713–719, 1993

211. Dougherty D, Shin LM, Alpert NM, et al: Anger in healthy men: a PET study using script-driven imagery: Biol Psychiatry 46:466–472, 1999

212. Rauch SL, Savage CR, Alpert NM, et al: A positron emission tomographic study of simple phobic symptom provocation. Arch Gen Psychiatry 52:20–28, 1995

213. Rauch SL, Jenike MA, Alpert NM, et al: Regional cerebral blood flow measured during symptom provocation in obsessive-compulsive disorder using oxygen 15–labeled carbon dioxide and positron emission tomography. Arch Gen Psychiatry 51:62–70, 1994

214. Rauch SL, van der Kolk BA, Fisler RE, et al: A symptom provocation study of posttraumatic stress disorder using positron emission tomography and script-driven imagery. Arch Gen Psychiatry 53:380–387, 1996

215. Shin LM, McNally RJ, Kosslyn SM, et al: Regional cerebral blood flow during script-driven imagery in childhood sexual abuse-related PTSD: a PET investigation. Am J Psychiatry 156:575–584, 1999

216. Johanson A, Smith G, Risberg J, et al: Left orbital frontal activation in pathological anxiety. Anxiety, Stress and Coping 5:313–328, 1992

217. McGuire PK, Bench CJ, Frith CD, et al: Functional anatomy of obsessive-compulsive phenomena. Br J Psychiatry 164:459–468, 1994

218. Cottraux J, Gerard D, Cinnoti L, et al: A controlled positron emission tomography study of obsessive and neutral auditory stimulation in obsessive-compulsive disorder with checking rituals. Psychiatry Res 60:101–112, 1996

219. Fredrikson M, Wik G, Greitz T, et al: Regional cerebral blood flow during experimental phobic fear. Psychophysiology 30:126–130, 1993

220. Fredrikson M, Wik G, Annas P, et al: Functional neuroanatomy of visually elicited simple phobic fear—additional data and theoretical analysis. Psychophysiology 32:43–48, 1995

221. Wik G, Fredrikson M, Ericson K, et al: A functional cerebral response to frightening visual stimulation. Psychiatry Res 50:15–24, 1993

222. Shin LM, Kosslyn SM, McNally RJ, et al: Visual imagery and perception in posttraumatic stress disorder: a positron emission tomographic investigation. Arch Gen Psychiatry 54:233–241, 1997

223. Volkow ND, Fowler JS, Wolf AP, et al: Changes in brain glucose metabolism in cocaine dependence and withdrawal. Am J Psychiatry 148:621–626, 1991

224. Grant S, London E, Newlin DB, et al: Activation of memory circuits during cue-elicited cocaine craving. Proc Natl Acad Sci U S A 93:12040–12045, 1996

225. Bachevalier J, Mishkin M: Visual recognition impairment follows ventromedial but not dorsolateral prefrontal lesions in monkeys. Behav Brain Res 20:249–261, 1986

226. Kowalska DM, Bachevalier J, Mishkin M: The role of the inferior prefrontal convexity in performance of delayed nonmatching-to-sample. Neuropsychologia 29:583–600, 1991

227. Quintana J, Fuster JM: Spatial and temporal factors in the role of prefrontal and parietal cortex in visuomotor integration. Cereb Cortex 3:122–132, 1993

228. Mishkin M: Memory in monkeys severely impaired by combined but not by separate removal of amygdala and hippocampus. Nature 273:297–298, 1978

229. Goldman PS, Rosvold HE, Mishkin M: Evidence for behavioral impairment following prefrontal lobectomy in the infant monkey. Journal of Comparative and Physiological Psychology 70:454–463, 1970

230. Jones B, Mishkin M: Limbic lesions and the problem of stimulus-reinforcement associations. Exp Neurol 36:362–377, 1972

231. Passingham RE: Visual discrimination learning after selective prefrontal ablations in monkeys (*Macaca mulatta*). Neuropsychologia 10:27–39, 1972

232. Passingham RE, Ettlinger G: Tactile discrimination learning after selective prefrontal ablations in monkeys (*Macaca mulatta*). Neuropsychologia 10:17–26, 1972

233. Anderson SW, Damasio H, Tranel D, et al: Cognitive sequelae of focal lesions in ventromedial frontal lobe (abstract). J Clin Exp Neuropsychol 14:83, 1992

234. Stuss DT, Kaplan EF, Benson DF, et al: Evidence for the involvement of orbitofrontal cortex in memory functions: an interference effect. Journal of Comparative and Physiological Psychology 96:913–925, 1982

235. Freedman M, Oscar-Berman M: Bilateral frontal lobe disease and selective delayed response deficits in humans. Behav Neurosci 100:337–342, 1986

236. Gold JM, Berman KF, Randolph C, et al: PET validation of a novel prefrontal task: delayed response alternation. Neuropsychology 10:3–10, 1996

237. Paradiso S, Facorro SC, Andreasen NC, et al: Brain activity assessed with PET during recall of word lists and narratives: Neuroreport 8:3091–3096, 1997

238. Andreasen KC, O'Leary DS, Arntdt S, et al: Short-term and long-term verbal memory: a positron emission tomography study. Proc Natl Acad Sci U S A 92:5111–5115, 1995

239. Nyberg L, Tulving E, Habib R, et al: Functional brain maps of retrieval mode and recovery of episodic information. Neuroreport 7:1249–1252, 1995

240. Stuss DT, Benson DF, Kaplan EF, et al: Leucotomized and nonleucotomized schizophrenics: comparison on tests of attention. Biol Psychiatry 16:1085–1100, 1981

241. Stuss DT, Benson DF, Kaplan EF, et al: The involvement of orbitofrontal cerebrum in cognitive tasks. Neuropsychologia 21:235–248, 1983

242. Wise RA: Addictive drugs and brain stimulation reward. Annu Rev Neurosci 19:319–340, 1996

243. Berridge KC: Food reward: brain substrates of wanting and liking. Neurosci Biobehav Rev 20:1–25, 1996

244. Blumberg HP, Stern E, Ricketts S, et al: Rostral and orbital prefrontal cortex dysfunction in the manic state of bipolar disorder. Am J Psychiatry 156:1986–1988, 1999

245. Bremner JD, Innis RB, Salomon RM, et al: Positron emission tomography measurement of cerebral metabolic correlates of tryptophan depletion-induced depressive relapse. Arch Gen Psychiatry 54:364–374, 1997

246. Baxter LR Jr, Phelps ME, Mazziotta JC, et al: Local cerebral glucose metabolic rates in obsessive-compulsive disorder: a comparison with rates in unipolar depression and in normal controls. Arch Gen Psychiatry 44:211–218, 1987

247. Baxter LR Jr, Schwartz JM, Mazziotta JC, et al: Cerebral glucose metabolic rates in nondepressed patients with obsessive-compulsive disorder. Am J Psychiatry 145:1560–1563, 1988

248. Nordahl TE, Benkelfat C, Semple WE, et al: Cerebral glucose metabolic rates in obsessive compulsive disorder. Neuropsychopharmacology 2:23–28, 1989

249. Swedo SE, Schapiro MB, Grady CL, et al: Cerebral glucose metabolism in childhood-onset obsessive-compulsive disorder. Arch Gen Psychiatry 46:518–523, 1989

250. Breiter HC, Kwong KK, Baker JR, et al: Functional magnetic resonance imaging of symptom provocation in patients with obsessive-compulsive disorder versus controls. Arch Gen Psychiatry 53:595–606, 1996

251. Benkelfat C, Nordahl TE, Semple WE, et al: Local cerebral glucose metabolic rates in obsessive-compulsive disorder: patients treated with clomipramine. Arch Gen Psychiatry 47:840–848, 1990

252. Swedo SE, Pietrini P, Leonard HL, et al: Cerebral glucose metabolism in childhood-onset obsessive-compulsive disorder: revisualization during pharmacotherapy. Arch Gen Psychiatry 49:690–694, 1992

253. Baxter LR Jr, Schwartz JM, Bergman KS, et al: Caudate glucose metabolic rate changes with both drug and behavior therapy for obsessive-compulsive disorder. Arch Gen Psychiatry 49:681–689, 1992

254. Schwartz JM, Stoessel PW, Baxter LR: Systematic changes in cerebral glucose metabolic rate after successful behavior modification treatment of obsessive-compulsive disorder. Arch Gen Psychiatry 53:109–113, 1996

255. Baxter LR: Brain imaging as a tool in establishing a theory of brain pathology in obsessive compulsive disorder. J Clin Psychiatry 51 (suppl):22–26, 1990

256. Modell JG, Mountz JM, Curtis GC, et al: Neurophysiologic dysfunction in basal ganglia/limbic striatal and thalamocortical circuits as a pathogenetic mechanism of obsessive-compulsive disorder. J Neuropsychiatry Clin Neurosci 1:27–36, 1989

257. Rapoport JL, Wise SP: Obsessive-compulsive disorder: evidence for basal ganglia dysfunction. Psychopharmacol Bull 24:380–384, 1988

258. Hodgson RJ, Rachman S: The effects of contamination and washing in obsessional patients. Behav Res Ther 10:111–117, 1972

259. Hornsveld RHJ, Kraaimaat FW, van Dam-Baggen RMJ: Anxiety/discomfort and handwashing in obsessive-compulsive and psychiatric control patients. Behav Res Ther 17:223–228, 1979

260. Salkovskis PM: Obsessional-compulsive problems: a cognitive-behavioural analysis. Behav Res Ther 23:571–583, 1985

261. Rachman S: Obsessions, responsibility and guilt. Behav Res Ther 31:149–154, 1993

262. The Clomipramine Collaborative Study Group: Clomipramine in the treatment of patients with obsessive-compulsive disorder. Arch Gen Psychiatry 48:730–738, 1991

263. Depue RD, Zald DH: Biological and environmental processes in nonpsychotic psychopathology, in Basic Issues in Psychopathology. Edited by Costello CG. New York, Guilford, 1993, pp 127–237

264. Doudet D, Hommer D, Higley JD, et al: Cerebral glucose metabolism, CSF 5-HIAA levels and aggressive behavior in rhesus monkeys. Am J Psychiatry 152:1782–1787, 1995

265. Chevalier G, Deniau JM: Disinhibiton as a basic process in the expression of striatal functions. Trends Neurosci 13:277–280, 1990

266. Penney JB Jr, Young AB: Speculations on the functional anatomy of basal ganglia disorders. Annu Rev Neurosci 6:73–94, 1983

267. Nishino H, Hattori S, Muramoto K, et al: Basal ganglia neural activity during operant feeding behavior in the monkey: relation to sensory integration and motor execution. Brain Res Bull 27:463–468, 1991

268. Cromwell HC, Berridge KC: Implementation of action sequences by a neostriatal site: a lesion mapping study of grooming syntax. J Neurosci 16:3444–3458, 1996

269. Aldrige JW, Berridge KC, Herman M, et al: Neuronal coding of serial order: syntax of grooming in the neostriatum. Psychological Science 4:391–395, 1993

270. Andreasen NC, O'Leary DS, Cizadlo T, et al: Remembering the past: two facets of episodic memory explored with positron emission tomography. Am J Psychiatry 152:1576–1585, 1995

5

Working Memory Dysfunction in Schizophrenia

Patricia S. Goldman-Rakic, Ph.D.

The prefrontal cortex has been directly or indirectly implicated in many neurological and psychiatric diseases; among these, schizophrenia is the mental illness that has most often been related to the prefrontal cortex.[1–6] The argument that prefrontal dysfunction is important in schizophrenia has been made on many grounds—pharmacological, developmental, neuropsychological, and electrophysiological—as well as on the basis of recent imaging studies of cortical blood flow and activation. In this chapter, I make the case for a connection solely on the basis of symptomatology, as Levin[4] and others have done before me. However, my goal is to take the argument further, to suggest that there may be a singular cognitive operation, working memory, the disruption of which could account for the cardinal feature of thought disorder.

Pinpointing the basic psychological defects in thought disorder would be an important step toward analyzing its biological basis. In our work, schizophrenic thought disorder is conceptualized as an impairment in a process called working memory that melds concepts, ideas, memories, and other symbolic representations.[6] This viewpoint focuses on information processing and not on the information itself.

Thus, the content of a person's mental life or verbal output may be expected to be idiosyncratic, but how that content is processed may depend on a fundamental mechanism common to all individuals. At the biological level, the neural circuitry and physiological mechanisms underlying the working memory functions of the prefrontal cortex could be essential for understanding schizophrenia and ultimately for developing rational approaches to its treatment.

I first describe studies, primarily from my own laboratory, concerned with prefrontal function in nonhuman primates. I then attempt to relate the studies in nonhuman primates to an understanding of deficits in patients with prefrontal damage and patients with schizophrenia.

THE CONCEPT OF WORKING MEMORY

Working memory is the term applied by cognitive psychologists and theorists to the type of memory that is active and relevant only for a short time, usually on the scale of seconds.[7] A common trivial example of working memory is keeping in mind a newly read telephone number until it is dialed and then immediately forgotten. Another common example is recall of the contents of a meal just devoured or the names of several individuals to whom one has just been introduced. The criterion "useful or relevant only transiently" distinguishes working memory from the processes that have been termed *reference memory,*[8] *semantic memory,*[9] and *procedural memory,*[10] all of which have in common that their contents are always true and, in principle, remain stable over time—for example, someone's name, the date of Independence Day, the shape of an apple. In contrast to working memory, all of these other forms of memory can be considered associative in the traditional sense; that is, information is acquired by the repeated contiguity between stimuli and responses.

If associative memory is the process by which stimuli and events acquire permanent meaning, working memory is the process for the proper use of acquired knowledge. Working memory confers the ability to guide behavior by representations of the outside world rather than by immediate stimulation and thus to base behavior on ideas and thoughts.

The implications for cognitive function of the guidance of behavior by symbolic representations versus by external stimuli cannot be overemphasized. At the most elementary level, our basic conceptual ability to appreciate that an object exists when out of view depends on the capacity to keep events in mind beyond the direct experience of those events. For some organisms, including most humans under certain conditions, "out of sight" is equivalent to "out of mind." However, working memory is generally available to provide the temporal and spatial continuity between our past experience and present actions.[7,10–13] Working memory has been invoked in all forms of cognitive processing, including linguistic processing.[7,11,12] It is certainly essential for performing mathematical operations (such as carrying over), playing chess, playing bridge, playing the piano from memory, and delivering a speech extemporaneously, as well as for fantasizing and planning.

Considerable evidence now shows that the brain obeys the distinction between working and other forms of memory and that the prefrontal cortex has a specialized, perhaps even preeminent, role in working memory processes.[6] Furthermore, several lines of evidence suggest that multiple working memory domains may exist in the prefrontal cortex, all organized according to a common functional principle but each dedicated to a different information-processing system.

COGNITIVE PROCESSING IN NONHUMAN PRIMATES

Working Memory in Nonhuman Primates

If working memory is so basic a process for cognition, can it be studied in animals? The capacity to keep events "in mind" for short periods actually has been studied in nonhuman primates by delayed-response paradigms for many decades. The classic delayed-response task was designed and introduced to psychology for that very purpose by the comparative psychologist Walter Hunter.[14] His intention was to devise a test that would differentiate among animals (including humans) in "intelligence," which he defined as the ability to respond to situations on the basis of stored information rather than on the basis of immediate stimulation.

The classic version of the delayed-response test is well known: the subject is shown the location of a food morsel that is then hidden from view by an opaque screen. After a delay period of several seconds, the subject must choose the correct location from two or more choices. In this situation, the subject must remember where the bait had been placed a few seconds earlier. A crucial feature of the delayed-response task is that the correct response is different on every trial, so that information relevant to the response on one trial is irrelevant on the next and is actually best forgotten because it could interfere with the current response. This differentiates the delayed-response task from associative learning or conditioning paradigms, in which the correct response is the same on each subsequent trial. The underlying principle of delayed response operates in other behavioral paradigms commonly used with monkeys, including spatial delayed alternation, object alternation, and matching-to-sample or nonmatching-to-sample tasks.

Cellular Analysis of Working Memory

A major advance in our understanding of delayed-response tasks and the prefrontal cortex came in the early 1970s when electrophysiological studies were performed for the first time in awake, behaving monkeys trained on delayed-response tasks.[15,16] These studies found that neurons in and around the principal sulcus in the prefrontal cortex (Walker's area 46, Figure 5–1) became activated during the delay period of a delayed-response trial. It was difficult to resist the hypothesis that the prefrontal neurons examined were

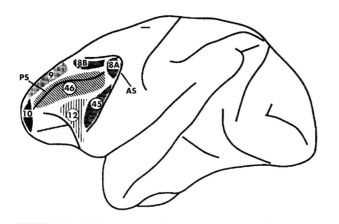

FIGURE 5–1. Diagram of rhesus monkey brain showing its basic divisions into prefrontal areas based on Walker's mapping system (1940).

The principal sulcus (PS; area 46) and other areas on the dorsolateral surface are indicated by shading. The prefrontal cortex has been divided into a number of cytoarchitectonic areas on its ventral and medial surfaces, but these are not shown. AS=arcuate sulcus.

Source. Adapted from Goldman-Rakic PS: "Circuitry of the Prefrontal Cortex and the Regulation of Behavior by Representational Knowledge," in *Handbook of Physiology, Vol 5.* Edited by Plum F, Mountcastle V. Bethesda, MD, American Physiological Society, 1987, pp. 373–417. Used with permission.

the cellular correlate of a mnemonic event—that cellular activation in the delay period is a means of keeping information in mind when it goes out of view.

Earlier studies on the behavioral effects of selective lesions of the prefrontal cortex had already indicated that the cortex in and around the principal sulcal cortex was involved in what we termed at the time *modality-specific* memory.[17,18] Our studies showed that monkeys with lesions of the principal sulcus were impaired on tasks that contained both spatial cued responses *and* a delay but performed well on tasks that contained only a delay or only a spatial cued response. These experiments provided early evidence of a working memory system dedicated to spatial vision that did not overlap with memory mechanisms for other domains of knowledge.

The evidence from neurophysiological studies of prefrontal neurons has been steadily accumulating since the early 1970s. Since that time, numerous studies have provided evidence that certain classes of dorsolateral prefrontal neurons are selectively activated during delay periods.[6,13] Yet the interpretation that such activity reflected a memory process was and sometimes still is resisted. Perhaps one reason is the be-

lief that neurons activated during the delay of a delayed-response trial are not necessarily holding specific information "on-line" but rather are engaged in some sort of general preparatory or motor set to respond.

A "preparation to respond" interpretation would invoke postural or motor mechanisms rather than a mnemonic process. However, our studies at Yale have provided the most convincing evidence yet of mnemonic processing in the prefrontal cortex. Shintaro Funahashi, Charles Bruce, and I[19] have been using an oculomotor delayed-response paradigm to study prefrontal function. This paradigm has many advantages over traditional methods of studying delayed-response performance. We require the animal to fixate a spot of light on a television monitor and maintain fixation during the brief (0.5-second) presentation of a stimulus and a subsequent delay period of variable length. Visual stimuli can be presented in any part of the visual field, and, importantly, we have complete control over the specific information that the animal has to remember on any given trial. The fixation spot is turned off only at the end of the delay period, and its offset is our instruction to the animal to break fixation and direct its gaze to where the target had been. Because the animal's behavior is strictly controlled in all phases of a trial, the animal can perform correctly only if it uses mnemonic processing.

In the oculomotor task, as in manual delayed-response tasks, prefrontal neurons increase (or often decrease) their discharge rate during the delay period of a trial. The neuronal activity shown in the center of Figure 5–2 (delay-selective activity) is an example: activity rises sharply at the end of the stimulus, remains tonically active during the delay (in the absence of the stimulus and before a response), and then ceases rather abruptly at the end of the delay.

The activation of prefrontal neurons when a stimulus disappears from view and the maintenance of that activation until a response is executed are highly suggestive of a working memory process. It cannot easily be argued that the delay period activity reflects simply the general motor set of the animal to respond at the end of the delay—as has been described by many authors for neurons in premotor fields—because we have shown that individual prefrontal neurons have increased or decreased discharge only for targets in specific locations within the visual field.[19] We have termed this directionally specific activity of individual cells the *memory field* of a prefrontal neuron. Thus, even though an animal is set to respond, and does respond, correctly at the end of the delay period on

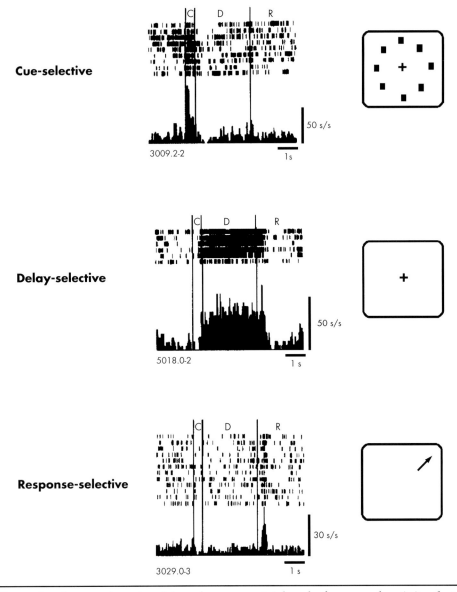

Cue-selective

Delay-selective

Response-selective

FIGURE 5–2.   Example of an oculomotor delayed-response trial and of neuronal activity that can be recorded from individual neurons while monkeys are performing the task.

Procedure: the monkey is required to fixate on a central spot on a television monitor. A target is presented for 0.5 s in one of eight locations (*top right*); after a delay of 3–6 s (*middle right*), the fixation spot disappears, and this is the instruction to the monkey to move its eyes to where the target had been (*bottom right*). One class of prefrontal neurons (cue-selective) shows a phasic response at the beginning of a trial when a stimulus is presented; a second class (delay-selective), activated after cue offset, maintains an elevated state until the end of the delay; a third class (response-selective) responds phasically shortly before the response is initiated, possibly in preparation for the response. Many prefrontal neurons show combinations of the pure activation patterns shown.

every trial regardless of target location, any given neuron is tuned to only one or a few locations. A general motor set explanation cannot easily explain this result.

If prefrontal neurons were involved in mnemonic processing, one would expect their activity to be sensitive to changes in the duration of the delay period. Indeed, the activity of prefrontal neurons that occurs during the delay period does expand and contract as the delay is lengthened or shortened.[19] Again, this would be expected if the neuron was holding information on-line that was to be retained until the end of the delay period.

Finally, if prefrontal neurons were coding only a preparatory set to respond, they would be expected to be activated before incorrect as well as correct responses. However, neurons that have memory fields—that is, those that have a "best direction" of discharge—falter in activity during the delay, or even completely fail to increase their rate, preceding responses in the nonpreferred, incorrect direction.[19] The fact that incremental firing precedes only correct responses indicates that the activity may be part of the internalized code needed to guide the correct response. Thus, it would serve a mnemonic function.

Anatomical Circuits for Spatial Working Memory

The principal sulcus in the prefrontal cortex is the anatomical focus for spatial delayed-response function, and knowledge of its connections with other structures is helping us to understand the circuit and cellular basis of working memory. It has become clear from our anatomical investigations that this prefrontal subdivision has reciprocal connections with more than a dozen distinct cortical association regions, including premotor centers, as well as with the caudate nucleus, superior colliculus, and brain stem centers.[6] Each of these connections presumably contributes different subfunctions to the overall capacity to guide a response by the mental representation of a stimulus. It is widely accepted that the reciprocal connections between the prefrontal and parietal cortex carry information about the spatial aspects of the outside world.[20] In our studies, we have traced several pathways from distinct visual centers concerned with peripheral vision to the principal sulcus via relays in the posterior parietal cortex[20–22] (Figure 5–3). By our anatomical account, prefrontal neurons in and around the principal sulcus are but two synapses removed from the primary visual cortex.

The mechanism for holding information on-line in the short-term memory buffer is not known at this point, and it is unclear what role is played in this process by the many connections that the prefrontal cortex has with limbic memory centers. We have described several multisynaptic routes of connectivity between the prefrontal cortex and the hippocampal formation and have speculated that these connections subserve a cooperative relationship between the hippocampus and the prefrontal cortex with regard to working memory[23,24] (Figure 5–4A). Evidence of elevated metabolic activity in the dentate gyrus and the several fields of Ammon's horn of monkeys performing working memory tasks support this line of think-

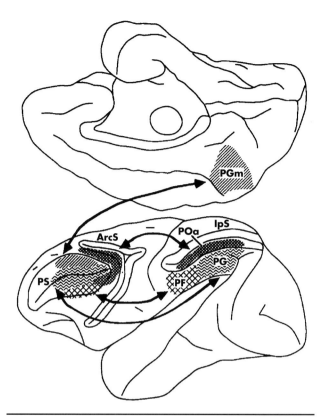

FIGURE 5–3. Transcortical pathways by which visuospatial information arriving at the primary visual cortex (not labeled) is transmitted via the posterior parietal cortex (PG, PF, PO_a, PG_m) to the prefrontal cortex.

PS=principal sulcus; ArcS=arcuate sulcus; IpS=inferior parietal sulcus.

Source. Adapted from Goldman-Rakic PS: "Circuitry of the Prefrontal Cortex and the Regulation of Behavior by Representational Knowledge," in *Handbook of Physiology, Vol 5.* Edited by Plum F, Mountcastle V. Bethesda, MD, American Physiological Society, 1987, pp. 373–417. Used with permission.

ing.[24] In further support for this linkage, neuronal activity during the delay period of delayed-response tasks has been recorded in Ammon's horn,[25] suggesting that hippocampal and prefrontal neurons are in the same circuit. Moreover, working memory tasks such as nonmatching-to-sample are exactly the types of tasks on which monkeys with lesions of the hippocampus are impaired. In the matching tasks, as in delayed-response tasks, information (the sample) is relevant for only one trial, and each trial is independent from the last. One conclusion that can be drawn from the literature is that the hippocampus and prefrontal cortex are functionally and anatomically related and, in general, that the prefrontal cortex regulates behav-

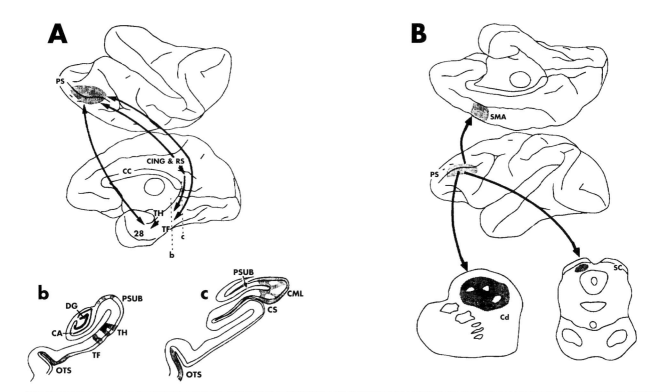

FIGURE 5–4. **A:** Summary of multiple pathways connecting the hippocampal formation with the prefrontal cortex. **B:** Summary of major output pathways from the principal sulcus (PS) to motor centers, including the caudate nucleus (Cd), the superior colliculus (SC), and the supplementary motor area (SMA), as well as other premotor centers.

CA=hippocampus; CC=corpus callosum; CING & RS=cingulate and retrosplenial cortex; CML=caudomedial lobule; CS=collateral sulcus; DG=dentate gyrus; OTS=occipitotemporal sulcus; PSUB=presubiculum; TF and TH=parahippocampal gyrus.

Source.   Adapted from Goldman-Rakic PS: "Circuitry of the Prefrontal Cortex and the Regulation of Behavior by Representational Knowledge," in *Handbook of Physiology, Vol. 5.* Edited by Plum F, Mountcastle V. Bethesda, MD, American Physiological Society, 1987, pp. 373–417. Used with permission.

ior in collaboration with a large set of other cortical and subcortical structures, which together constitute the brain's machinery for spatial cognition.

Finally, connections with the caudate nucleus[26] and superior colliculus,[27] among other motor centers, are thought to play a role in transmitting response commands to the motor centers (Figure 5–4B). The principal sulcus projects to premotor centers, including the supplementary motor areas[28,29] and cingulate motor areas,[29] and through these centers has access to the primary motor cortex. Again, therefore, with respect to motor control, the principal sulcus is but two synapses removed from primary motor neurons.

Multiple Working Memory Domains

Our previous studies have examined area 46 and its role in spatial delayed-response tasks. We have now

identified at least one other working memory domain in areas 12 and 45 of the prefrontal cortex[30] (Figure 5–1). Recordings were obtained from neurons in these areas in the inferior convexity region of the prefrontal cortex in monkeys trained to perform delayed-response tasks in which spatial or feature memoranda had to be recalled on independent, randomly interwoven trials. Although spatial and feature trials required exactly the same eye movements at the end of the delay, they differed in the nature of the mnemonic representation that guided those responses. Our major finding was that most of the inferior convexity neurons, unlike those in the principal sulcus (area 46), encode the features of visual stimuli rather than their locations.[30] Moreover, the areas from which such neurons are recorded are interconnected with the inferotemporal areas of the temporal lobe where object vision is represented. The results of studies thus provide strong evidence that information about the features of objects and information about their spatial location may be processed separately.

The finding that the prefrontal cortex contains a second area with working memory functions supports the prediction that prefrontal areas are specialized for working memory function and that the subdivisions represent different informational domains rather than different processes.[6] We also can infer that areas 12 and 45 in humans may be the areas most relevant for performance on tasks such as the Wisconsin Card Sorting Test (WCST; see WCST subsection in this chapter).

SCHIZOPHRENIA: CHARACTERIZATION OF THE COGNITIVE PROCESS IN THE DISEASE

Clinical Observations

The catalogue of symptoms that define schizophrenia is a subject of continuing discussion and research in psychiatry, one that is complicated by the heterogeneity of the disease. The question I wish to raise here is whether and to what extent the thought disorder expressed in schizophrenia reflects a basic underlying cognitive dysfunction, specifically in the process of working memory.

Several distinguished experts on schizophrenia have commented on the central features of the cognitive disorder observed in schizophrenia. These observations are not only highly consistent with one another but also compatible with the presence of an underlying deficit in working memory processes. According to Shakow,[31] the schizophrenic patient, like the frontal lobe patient, has reasonable basic sensorimotor skills, and performance falls within the normal range on simple associative tasks. However, these intact functions coexist with fragmentation, stereotypy, and disorganization of types of behavior that require symbolic or verbal representation. Shakow summarized his views after 30 years of research on the cardinal psychological deficits in schizophrenia: the schizophrenic patient "reacts to old situations as if they were new ones, and to new situations as if they were recently past ones" (p. 303). According to Schmolling,[32] the schizophrenic thought process often exhibits "a strong focus on the irrelevant and a weak focus on the relevant," and abstractions and verbal productions tend to be "autistic, idiosyncratic, tangential and bizarre" (p. 253). Similarly, Salzinger[33] characterized schizo-

phrenic behavior as excessively dominated by immediate stimulation rather than by a balance of current, internal, and past information. Cohen and Servan-Schreiber[34] argued that "word salad" in schizophrenia could reflect the failure to keep a word in mind (their term is *stimulus persistence*) after it has been uttered, leading to a grave restriction in the span over which contextual interactions can occur. Anscombe[35] discussed the schizophrenic thought disorders in terms of selective attention. However, the descriptions that support an attention deficit are entirely compatible with the lack of ability to guide behavior by representations and attendant susceptibility to environmental control and distractibility. Thus, Anscombe focused on the capture of the schizophrenic patient's attention by incidental or irrelevant details and explained how this process can lead to dissociated states: "Intentional actions are brought into being by means of active mental operations, and they confer upon the thinker a sense of personal urgency.... Without this capacity to shape and to direct thought, the person cannot give coherence to his behavior and remains at the mercy of his surroundings or impulse" (p. 246). I argue that the ability to keep ideas in mind—working memory—is the basic psychological process that allows "active mental operations" and prevents the tyranny of external stimuli.

Spatial Delayed-Response Tasks

Impairments on classic spatial delayed-response tasks, analogous to those found in monkeys with prefrontal lesions, have been reported in human patients with prefrontal lesions,[36–39] and considerable evidence of defective use of visuospatial coordinate systems is also seen in such patients.[40,41]

Oculomotor working memory tasks, too, have been explored with schizophrenic patients. Park and Holzman[42] employed a modified version of the oculomotor task from our electrophysiological study performed on rhesus monkeys.[19] In the modified task, the target was presented for only 200 milliseconds, and two delays—5 seconds and 30 seconds—were used. Also, the human subjects performed a distracter task during the delay; this distracter was essential to prevent the subject from transforming the spatial memorandum into a verbal mediator that would obviate the visuospatial character of the memory and bridge the delay. Schizophrenic patients were impaired on the oculomotor delayed-response task, and, as in monkeys with dorsolateral prefrontal lesions,[43] the deficit observed in the patients was most prominent on the memory-guided tasks, with much slighter impairments on a sensory-guided control task. The pattern of results represents a remarkable correspondence between the results in schizophrenic patients and those obtained in monkeys with prefrontal lesions.

Wisconsin Card Sorting Test

The neuropsychological deficit most widely recognized as being associated with prefrontal dysfunction in humans is that identified by the WCST.[44] In this task, the subject is asked to sort a deck of cards bearing stimuli that vary in number, color, and shape. As each card in the stack comes up, the subject has to match it to a set of reference cards on the basis of one dimension (e.g., color) that is arbitrarily selected by the experimenter. The experimenter then informs the subject whether he or she is "right" or "wrong," and the patient tries to get as many correct matches as possible. After the patient achieves a specified number of consecutive correct matches, the sorting principle is shifted without warning (e.g., from color to shape), and the patient must modify his or her responses accordingly. Patients with prefrontal damage show difficulty in switching from one category to another.[45,46]

At first glance, there seems little reason to believe that the function identified by the WCST in frontal lobe patients is the same as or similar to that measured by spatial delayed-response tasks in monkeys. Commonalities between these two tasks have rarely been claimed. However, the WCST does resemble the delayed-response tasks in one essential respect. Although the relevant features of the stimuli (color, shape, number) are all present in the environment at the time of response, the environmental stimuli contain no information about the correct response. That information must be provided from representational memory—in this case, the instruction or concept "color," "shape," or "number" guides the response choice. Although the capacity for this type of higher order representational system appears to be a unique acquisition of human intelligence, undoubtedly linked to the emergence of language, it clearly must be built on a lower order representational capacity shared with other mammals. The inability to keep the concept or category in mind reduces the patient to reliance on external cues or to associative conditioning whereby each instance of a color that was previously reinforced is repeated until a conditional response repertoire based on stimulus-response principles is built up.

According to this view, switching categories poses a problem precisely because the patient has no deficit in associative learning; he or she has learned the discrimination task well, and that learning now must be extinguished. Likewise, monkeys with prefrontal lesions and even hippocampal lesions perform excellently on associative tasks such as visual discrimination problems because the prefrontal cortex is not essential for such behavior.[6] Schizophrenic subjects are impaired on the WCST,[5] and their behavior is strongly reminiscent of that of a frontal patient who latches onto a stimulus dimension in the WCST and perseverates this choice when it is no longer correct or of a monkey with a prefrontal lesion that responds to the same location that happened to be rewarded on the preceding trial.

Moreover, direct evidence for a functional alteration in the prefrontal cortex in schizophrenia comes from studies reporting that schizophrenic subjects did not show the pattern of an increased, "hyperfrontal" blood flow that characterizes nonschizophrenic persons studied at rest.[3,47] Additional studies that used positron-emission tomography have independently reported slight to moderate decreases in blood flow or metabolism to the prefrontal cortex in schizophrenic patients.[47–49] Berman, Zec, and Weinberger's study[49] is notable for studying medication-free patients and for assessing blood flow under various conditions: at rest, during performance of the WCST, and during performance of a number-matching task that controlled for attentional and nonspecific behavioral variables. In that study, blood flow to the prefrontal cortex of schizophrenic patients was decreased in the at-rest condition; however, more important, blood flow to the dorsolateral prefrontal cortex did not increase in the schizophrenic patients as it did in the nonschizophrenic control subjects during the performance of the sorting task. Furthermore, the prefrontal cerebral blood flow in patients correlated positively with performance on the WCST. Finally, a variety of control tests, including the Continuous Performance Test and Raven's Progressive Matrices, which require attention and mental effort and also elicit poor performance from schizophrenic patients, did not produce differential blood flow patterns in schizophrenic patients relative to age-matched control subjects. Further evidence that the prefrontal cortex is a potentially important pathogenic area in schizophrenia can be derived from studies of electroencephalographic abnormalities[50] and of frontal eye field function in schizophrenic subjects.[51]

In addition to the WCST, various other tests reflect prefrontal dysfunction. These include the Stroop Test,[52] in which the names of colors are printed in the ink of another color (the word *yellow* is printed in red), and subjects are instructed to report the color of the word while suppressing the natural or prepotent tendency to report the written content of the word. Here again the subject must ignore the immediate stimuli and instead guide his or her response by a representational memory, in this case the memory of an instruction. Patients with prefrontal lesions are also impaired on tasks in which they must both keep track of the recency or order of their previous responses[46,53] and project sequences of future responses, as required on "look-ahead" puzzles such as the Tower of London test.[11] In that task, a goal has to be decomposed into subgoals that must then be tackled in the correct order. Such tasks, like delayed-response tasks, require an ability to base current responses on representations of past or future events. A report by Andreasen et al.[54] indicated that nonmedicated schizophrenic patients are impaired on the Tower of London task and show hypofrontal blood flow while performing it.

Future studies should determine the extent to which these impairments are specifically related to prefrontal dysfunction rather than reflecting a generalized impairment. For now, the data drawn from this brief survey provide support for the thesis of this chapter: that deficits shown by schizophrenic patients on a variety of neuropsychological tests may be reducible to impairment of the mechanisms by which symbolic representations are accessed and held "on line" to guide behavior in the absence of, or even in spite of, discriminative stimuli in the outside world.

CONCLUSIONS

I have emphasized the possibility that many cardinal cognitive symptoms associated with schizophrenia bear strong resemblance to the thought disorders, attentional problems, and lack of initiative, plans, and goals that characterize patients with physical prefrontal damage. If, as numerous findings suggest, the prefrontal cortex is centrally involved in schizophrenia, we can begin to think of some aspects of the disorder as constituting a breakdown in the processes by which representational knowledge governs behavior. An implication of the neurobehavioral analysis presented here is that the most likely focus of a lesion in this disorder may be the cortical processing networks by which the prefrontal cortex "accesses" and holds "online" representational knowledge of the outside world through its connections with parietal and limbic centers. A defective ability to keep instructions, concepts, and goals in mind would necessarily lead to confusion, distractibility, attentional disturbance, misinterpretation of causality, and so forth.

The positive symptoms of the disorder lead us to believe that cortical feedback pathways may be particularly important for bringing representational data into line with reality via the anatomical mechanisms discussed in Goldman-Rakic.[6] For example, prefrontal projections to the parietal (and temporal) association areas may be able to gate sensory (real-world) information that these areas receive from the thalamus and secondary sensory areas. An impairment in this mechanism could lead to altered consciousness of sensory experience. Impairment in some of the feed-forward projections to and from the prefrontal cortex also may be important in certain negative symptoms: lack of initiative, poverty of speech, and lack of goal-directed behavior or initiative.

In schizophrenia, we cannot yet pinpoint a lesion, but the disruption of cognitive ability must either directly or indirectly involve the corticocortical and corticosubcortical pathways that establish the inner models of reality and adjust them to contemporary demands. This information-processing network may be the system that is most severely influenced by dopamine hyperactivity and that is acted on by neuroleptic medication.

It is important to underscore that the prefrontal cortex is a component of a larger network of cortical areas,[55] and symptoms may reflect dysfunction in any part of the network, giving rise to much heterogeneity in the expression of schizophrenia. At the same time, because this network is crucial for memory-guided behavior, it would not be surprising to find common neuropsychiatric symptoms and common involvement of corticocortical processing between schizophrenia and other diseases that affect cognitive processes. Thus, future efforts to understand the frontal lobe may pay dividends by contributing to the understanding of a family of mental disorders that reflect breakdown in its circuitry.

REFERENCES

1. Alzheimer A: Beitrage zur pathologischen Anatomie der Dementia Praecox. Allgemeine Zeitschrift für Psychiatrie 70:810–812, 1913

2. Moniz E: Les première tentatives opératoires dans le traitement de certaines psychoses. Encéphale 31:1–29, 1936

3. Franzen G, Ingvar DH: Absence of activation in frontal structures during psychological testing of chronic schizophrenics. J Neurol Neurosurg Psychiatry 38:1027–1032, 1975

4. Levin S: Frontal lobe dysfunctions in schizophrenia, II: impairments of psychological and brain functions. J Psychiatr Res 18:57–72, 1984

5. Weinberger DR, Berman KF, Zec RF: Physiological dysfunction of dorsolateral prefrontal cortex in schizophrenia, I: regional cerebral blood flow (rCBF) evidence. Arch Gen Psychiatry 43:114–125, 1986

6. Goldman-Rakic PS: Circuitry of the prefrontal cortex and the regulation of behavior by representational knowledge, in Handbook of Physiology, Vol 5. Edited by Plum F, Mountcastle V. Bethesda, MD, American Physiological Society, 1987, pp 373–417

7. Baddeley A: Working Memory. London, Oxford University Press, 1986

8. Olton DS, Papas BC: Spatial memory and hippocampal function. Neuropsychologia 17:669–682, 1979

9. Tulving E: Episodic and Semantic Memory. New York, Academic Press, 1972, pp 381–403

10. Squire L, Cohen NJ: Human memory and amnesia, in Neurobiology of Memory and Learning. Edited by Lynch G, McGaugh JL, Weinberger NM. New York, Guilford, 1984, pp 3–64

11. Shallice T: Specific impairments in planning. Philos Trans R Soc Lond B Biol Sci 298:199–209, 1982

12. Ingvar DH: Several aspects of language and speech related to prefrontal cortical activity. Human Neurobiology 2:177–189, 1983

13. Fuster JM: The prefrontal cortex and temporal integration, in Cerebral Cortex. Edited by Jones EG, Peters A. New York, Plenum, 1985, pp 151–177

14. Hunter WS: The delayed reaction in animals and children. Behavior Monographs 2:1–86, 1913

15. Kubota K, Niki H: Prefrontal cortical unit activity and delayed cortical unit activity and delayed alternation performance in monkeys. J Neurophysiol 34:337–347, 1971

16. Fuster JM, Alexander GE: Neuron activity related to short-term memory. Science 173:652–654, 1971

17. Goldman PS, Rosvold HE: Localization of function within the dorsolateral prefrontal cortex of the rhesus monkey. Exp Neurol 27:291–304, 1970

18. Goldman PS, Rosvold HE, Vest B, et al: Analysis of the delayed alternation deficit produced by dorsolateral prefrontal lesions in the rhesus monkey. Journal of Comparative and Physiological Psychology 77:212–220, 1971

19. Funahashi S, Bruce CJ, Goldman-Rakic PS: Mnemonic coding of visual space in the monkey's dorsolateral prefrontal cortex. J Neurophysiol 61:1–19, 1989

20. Cavada C, Goldman-Rakic PS: Posterior parietal cortex in rhesus monkey, I: parcellation of areas based on distinctive limbic and sensory cortico-cortical connections. J Comp Neurol 287:393–421, 1989

21. Cavada C, Goldman-Rakic PS: Posterior parietal cortex in rhesus monkey, II: evidence for segregated cortico-cortical networks linking sensory and limbic areas with the frontal lobe. J Comp Neurol 287:422–445, 1989

22. Goldman-Rakic PS: Changing concepts of cortical connectivity: parallel distributed cortical networks, in Neurobiology of Neocortex. Edited by Rakic P, Singer W. New York, Wiley, 1988, pp 177–202

23. Goldman-Rakic PS, Selemon LD, Schwartz ML: Dual pathways connecting the dorsolateral prefrontal cortex with the hippocampal formation and parahippocampal cortex in the rhesus monkey. Neuroscience 12:719–743, 1984

24. Friedman HR, Goldman-Rakic PS: Activation of the hippocampus by working memory: a 2–deoxyglucose study of behaving rhesus monkeys. J Neurosci 8:4693–4706, 1988

25. Watanabe T, Niki H: Hippocampal unit activity and delayed response in the monkey. Brain Res 325:241–254, 1985

26. Selemon LD, Goldman-Rakic PS: Common cortical and subcortical target areas of the dorsolateral prefrontal and posterior parietal cortices in the rhesus monkey (abstract). Society for Neuroscience Abstracts 11:323, 1985

27. Goldman PS, Nauta WJH: Autoradiographic demonstration of a projection from prefrontal association cortex to the superior colliculus in the rhesus monkey. Brain Res 116:145–149, 1976

28. McGuire PK, Bates JF, Goldman-Rakic PS: Interhemispheric integration, I: symmetry and convergence of the corticocortical connections of the left and the right principal sulcus (PS) and the left and the right supplementary motor area (SMA) in the rhesus monkey. Cereb Cortex 1:390–407, 1991

29. Bates JF, Goldman-Rakic PS: Prefrontal connections of medial motor areas in the rhesus monkey. J Comp Neurol 335:1–18, 1993

30. Wilson FAW, O'Scalaidhe SP, Goldman-Rakic PS: Dissociation of object and spatial processing domains in primate prefrontal cortex. Science 260:1955–1958, 1993

31. Shakow D: Psychological deficit in schizophrenia. Behav Sci 8:275–305, 1963

32. Schmolling P: A systems model of schizophrenic dysfunction. Behav Sci 28:253–267, 1983

33. Salzinger K: An hypothesis about schizophrenic behavior. Am J Psychother 25:601–614, 1971

34. Cohen JD, Servan-Schreiber D: A parallel distributed processing approach to behavior and biology in schizophrenia (Technical Report AIP-100). Pittsburgh, PA, Carnegie-Mellon University, 1989

35. Anscombe R: The disorder of consciousness in schizophrenia. Schizophr Bull 13:241–260, 1987

36. Chorover SL, Cole M: Delayed alternation performance in patients with cerebral lesions. Neuropsych 4:1–7, 1966

37. Verin M, Partiot A, Pillon B, et al: Delayed response tasks and prefrontal lesions in man: evidence for self generated patterns of behaviour with poor environmental modulation. Neuropsychologia 31:1379–1396, 1993

38. Freedman M, Oscar-Berman M: Bilateral frontal lobe disease and selective delayed-response deficits in humans. Behav Neurosci 100:337–342, 1986

39. Pribram KH, Ahumada A, Hartog J, et al: A progress report on the neurological processes disturbed by frontal lesions in primates, in The Frontal Granular Cortex and Behavior. Edited by Warren JM, Akert K. New York, McGraw-Hill, 1964, pp 28–55

40. Teuber HL, Mishkin M: Judgement of visual and postural vertical afterbrain injury. J Psychol 38:161–175, 1954

41. Semmes JS, Weinstein S, Ghent L, et al: Correlates of impaired orientation in personal and extrapersonal space. Brain 86:747–772, 1963

42. Park S, Holzman PS: Schizophrenics show spatial working memory deficits. Arch Gen Psychiatry 49:975–982, 1992

43. Funahashi S, Chafee MV, Goldman-Rakic PS: Prefrontal neuronal activity in rhesus monkeys performing a delayed anti-saccade task. Nature 365:753–756, 1993

44. Milner B: Effects of different brain lesions on card sorting. Arch Neurol 9:100–110, 1963

45. Kolb B, Whishaw IQ: Performance of schizophrenic patients on tests sensitive to left or right frontal, temporal, or parietal function in neurological patients. J Nerv Ment Dis 171:435–443, 1983

46. Milner B, Petrides M: Behavioral effects of frontal-lobe lesions in man. Trends Neurosci 7:403–406, 1984

47. Buchsbaum MS, DeLisi LE, Holcomb HH: Anteroposterior gradients in cerebral glucose use in schizophrenia and affective disorders. Arch Gen Psychiatry 41:1159–1166, 1984

48. Farkhas T, Wolf AP, Jaeger J, et al: Regional brain glucose metabolism in chronic schizophrenia. Arch Gen Psychiatry 41:293–300, 1984

49. Berman KF, Zec RF, Weinberger DR: Physiological dysfunction of dorsolateral prefrontal cortex in schizophrenia, II: regional cerebral blood flow (rCBF) evidence. Arch Gen Psychiatry 43:126–135, 1986

50. Morihisa JM, Duffy FH, Wyatt RJ: Brain electrical activity mapping (BEAM) in schizophrenic patients. Arch Gen Psychiatry 40:719–728, 1983

51. Levin S: Frontal lobe dysfunctions in schizophrenia, I: eye movement impairments. J Psychiatr Res 18:27–55, 1984

52. Perret E: The left frontal lobe of man and the suppression of habitual responses in verbal categorical behaviour. Neuropsychologia 12:323–330, 1974

53. Petrides M, Milner B: Deficits on subject-ordered tasks after frontal- and temporal-lobe lesions in man. Neuropsychologia 20:249–262, 1982

54. Andreasen NC, Rezai K, Alliger R, et al: Hypofrontality in neuroleptic-naive patients and in patients with chronic schizophrenia: assessment with xenon 133 single-photon emission computed tomography and the Tower of London. Arch Gen Psychiatry 49:943–958, 1992

55. Goldman-Rakic PS: Topography of cognition: parallel distributed networks in primate association cortex. Annu Rev Neurosci 11:137–156, 1988

EDITOR'S COMMENTS

In this chapter, Dr. Goldman-Rakic has presented the groundwork for understanding the complex cognitive system involved in working memory. Recent work by her group and others has begun to elucidate the pharmacological mechanisms regulating spatial working memory. Rhesus monkeys with prefrontal dopamine depletion and patients with Parkinson's disease have impaired working memory, which implicates dopamine in working memory.[1–3] In a series of elegant studies, Dr. Rakic and her colleagues have reported that the D_1 dopamine receptor plays a key role in the activation patterns of neurons in the prefrontal cortex specialized for firing during the delay period in spatial working memory tasks. Iontophoresing drugs onto neurons in single-unit studies showed that the selective D_1 antagonist Sch 39166 enhanced neuronal firing in the isodirectional pyramidal cell and inhibited firing in the corresponding cross-directional pyramidal neuron during the delay phase of spatial working memory.[4–6] No change in these neurons occurred during the cue or response periods of the working memory task. The enhancing effect of the selective D_1 antagonist was reversed by treatment with a partial D_1 agonist.

D_1 receptors are 20 times more abundant in the prefrontal cortex than are D_2 receptors. The D_1 receptors are localized on the distal spines of pyramidal cell dendrites near glutamate receptors. The principal mechanism to explain this faciliatory effect is that D_1 blockade augments neuronal firing by enhancing *N*-methyl-D-aspartate receptor excitability. The close interaction of dopamine and glutamate receptors on pyramidal cell dendrites appears to exert a "tuning" of activity during spatial working memory tasks.

Enhancement of the neuron's memory field or spatial tuning is observed only at low doses of the antagonist. D_1 blockade at higher doses suppresses neuronal firing, which may explain why D_1 antagonists with a high degree of D_1 blockade used in the treatment of schizophrenia may have a negative effect on working memory functions.[7,8] D_2 blocking agents have a negative effect on neuronal firing during spatial working memory tasks.

γ-Aminobutyric acid (GABA)ergic interneurons and serotonergic inputs also modify spatial tuning of prefrontal neurons. GABAergic interneurons may play a powerful role in the activity of memory fields primarily through feed-forward disinhibition at the soma and axon hillock of pyramidal cells. Dopamine also may facilitate firing by inhibiting GABAergic interneurons. Low doses of serotonin enhance memory fields possibly through serotonin type 2A ($5\text{-}HT_{2A}$) receptors on proximal dendrites of pyramidal neurons or by binding to the $5\text{-}HT_{2A}$ receptor on GABAergic interneurons.

In summary, Dr. Goldman-Rakic and colleagues are to be lauded for making important strides in characterizing the pharmacological control of spatial working memory. Their work highlights the key role of prefrontal pyramidal neurons in specific working memory tasks and has shown that mnemonic processes are sculpted by GABAergic actions at the soma of pyramidal cells, serotonergic input at the $5\text{-}HT_2$ receptors on proximal dendrites, and D_1 action on pyramidal spines at the site of glutamatergic excitatory input. This approach should provide the framework for a rational approach to drug design to enhance working memory in aging and disease.

Stephen P. Salloway, M.D., M.S.

REFERENCES

1. Brozoski T, Brown RM, Rosvold HE, et al: Cognitive deficit caused by regional depletion of dopamine in prefrontal cortex of rhesus monkey. Science 205:929–932, 1979
2. Brown RG, Marsden CD: Internal vs external cues and the control of attention in Parkinson's disease. Brain 111:323–345, 1988
3. Gotham AM, Brown RG, Marsden CD: Frontal cognitive function in patients with Parkinson's disease on and off levodopa. Brain 111:299–321, 1988
4. Goldman-Rakic PS: The "psychic" neuron of the cerebral cortex. Ann N Y Acad Sci 868:13–26, 1999
5. Williams GV, Goldman-Rakic PS: Modulation of memory fields by dopamine D1 receptors in prefrontal cortex. Nature 376:572–575, 1995
6. Goldman-Rakic PS: Regional and cellular fractionation of working memory. Proc Natl Acad Sci U S A 92:13473–13480, 1996
7. Youngren KD, Inglis FM, Pivirotto PL, et al: Clozapine preferentially increases dopamine release in the rhesus monkey prefrontal cortex compared with the caudate nucleus. Neuropsychopharmacology 20:403–412, 1999
8. Goldman-Rakic PS, Selemon LD: Functional and anatomical aspects of prefrontal pathology in schizophrenia. Schizophr Bull 23:437–458, 1997

6

Lateralization of Frontal Lobe Functions

Kenneth Podell, Ph.D., Mark Lovell, Ph.D., Elkhonon Goldberg, Ph.D., A.B.C.N.

Historically, hemispheric specialization has been cast in categorical and static terms: the left hemisphere is the linguistic one, and the right hemisphere is the visuospatial one. Although this premise has become extremely influential, significant developments have taken place in cognitive neuroscience that challenge this classic dichotomy. It is important to bring these developments to the attention of clinical neuroscientists.

The traditional assumption holds that the left cerebral cortex of the human brain controls the processing of linguistic information, whereas the right hemisphere controls the processing of information for which language encoding is less feasible. The available data suggest, however, that the actual distribution of hemispheric responsibilities is not so clear-cut: the right hemisphere is not irrelevant to language nor is the left hemisphere irrelevant to processing nonlinguistic information.[1]

In this chapter, we introduce a distinct approach to hemispheric specialization called the *novelty-routinization continuum,* which argues for a more fundamental basis for lateralization of cerebral functions and how this is particularly expressed in regard to prefrontal systems functioning. We review evidence relating to anatomy, neurochemistry, neuroimaging, cognitive processes in healthy control subjects and brain-lesioned subjects, novel cognitive tasks, and neuropsychiatric disorders.

THE NOVELTY-ROUTINIZATION THEORY OF HEMISPHERIC SPECIALIZATION

Goldberg and colleagues[1,2] have proposed a theory of hemispheric specialization that is considered a more fundamental explanation of the functional differences between the two hemispheres. They proposed that the right hemisphere is critical for the exploratory processing of novel cognitive situations to which none of the codes or strategies preexisting in the individual's cognitive repertoire readily apply. The left hemisphere is critical for processing based on preexisting representations and routinized cognitive strategies. The traditional language/nonlanguage dichotomy then becomes a special case of this more fundamental principle.

This principle of hemispheric specialization is intriguing and addresses many shortfalls of the more traditional language/nonlanguage distinction. First, the distinction between cognitive novelty and cognitive routinization is not limited to humans. It can be meaningfully applied to any species capable of learning. Because language is unique to humans, the assumption of the primacy of the linguistic/nonlinguistic dichotomy emphasizes the uniqueness of hemispheric specialization to humans and emphasizes an evolutionary discontinuity in cerebral functional organization. Lateralized asymmetries have been noted in other species, but they do not permit meaningful homologies with humans within this framework. By divesting natural language of its cardinal role in hemispheric specialization, the novelty-routinization approach opens the avenue for tracing the evolutionary continuity in the development of cerebral lateralization and for the search of homologies across species through parallel experimentation. This position has the epistemological appeal of being more consistent with general biological assumptions.

In addition, the novelty-routinization approach emphasizes individual differences and argues against the fixed assignment of particular materials and tasks to one or the other hemisphere. What is cognitively novel to one individual is familiar and routinized to another.

Finally, the novelty-routinization hypothesis offers a dynamic rather than a static view of hemispheric specialization. It implies that the pattern of hemispheric specialization is different in a given individual at different developmental stages. Specifically, it implies that the locus of cortical control shifts from the right to the left hemisphere in the course of cognitive skill development.

Evidence Supporting the Novelty-Routinization Theory of Hemispheric Specialization

Evidence supporting the novelty-routinization theory of hemispheric specialization can be found in a large and expansive body of research covering several different areas. The body of evidence in support of this theory will cover atypical lateralization of linguistic and nonlinguistic processes, agnosias, biochemical (catecholamines) distribution and function, cross-sectional and quasi-longitudinal tachistoscopic studies, early-onset hemispheric lesion and cognitive development, and computational modeling.

The Right Hemisphere and Linguistic Processes

Left hemispheric dominance is not equally strong for all aspects of language processing. The left hemispheric advantage is more evident for consonants than for vowels, for long words than for short words, for ab-

stract words than for concrete words, and for lower frequency words than for higher frequency words.[3–8] When learning taxonomically similar words in a word-pair learning paradigm, a strong right frontal hypermetabolism is found during single photon emission computed tomography (SPECT).[9] Also, when inferring the moral of a story, right hemisphere activation (frontotemporal) is detected on regional cerebral blood flow (rCBF),[10] whereas the left hemisphere is activated for semantic components of the task.

The effects of early hemidecortication also suggest that the left hemisphere is not equally necessary for the development of all verbal skills. Early left hemidecortication permits the subsequent development of phonemic discrimination between real words but not between paralogs or phonologs (pseudowords).[11,12] Early left hemidecortication permits the development of propositional analysis, but it is limited to inference based on lexical information and general logical constraints, as opposed to the explicit appreciation of syntax.[13–15] Early left hemidecortication permits the development of a large auditory lexicon but of only limited categorical links between lexical items.[13,15]

It has been concluded that the right hemisphere plays a significant role in the formation of the referential basis of the code, but the left hemisphere is particularly important for the rule-based internal derivations within the code.[2]

The Left Hemisphere and Nonlinguistic Processes

A body of evidence indicates that the left hemisphere plays a role in the processing of nonlinguistic information, including visuospatial information. Lateralized damage to the left hemisphere may produce a severe perceptual deficit in the relative absence of a language deficit. Two families of agnosias exist: associative and apperceptive. They have opposite, complementary patterns of localization relative to the two cerebral hemispheres.

Associative agnosias. In associative agnosias, a patient cannot recognize an object as a member of a generic category, even though elementary perceptual analysis of its physical components and the ability to copy it may be relatively spared. Associative agnosias involve the degradation of, or impaired access to, the generic knowledge base—the long-term, categorical representations that normally allow us to perceive the world in terms of prespecified, invariant classes.[16] Teuber[17] referred to associative agnosias as "percepts stripped of their meaning."

Associative agnosias may be caused by bilateral or unilateral damage to the posterior association cortices. Unilateral lesions producing these syndromes invariably involve the left hemisphere and not the right hemisphere. Associative agnosias may exist in the absence of comparably severe language deficit.

Associative agnosias are modality-specific. The visual form of this syndrome is known as *visual object agnosia*.[18–26] The neuroanatomy of visual object agnosia involves damage to the occipital/occipitotemporal regions bilaterally or in the left hemisphere. The tactile form of this syndrome is known as *pure astereognosia*.[21,27–29] The neuroanatomy of pure astereognosia involves damage to the temporoparietal regions bilaterally or in the left hemisphere. The auditory form of this syndrome (an inability to understand the meaning of nonverbal sounds and noises and to associate them with the correct source) is known as *semantic associative agnosia*.[30–33] The neuroanatomy of semantic associative agnosia involves damage to the region of the superior temporal gyrus bilaterally or in the left hemisphere. Thus, it appears that some aspects of perceptual analysis, those impaired in associative agnosias, are linked to the left hemisphere.

Apperceptive agnosias. In apperceptive agnosias, the physical rather than categorical object identification is impaired. Although there is no elementary sensory deficit, the patient loses the ability to identify an object as being the same one under diverse conditions of observation, such as differing levels of brightness.[34,35] In associative agnosias, the ability to relate on-line percepts to preexisting generic representations is impaired. By contrast, the processes affected in apperceptive agnosia do not appear to involve long-term storage.

The neuroanatomy of apperceptive agnosias is different from, and in fact complementary to, that of associative agnosias. Apperceptive agnosias may be caused by bilateral or unilateral damage to the posterior association cortices. Unilateral lesions producing apperceptive agnosia invariably involve the right and not the left hemisphere.

Lateralization of Catecholamines

Norepinephrine and dopamine are preferentially abundant and lateralized within the prefrontal cortex in terms of concentration levels.[36–41] Additionally, ample evidence indicates that norepinephrine and dopamine are responsible for complementary behaviors. Norepinephrine is critical for orienting to novel stimuli and exploratory behavior, whereas dopamine is critical in redundant and stereotypic behavior.[42–47] This implies a link between the right hemisphere, norepinephrine, and cognitive novelty and between the left hemisphere, dopamine, and cognitive routinization.[45]

The Right-to-Left Shift of Hemispheric Control in Cognitive Learning

The novelty-routinization hypothesis constitutes a major change in understanding hemispheric specialization. It emphasizes the dynamic nature of hemispheric specialization. It predicts that the function of task acquisition is a unidirectional shift of hemispheric control from the right hemisphere to the left hemisphere.

The unidirectional nature of the shift of hemispheric involvement in the course of learning makes the novelty-routinization hypothesis testable and falsifiable. It is supported by a large body of experimental studies, which fall within several groups.

Cross-sectional evidence. In tachistoscopic and dichotic paradigms, task-naive healthy subjects show a right hemisphere advantage, and task-experienced subjects show a left hemisphere advantage. This difference has been reported for various nonverbal tasks in adults.[48–51] In healthy children, the increase in the degree of left hemisphere advantage with age and task proficiency has been shown for several language tasks.[52–56] This relation suggests a decreasing role of the right hemisphere in language as the function of the development of linguistic skills.

Quasi-longitudinal evidence. In healthy subjects introduced to a novel task tachistoscopically presented over blocks of trials, a right hemisphere advantage exists during early blocks of trials, and a left hemisphere advantage exists during late blocks. This has been shown both for nonverbal tasks[57–62] and for verbal tasks that entail uncommon use of language.[62–64] The right-to-left shift of hemispheric advantage as the function of learning appears to be universal and independent of stimulus modality. The novelty-routinization distinction overrides the linguistic/nonlinguistic distinction in determining the pattern of hemispheric involvement in a given cognitive task.

Early lesion effects. The effects of early hemidecortication on cognition are not symmetric. Early right hemispherectomy has subtle adverse effects on the subsequent acquisition of both nonlinguistic and linguistic cognitive skills. The earlier the age at which the right hemispherectomy was conducted, the greater the effect. Early left hemispherectomy has a significant adverse effect on the subsequent acquisition of linguistic skills but little adverse effect on the acquisition of nonverbal skills, and there is no interaction with age at hemispherectomy.[65,66] This suggests that the right hemisphere plays a major role at early stages of language acquisition and that this role decreases with age.

Computational evidence. Grossberg[67] draws the distinction between computational "stability" and computational "plasticity" in ways similar to the distinction between the exploratory and routinized behaviors. Grossberg suggested that to enhance the computational efficiency of a neural net, the stability and plasticity subsystems must be separate.

Frontal Lobes and Cognitive Novelty

The prefrontal cortex is presumed to be singularly important in cognitive control over situations for which no set solutions are available in the organism's cognitive repertoire. The role of the prefrontal cortex is believed to be particularly great when the organism is challenged with a novel task that requires that the pre-existing cognitive routines be accessed and configured in a new way.[23] On the other hand, the posterior association cortices are thought to provide the storage of cognitive routines and preexisting cognitive representations.[68]

Therefore, the prefrontal cortex has a particular affinity for cognitive novelty, and the posterior association cortex has an affinity for cognitive routinization. This points to an interesting implication of the novelty-routinization hypothesis: the left-right and anterior-posterior dimensions of cortical functional organization are not functionally orthogonal. In a sense, the left hemisphere is functionally dominated by the posterior association cortex and the right hemisphere is dominated by the prefrontal cortex. In terms of the novelty-routinization model advanced here, the nonorthogonal relation between the left-right and anterior-posterior cortical dimensions suggests that the shift of the locus of cortical control as a function of learning involves both dimensions: from the right prefrontal systems to the left posterior systems.

It is curious that the left-right and anterior-posterior cortical dimensions are not entirely orthogonal in a structural sense either. The cerebral hemispheres are

characterized by the Yakovlevian torque: the right frontal pole is thicker than, and protrudes over, the left frontal pole, and the left occipital pole is thicker than, and protrudes over, the right occipital pole.[69,70] The structural affinity between the frontal lobes and the right hemisphere captured in the Yakovlevian torque is consonant with the functional affinity between the frontal lobes, cognitive novelty, and the right hemisphere.

Internal and External Determinants of Cognitive Control: Are They Lateralized in the Frontal Lobes?

Historically, research into hemispheric specialization has emphasized the posterior cortex. It was implicitly assumed that the hemispheric differences were less pronounced in the frontal lobes. A growing body of evidence, however, indicates that significant functional lateralization is found in the frontal lobes as well.

The earlier studies driven by the traditional language-versus-visuospatial distinction of hemispheric specialization had already provided evidence for a functional dissociation between the left and right prefrontal cortex. Such a dissociation was found on the "generation" tasks, in which subjects were asked to generate as many different responses as possible according to specific rules. Performance by subjects with lateralized left or right prefrontal lesions was impaired relative to control subjects without lesions in both the verbal and the nonverbal generation tasks. When the two lesion groups were compared, the left prefrontal lesion group was more impaired on verbal generation tasks,[71–73] and the right prefrontal lesion group was more impaired on nonverbal generation tasks.[74,75]

Increasing evidence exists, however, that the functional differences between the left and right prefrontal systems are not limited to the verbal-nonverbal distinctions. Prefrontal cortex is critical for the selection of task-appropriate cognitive routines and representations.[23,76,77] This selection may be guided by internal contingencies represented in working memory[77] or by external contingencies reflecting environmental changes.[72,78] A preliminary but growing body of evidence suggests that the contributions of the prefrontal systems in executing the two types of cognitive control are lateralized in right-handed individuals. The left prefrontal system appears to be particularly important for guiding cognitive selection by working memory–mediated internal contingencies. The right prefrontal system appears to be particularly important for guiding cognitive selection by environmental external contingencies. The evidence of the lateralization of frontal lobe control over these functions is based on the functional neuroimaging of activation patterns in healthy volunteers and in patients and on the observations of frontal lesion effects on behavior.

Functional Neuroimaging in Healthy Volunteers

The techniques of functional neuroimaging have allowed us to study the role of prefrontal systems in cognition directly in healthy control subjects. This has resulted in a wide range of new findings regarding the role of prefrontal systems in cognition. We believe that this evidence supports our idea that the left prefrontal system is important in processing guided by internal representations and that the right prefrontal system is critical in processing guided by external contingencies.

A lateralized increase in the activation of the left superior prefrontal region occurs on both positron-emission tomography (PET) and measures of rCBF when subjects perform a task based on prior instructions.[79–85] Electrophysiological studies offer similar results. Gevins and colleagues[86–88] found a consistently lateralized, left frontal "preparatory set" by use of electroencephalogram measurement and analyses. Subjects were given verbal instructions and practice on a visuomotor task. Between the presentation of a stimulus (a slanted line on a computer screen) and the response (pressing a switch with the left or right index finger), a focal activation of the left dorsolateral prefrontal cortex region was consistently present, regardless of the response hand. More recently, Ruchkin et al.[89] used event-related potential methodology and reported a left frontal activation in a working memory task, both for verbal and for visuospatial representations. By contrast, tasks requiring orientation to unexpected external events and attention to external stimuli (without a preestablished "preparatory set") produce greater activation of the right than left prefrontal areas. These effects have been reported with PET,[90] rCBF measures,[91,92] and event-related potentials.[93]

Roland[92] found that during selective attention to a sensation (auditory, visual, or somatosensory), right prefrontal rCBF was significantly higher than left prefrontal rCBF. Pardo et al.[90] found a consistent right prefrontal activation on PET, regardless of the laterality of stimulus presentation, in subjects asked to sustain their attention to a particular sensory stimulus (visual or somatosensory). Nishizawa et al.[91] found a trend for increased right prefrontal rCBF activation

when the subject was told to "just listen" to spoken words.

The above studies are particularly interesting in that the selective activation of the left or right prefrontal region depends solely on the nature of the task (following internalized instructions vs. attending to external stimuli) and not on the side of stimulus delivery or stimulus modality. The type of material (verbal or nonverbal) does not seem to matter either, nor does the response hand.

Several tasks particularly sensitive to frontal lobe functions are commonly used to assess the integrity of the frontal lobes. Some of these tasks are dependent on the changing content of working memory (e.g., Wisconsin Card Sorting Test [WCST] and The Tower of London [TL]), whereas others require selective attention to external stimuli (Continuous Performance Task [CPT]). Distinct, complementary lateralized activation patterns have been elicited by these tasks in healthy volunteers on PET and SPECT: WCST and TL activated the left frontal systems, and CPT activated the right frontal systems.[94–96] However, the findings are not entirely consistent, because other studies have found selective activation of the right prefrontal region during the WCST.[97] It is quite possible that these discrepancies can be accounted for by methodological differences.

Furthermore, the degree of focality of activation was different in the two hemispheres. Roland and colleagues[80–85] found a more focal activation in the left hemisphere (probably the superior portion of Brodmann's area 10 and/or inferior portion of area 9). Pardo et al.[90] and Mazziotta et al.[98] found a more diffuse activation in the right prefrontal region. Pardo et al. described it as "a variable coronal band of activity along the right dorsolateral convexity, corresponding to Brodmann's areas 8, 9, 44, 46 (with concentration in area 9)"(p. 63).

Consistent with these findings was the work of Mazziotta et al.,[98] who found that the right prefrontal region was more sensitive than the left prefrontal region to the effects of sensory deprivation. As the degree of sensory deprivation increased (from the eyes open/ears open, to the eyes closed/ears open, to the eyes closed/ears closed condition), the decrease in activation was more pronounced in the right than in the left frontal regions.

Odor recognition memory may be lateralized within the prefrontal region as well. Recall for odors presented birhinally (half having a verbal label) was selectively impaired following right, but not left, orbitofrontal or temporal lesions.[99]

Neuropsychological and Functional Neuroimaging Findings Following Focal Prefrontal Lesions

Normally the two types of cognitive control, one guiding behavior by internal cues and the other guiding behavior by external cues, operate in concert and are in dynamic balance. Damage to the frontal lobes may disrupt this balance, and this disruption may result in two extreme types of behavior.

The first type is *perseveration*,[100] an inability to extinguish the representations evoked in the context of a prior cognitive task. Perseveration can be thought of as a diminished ability to switch behaviors in response to changing demands.

The second type is *environmental dependency*,[100–102] in which the subject's behavior becomes dependent on incidental, external factors. Environmental dependency can be thought of as a diminished capacity for internally generated planning to guide behavior.

There appears to be a relation between the side of lateralized frontal lesions and the type of extreme behavior caused by them. This relation was apparent in two studies of the effects of lateralized frontal lesions on WCST performance. Drewe[103] found that although both the left and the right prefrontal lesion groups performed worse than healthy volunteers on the number of categories sorted, the right prefrontal lesion group made more perseverative errors, and the left prefrontal lesion group made more nonperseverative errors. Robinson et al.[104] found that even when the left and right frontal lesion groups had equivalent scores on the Halstead-Reitan Average Impairment Rating, the right frontal lesion group made more perseverative responses on the WCST. By contrast, the patients with left prefrontal lesions were unable to maintain the correct pattern of response and kept switching between the different possible categories. These findings are tempered, however, by the failure to find lateralized effects of frontal lobe lesions on WCST performance in other studies.[105,106]

Milner and Petrides[107–109] also reported findings not easily understood in terms of the verbal/nonverbal distinction. On the basis of their work with recency memory tests and subject-ordering tasks in patients with lateralized frontal lesions, they concluded that the left prefrontal cortex was important for "programming" internally ordered events and that the right prefrontal cortex was important for "programming" externally ordered events, regardless of whether the stimulus was verbal or nonverbal.

McCarthy and Warrington[110] reached a similar conclusion. They proposed that "failure on those tasks which require internal generation of strategies and/or control of motor-executive functions shows a greater tendency to be associated with damage to the left frontal lobe rather than the right" (p. 356). McCarthy and Warrington also concluded that very few tasks are both sensitive and specific to unilateral right frontal lobe lesions.

Context-Dependent and Context-Independent Response Selection Bias and the Effects of Lateralized Prefrontal Lesions

The expression of the novelty-routinization theory within the prefrontal system has been well articulated by Goldberg and colleagues.[111,112] It is hypothesized that the left prefrontal system is critical to the organism's ability to guide behavior by a current cognitive context. In contrast, the right prefrontal system is critical to the organism's ability to alter the cognitive context in response to ongoing events by defaulting on context-invariant responses to the environmental stimuli present at the time. The left prefrontal system emphasizes a context-dependent response selection bias, and the right prefrontal system emphasizes a context-independent response selection bias.

To test this hypothesis, Goldberg et al.[111] developed the Cognitive Bias Task. The Cognitive Bias Task is an inherently ambiguous, multiple-choice task in which a subject is presented with cards that have geometric designs on them. Each design is characterized along five binary dimensions. Thus, a comparison in dimensional similarity can be made between any two cards. The subject is first presented with a target card, followed by the simultaneous presentation of two choice cards vertically aligned below the target card. The instructions ask the subject to look at the target card and then choose one of the two choice cards that he or she likes the best. The two choice cards are characterized by different degrees of dimensional similarity to the target card. Thus, the subject must select a choice card that is more similar to, or more different from, the target card.

The subject's choice pattern across 60 trials is quantified. The Cognitive Bias Task has two patterns of response. The subject can respond in a highly context-dependent pattern (e.g., the subject consistently chooses either the most similar choice card or the most different choice card) or a context-invariant pattern (e.g., the subject's choice is not based on a consistent comparison to the target [i.e., disregard for context] but rather some subjective dimensional, sensory preference).

Results on the Cognitive Bias Task indicated two different, and opposite, response selection patterns following left and right prefrontal lesions in right-handed males. Left prefrontal lesions produced an extremely context-independent response selection bias, and right prefrontal lesions produced an extremely context-dependent response selection bias. Healthy male subjects performed in the middle of the response range. Lateralized posterior lesions showed the same general trend as their ipsilateral frontal lesions but not as robust.

Surprisingly, the pattern of performance in right-handed females was different from that found in males. In females, both left and right prefrontal lesions in females produced context-dependent response patterns. Conversely, the lateralized posterior lesions in right-handed females each produced context-independent patterns of responding on the Cognitive Bias Task. Thus, it appears that the axis of cortical functional differences in Cognitive Bias Task performance is sex-dependent—left versus right in males and anterior versus posterior in females.

Although the idea of a sex-specific nature of functional cortical differentiation is not universally accepted, ample evidence supports it, especially in regard to the prefrontal systems. Kimura[113] was one of the first to present evidence that the axis of differentiation differs between males and females in the direction consistent with the findings of Goldberg et al.[111] Language function in males is strongly lateralized to the left hemisphere but bilaterally represented in females following cerebrovascular accidents[113–115] and during functional magnetic resonance imaging in healthy subjects.[116] These findings are highly consistent with the sex differences on the Cognitive Bias Task.

Furthermore, a strong relation was found between the functional lateralization of the frontal lobes and handedness on the Cognitive Bias Task.[111] We found a complete reversal of performance patterns based on familial and individual handedness. Healthy control and frontal-lesioned subjects classified as non-right-handed (either individual left-handedness or first-degree familial left-handedness) produced completely opposite Cognitive Bias Task score patterns when compared with their right-handed counterparts. This may be the first demonstration of a strong relation between handedness and hemispheric specialization. That this relation involves the frontal lobes is particularly remarkable, given that the functional lateralization of the frontal lobes has been downplayed in the past.

The results of the study by Goldberg et al.[111] indicated that the Cognitive Bias Task is sensitive and specific to prefrontal dysfunction (as mentioned above, posterior lesion effects in males were of considerably less magnitude). Furthermore, the effects of lateralized prefrontal lesions on performance were directly dependent on the inherent ambiguity of the Cognitive Bias Task. In a control task in which the same stimuli were used, the lesioned subjects were given explicit instructions to choose either the most similar or the most different choice card. On such a disambiguated control task, any differences between the prefrontal-lesioned and healthy subjects were eliminated. The combination of the Cognitive Bias Task and the disambiguated control task lends itself as a natural subtraction paradigm for functional neuroimaging techniques.[106,112,117]

The inherent ambiguity of the Cognitive Bias Task makes it a novel approach that assesses actor-centered, adaptive decision making that is based on an individual's priorities. This is in comparison to veridical, actor-independent decision making that requires a correct response intrinsic to the external situation. Most purported tests of frontal lobe functioning (such as the WCST) depend on veridical decision making. The fact that the Cognitive Bias Task measures adaptive decision making may account for its robust lateralization and sex findings. Thus, innovative, actor-centered decision-making tasks, such as the Cognitive Bias Task, are required to better elucidate the functions of the frontal lobes and are probably more ecologically valid tests of frontal lobe functioning.[118,119]

GONADAL HORMONAL INFLUENCES ON SEX-SPECIFIC NEUROANATOMICAL DEVELOPMENT

Organizational Effects

What could account for the sex differences in performance on the Cognitive Bias Task and other cognitive tasks? One obvious area to explore would be the role of hormones, specifically testosterone. The "central hypothesis"[120] states that the gonadal hormones (primarily testosterone) produce sexual differentiation of the brain. A large body of animal (rat and nonhuman primate) and human research clearly indicates that sex-specific lateralization of the brain, especially prefrontal regions, is highly dependent on the pre- and perinatal organizational effects of the gonadal hormones. Whether the "initial" sex of the human brain is female[121–123] or androgenous[124] is not clear. However, it is clear that the masculinization of the brain is directly dependent on the presence of testosterone during development.[125] (In the brain, testosterone is aromatized into estradiol, an estrogenic compound. Estradiol exerts its effect on brain organization, at least in rats. In nonhuman primates, evidence indicates that testosterone is aromatized into estradiol but can also have a direct androgenic effect.) This suggests real neuroanatomical differences that are sex specific.

Several lines of evidence indicate testosterone's crucial role in shaping neuroanatomy, specifically the cerebral cortex. Estrogen receptors rapidly proliferate in embryonic development, which peaks within 3–10 weeks postnatally in mice,[126,127] rats,[128] and nonhuman primates.[129] Also, aromatase complex, which converts testosterone into estradiol in the brain, is prevalent in the frontal cortex of rats and human fetuses.[130]

Sex Differences in the Effects of Gonadal Hormones on Cortical Development

The development of the cerebral cortex in males and females is differentially affected by testosterone. Even though male and female rats have the greatest concentration of estrogen receptors soon after birth, males consistently have a high concentration in the left hemisphere. Females, however, have a varying ratio of estrogen concentration in the right and left hemispheres, with no clear pattern emerging.[128]

Estrogen (and estradiol) is believed to inhibit cortical growth. Male rats have a significantly thinner left than right cortical hemisphere, whereas female rats have equally thick cortical hemispheres. These differences are present at birth and until a very old age, when testosterone production decreases greatly. The effect was directly related to the amount of testosterone and estradiol receptors in the brain.[131–135]

Testosterone may not be the only hormone involved in the development of the cerebral cortex. Progesterone (considered to be "antiestrogenic" and a neuronal cell growth enhancer), when injected into ovariectomized female rats, produced a thickening of the cortex.[135] Also, adult female rats had a significantly higher concentration of progesterone receptors in the frontal cortex compared with males. The males, in fact, had their lowest concentration of cortical progesterone receptors in the frontal region. When gonadectomized females were masculinized (treated with testosterone propionate) immediately after birth, their

distribution of frontal progesterone receptors was equivalent to that of normal males.[136]

Effect of Gonadal Hormones on the Frontal Lobes

Evidence indicates that male rhesus monkeys have a complementary and lateralized relation between estradiol and androgen receptors in the frontal cortex, and female monkeys have no asymmetric pattern. The male monkeys have a greater number of androgen receptors in the right prefrontal region and a greater number of estradiol receptors in the left prefrontal region.[137] Estradiol inhibits growth, and androgen (testosterone is a form of androgen) enhances neuritic growth.

Also, the rate of development of the frontal cortex appears to be sex specific. In male rats, the frontal cortex develops particularly rapidly, but in female rats, the posterior cortex develops more rapidly,[138] and this effect is directly mediated by manipulation of testosterone.[131] Also, in nonhuman primates, the frontal lobes become functional sooner in males than in females (by 15–18 months on an object reversal task), and this can be altered by changing testosterone levels.[139–141]

Finally, some evidence indicated a sex difference in the development of the human fetal prefrontal cortex. In studying 21 fetal brains (from the Yakovlev series), de Lacoste, Horvath, and Woodward[142] performed volumetric analysis of several different cortical regions. The results indicated that males were more likely to have larger right than left prefrontal regions (frontal pole to genu of corpus callosum), whereas females tended to have more symmetrical prefrontal regions or slightly larger left than right prefrontal regions. The authors suggested that their findings were due, at least in part, to the effect of testosterone on fetal brain development.

NEUROPSYCHIATRIC DISORDERS AND LATERALIZED PREFRONTAL DYSFUNCTION

The role of prefrontal systems in neuropsychiatric disorders has taken center stage with the advent of modern neuroimaging techniques. For the first time, neuropsychiatric states producing positive symptomatology without any known brain lesion (e.g., obsessive-compulsive disorder and depression) have been shown to have direct prefrontal involvement. This has led to insight into the mechanisms of the disorders and has helped to define neuropsychiatry and its view of such disorders. In the following section, we briefly review some of the research indicating lateralized prefrontal activation/dysfunction in various neuropsychiatric states. However, because of the scope of this chapter, we do not discuss those disorders known to have a large bilateral prefrontal involvement (e.g., see Chapter 13), emphasizing only lateralized differences in the prefrontal system.

Depression

The involvement of prefrontal systems in depression has been extensively studied. Although there is no complete agreement with regard to laterality, most studies that use functional neuroimaging and electrophysiology point to a left inferior frontal dysfunction.

Studies examining secondary depression (depression following a primary neurological disorder such as stroke or neurodegenerative diseases) have indicated significant prefrontal dysfunction, but the presence of laterality may be dependent on etiology. The initial studies of secondary depression were performed in stroke patients. The results indicated that depression was most common following a left hemisphere lesion and was highly correlated with its proximity to the frontal pole.[143-148] However, not all studies were in agreement.[149] It appears that the left fronto-opercular region may be a "hot spot" for causing secondary depression in stroke patients.[145] Similar findings were reported for strokes following the head of the left caudate and anterior limb of the internal capsule,[145,150] areas with extensive prefrontal connections. Although depression following right hemisphere lesions does occur, it appears to be related to a positive history of familial depression, which is not the case in patients with left hemisphere cerebrovascular accidents.[151]

The findings of depression in neurodegenerative disorders such as Parkinson's and Huntington's disease are somewhat different. They indicate hypometabolism in limbic and orbitofrontal regions bilaterally (see Mayberg, Chapter 12, in this volume).

Findings in patients with primary depression also have implicated left prefrontal dysfunction based on PET[152-156] and electroencephalography.[157-160] However, some studies reported increased flow or no asymmetry.[160,161] These inconsistencies have been attributed to methodological differences between studies or regional differentiation in prefrontal recording sights.[161,162]

A related body of research has attempted to determine whether the left hypofrontality is secondary to the depressed state or may actually serve as a biological marker for predisposition to depression. Henriques and Davidson[163] reported a left hypofrontality by using electroencephalography in a group of formerly depressed euthymic subjects when compared with healthy control subjects without a history of affective disorders. They also found a right posterior hypoactivation, which may provide evidence for the right hemisphere dysfunction in depression.[164]

The left frontal hypoactivation has been found in individuals at risk for depression but who have never had a depressive episode. Children (adolescents and infants) of depressed mothers (considered at high risk for depression), when compared with healthy control subjects without a family history of depression (low risk), showed a left frontal hypoactivation during a resting electroencephalogram[165-167] and interactions with others.[168]

When asked to imagine a very sad situation, avoiding any feelings of anger or anxiety, psychiatrically healthy males showed a left orbitofrontal hypoactivation, whereas healthy females showed a bilateral orbitofrontal hypoactivation on rCBF.[169] Although few subjects were involved, the findings were consistent with those reported by Goldberg et al.[111] on the Cognitive Bias Task. The pattern of frontal lobe involvement in depression parallels the lesion effects: lateralized in males and bilateral in females. This finding also emphasizes the importance of gender in neuroimaging studies of neuropsychiatric diseases.

Although the above findings indicate left prefrontal dysfunction during depression, a body of evidence also implicates the right hemisphere in general, and the right prefrontal region in particular,[170] including alpha suppression (electroencephalogram activation) over the right frontal lobe when healthy subjects were in an induced depressed mood and visuospatial deficits.[171,172]

These findings may appear discrepant, but evidence suggests a consistent pattern of results. The literature indicates that positive affect and approach behaviors are associated with a relative increase in left prefrontal activation, whereas relative increases in right hemisphere activation are associated with negative affect or withdrawal behaviors.[173] This has been demonstrated ectrophysiologically[173] and during functional magnetic resonance imaging activation.[174] Evidence even suggests that lateralized prefrontal electroencephalogram activation in depressed subjects can be altered with music.[175] Depressed subjects show an attenuation of right frontal electroencephalographic activity and a concomitant decrease in cortisol levels during and immediately after listening to music.

Repetitive transcranial magnetic stimulation (rTMS) is one of the newest and most exciting areas of research and clinical treatment that addresses lateralized prefrontal functioning and treatment of neuropsychiatric disorders. A detailed review of rTMS is beyond the scope of this chapter,[176] but the evidence suggests that unilateral rTMS may be an efficacious and a safe form of treatment (with few side-effects) for several neuropsychiatric disorders, including depression, anxiety, and mania.

It is believed, although not definitively confirmed, that different forms of rTMS—fast versus slow frequency—may have opposite effects on neuronal functioning. Fast-frequency rTMS may produce neuronal excitation, whereas slow-frequency rTMS may produce neuronal inhibition. Therefore, unilateral left and right rTMS can produce the same relative change in the proportionate balance of right and left prefrontal activation depending on the type—fast or slow. Although not completely consistent and reproducible, mounting evidence suggests that unilateral left prefrontal fast-frequency rTMS[177,178] and unilateral right prefrontal slow-frequency rTMS[179–181] improve refractory depression. However, some findings by others are contradictory.[176] Complementary findings[182,183] have shown that right, rather than left, prefrontal fast-frequency rTMS was better in reducing manic symptoms in treating acute mania. Similarly, right prefrontal fast-frequency rTMS may increase anxiety and worsen mood in healthy control subjects.[176]

The rTMS findings to date, in combination with the evidence cited above, would be consistent with Davidson's[173] notion that relative right prefrontal activation is associated with negative affect or withdrawal, whereas relative left prefrontal activation is associated with positive affect or approach. It appears that any alteration in the balance of right and left prefrontal activation can produce different neuropsychiatric illness, depending on the direction of the imbalance, and that a relative balance between left and right frontal activation may be required for healthy emotional functioning.

Tucker et al.[170] presented evidence that explains most, but not all, of the findings of differential lateralization of the frontal lobes in neuropsychiatric disorders, especially depression. They suggested that the left prefrontal region is important in inhibiting the

negative affective state of the ipsilateral limbic region. Conversely, the right prefrontal region has inhibitory control over the positive emotional tone of the right limbic system. This would account for depression following left prefrontal lesions and hypoactivation in primary depression. It would also explain the increase in left orbitofrontal activity reported in obsessive-compulsive disorder and mania following right prefrontal lesions. The increase in left orbitofrontal activation in obsessive-compulsive disorder may actually reflect increased activity of the left anterior cingulate and caudate regions, which have extensive connections to the orbitofrontal region and have been implicated in obsessive-compulsive disorder (see following section, "Obsessive-Compulsive Disorder"). Conversely, the lack of inhibitory control following a right prefrontal lesion would allow the positive emotional tone of the right limbic system to go unchecked, causing a maniclike state.

Obsessive-Compulsive Disorder

The relation between obsessive-compulsive disorder and lateralized prefrontal systems is uncertain. It is clear that the orbitofrontal region, caudate nucleus, and anterior cingulate gyrus are involved,[184,185] but the question of a bilateral orbitofrontal hyperactivation,[186] greater left orbitofrontal activation,[184,187–191] or some variant thereof is still very controversial. Experts talk about methodological and imaging differences and defining neuroanatomical regions of interest as possible explanations for some of the discrepancies in the findings.[185]

The neuroimaging data on obsessive-compulsive disorder also point to sex differences.[185,192] Baxter et al.[185] reported opposite patterns of lateralization in male (left) and female (right) obsessive-compulsive disorder patients. As with the neuroimaging literature on depression, the obsessive-compulsive disorder literature indicates that gender is an important variable to study when assessing prefrontal systems, but it has rarely been incorporated as an independent variable.

Other Neuropsychiatric Disorders

Gilles de la Tourette's syndrome has been associated with an increased activation (SPECT) in the right orbitofrontal region.[193] If obsessive-compulsive disorder is truly characterized by an increase in left orbitofrontal activation, then it may serve as the complementary finding to the increased activation patterns reported in Gilles de la Tourette's syndrome. Whereas obsessive-compulsive disorder is usually characterized by perseveration-like, stereotypic behaviors, Gilles de la Tourette's syndrome is characterized by heterogeneous clinical presentations, some of which are dominated by excessive and forced exploratory behaviors.[194]

Some evidence indicates that mania or maniclike behavior is associated with impaired prefrontal functions, possibly greater in the right hemisphere. Some studies reported bilateral inferior frontal hypoactivation during rCBF in manic patients,[195] whereas others reported an association between manic symptoms and lesions in the right prefrontal region.[196] However, it appears that mania following acute central nervous system injury occurs with injury to the paleocortical pathway, usually with lesions to the basolateropolar temporal and orbitofrontal cortices.

Finally, content-specific delusions (monosymptomatic) occur in adult patients sustaining acute central nervous system dysfunction (typically vascular or head trauma) usually to the right hemisphere, particularly the right prefrontal region (see Malloy and Richardson, Chapter 15, in this volume).

Thus, lateralized prefrontal dysfunction is highly prevalent and differentially associated with several neuropsychiatric disorders. It becomes very important to understand the role of the left and right prefrontal systems to better understand neuropsychiatric disorders, which may lead to more precise diagnosis and treatment of these disabling conditions. With the neuroimaging of the frontal lobes gaining prominence in neuropsychiatric research, a test sensitive to lateralized prefrontal dysfunction would be of great value. As we have shown previously, the Cognitive Bias Task is particularly well suited to help elucidate some of the unanswered questions.[106,117] In the past, the WCST was used as a cognitive challenge test in neuropsychiatric disorders (see Chapter 13). Although the WCST is effective in eliciting bilateral prefrontal hypoactivation, only one neuroimaging study exists to date indicating lateralized activation and only in healthy control subjects.[97]

Podell et al.[106] directly compared performance on the Cognitive Bias Task and the WCST in right-handed male subjects with lateralized prefrontal lesions. The Cognitive Bias Task showed robust differences between the left and right prefrontal lesion groups, but no appreciable difference was shown on the WCST. Furthermore, the Cognitive Bias Task has been designed with appropriate subtraction tasks, which make it particularly well suited for functional neuroimaging in neuropsychiatric disorders.

CONCLUSIONS

It is becoming increasingly obvious that the frontal lobes are characterized by robust hemispheric specialization. This specialization is not adequately described by the classic distinction between linguistic and nonlinguistic processes. The right hemisphere appears to be critical for dealing with novel cognitive situations and the left hemisphere for the processes mediated by well-routinized representations and strategies. The left frontal systems appear to be crucial for cognitive selection driven by the content of working memory and for context-dependent behavior; the right frontal systems appear to be crucial for cognitive selection driven by the external environment and for context-independent behavior. The role of the right hemisphere in processing cognitive novelty highlights the importance of the right frontal systems in task orientation and the assembly of novel cognitive strategies. A sex difference in the functional lateralization of the frontal cortex exists, which may be mediated by the organizational effects of gonadal hormones.

REFERENCES

1. Goldberg E, Vaughan HG, Gerstman LJ: Nonverbal descriptive systems and hemispheric asymmetry: shape versus texture discrimination. Brain Lang 5:249–257, 1978
2. Goldberg E, Costa LD: Hemispheric differences in the acquisition and use of descriptive systems. Brain Lang 14:144–173, 1981
3. Cutting JA: A parallel between encodeness and the magnitude of the right ear effect. Haskins Laboratories Status Report on Speech Research SR-29/30:61–68, 1972
4. Ellis HD, Shepherd JW: Recognition of abstract and concrete words in left and right visual fields. J Exp Psychol 103(5):1035–1036, 1974
5. Gazzaniga MS: The Bisected Brain. New York, Appleton-Century-Crofts, 1970
6. Gibson AR, Dimond SJ, Gazzaniga MS: Left field superiority forward matching. Neuropsychologia 10:463–466, 1972
7. Hines D: Recognition of verbs, abstract nouns and concrete nouns from the left and right visual half-fields. Neuropsychologia 14:211–216, 1976
8. Shankweiler D, Stutart-Kennedy M: Identification of consonants and vowels presented to the left and right ears. Q J Exp Psychol 19:59–63, 1967
9. Uhl F, Podreka I, Deecke L: Anterior frontal cortex and the effect of proactive interference in word pair learning—results of brain-SPECT. Neuropsychologia 32:241–247, 1994

10. Nichelli P, Grafman J, Pietrini P, et al: Where the brain appreciates the moral of a story. Neuroreport 6:2309–2313, 1995

11. Dennis M, Lovett M, Wiegel-Crump CA: Written language acquisition after left or right hemidecortication in infancy. Brain Lang 12:54–91, 1981

12. Dennis M, Whitaker HA: Language acquisition following hemidecortication: linguistic superiority of the left over the right hemisphere. Brain Lang 3:404–433, 1976

13. Dennis M: Language acquisition in a single hemisphere: semantic organization, in Biological Studies of Mental Processes. Edited by Caplan D. Cambridge, MA, MIT Press, 1979

14. Dennis M: Capacity and strategy for syntactic comprehension after left or right hemidecortication. Brain Lang 10:287–317, 1980

15. Zaidel E: Lexical organization in the right hemisphere, in Cerebral Correlates of Conscious Experience. Edited by Buser P, Rougeul-Buser A. Amsterdam, The Netherlands, Elsevier, 1977, pp 177–198

16. Goldberg E: Associative agnosias and the functions of the left hemisphere. J Clin Exp Neuropsychol 12:467–484, 1990

17. Teuber H-L: Alteration of perception and memory in man, in Analysis of Behavioral Change. Edited by Weiskrantz L. New York, Harper & Row, 1968, pp 268–375

18. Albert ML, Reches A, Silverberg R: Associative visual agnosia without alexia. Neurology 25:322–326, 1975

19. De Renzi E, Spinnler H: Visual recognition in patients with unilateral cerebral disease. J Nerv Ment Dis 142:513–525, 1966

20. Hecaen H, Albert MJ: Human Neuropsychology. New York, Wiley, 1978

21. Hecaen H, Angelerques R: La cécité psychique. Paris, France, Masson, 1963

22. Hecaen H, Goldblum MC, Masure MC, et al: Une nouvelle observation d'agnocie d'object: déficit de l'association, ou de la catégorisation specifique de la modalité visuelle? Neuropsychologia 12:447–464, 1974

23. Luria AR: Higher Cortical Functions in Man, 2nd Edition. New York, Basic Books, 1980

24. McCarthy RA, Warrington EK: Visual associative agnosia: a clinico-anatomical study. J Neurol Neurosurg Psychiatry 49:1233–1240, 1986

25. Rubens AB, Benson DF: Associative visual agnosia. Arch Neurol 24:305–316, 1971

26. Warrington EK: The selective impairment of semantic memory. Q J Exp Psychol 27:635–657, 1975

27. Foix C: Sur une variété de troubles bilateraux de la sensibilité par lésion unilaterale du cerveau. Rev Neurol (Paris) 29:322–331, 1922

28. Goldstein K: Über kortikale sensibilitätsstärungen. Neurologisches Zentralblatt 19:825–827, 1916

29. Lhermitte J, de Ajuriaguerra J: Asymbolie tactile et hallucinations du toucher: étude anatomoclinique. Revue Neurologique 59:492–495, 1938

30. Faglioni P, Spinnler H, Vignolo LA: Contrasting behavior of right and left hemisphere–damaged patients on a discriminative and a semantic task of auditor recognition. Cortex 5:366–389, 1969

31. Kleist K: Gehirnpathologische und lokalisatorische ergebnisse über horstorungen, gerausch-taubheiten und amusien. Monatschrift für Psychiatrie und Neurologie 68:853–860, 1928

32. Spinnler H, Vignolo LA: Impaired recognition of meaningful sounds in aphasia. Cortex 2:337–348, 1966

33. Vignolo LA: Auditory agnosia. Philos Trans R Soc Lond B Biol Sci 298:49–57, 1982

34. Humphreys GW, Riddoch MJ: To See But Not to see: A Case Study of Visual Agnosia. London, UK, Lawrence Erlbaum, 1987

35. Kertesz A: The clinical spectrum and localisation of visual agnosia, in Visual Object Processing: A Cognitive Neuropsychological Approach. Edited by Humphreys GW, Riddoch MJ. London, Lawrence Erlbaum, 1987, pp 175–196

36. Glick SD, Meibach RC, Cox RD, et al: Multiple and interrelated functional asymmetries in rat brain. Life Sci 25:395–400, 1979

37. Glick SD, Ross DA, Hough LB: Lateral asymmetry of neurotransmitter in human brain. Brain Res 234:53–63, 1982

38. Oke A, Keller R, Mefford I, et al: Lateralization of norepinephrine in human thalamus. Science 200:1411–1413, 1978

39. Oke A, Lewis R, Adams RN: Hemispheric asymmetry of norepinephrine distribution in rat thalamus. Brain Res 188:269–272, 1980

40. Robinson RG: Differential and biochemical effects of the right and left hemispheric cerebral infarction in the rat. Science 205:707–710, 1979

41. Wagner HN, Burns DH, Dannals RF, et al: Imaging dopamine receptors in human brain by positron emission tomography. Science 221:1264–1266, 1983

42. Aston-Jones G, Bloom FE: Norepinephrine-containing locus coeruleus neurons in behaving rats exhibiting pronounced responses to non-noxious environmental stimuli. J Neurosci 1:887–900, 1981

43. Iversen SD: Brain dopamine systems and behavior, in Handbook of Psychopharmacology, Vol 8: Drugs, Neurotransmitters and Behavior. Edited by Iversen LL, Iversen SD, Snyder SH. New York, Plenum, 1977, pp 333–384

44. Lyons M, Robbins TW: The action of central nervous system drugs: a general theory concerning amphetamine effects, in Current Developments in Psychopharmacology, Vol 2. Edited by Essman W, Valzelli L. New York, Spectrum, 1975, pp 81–163

45. Tucker DM, Williamson PA: Asymmetric neural control systems in human self-regulation. Psychol Rev 91:185–215, 1984

46. Mason ST, Fibiger HC: NE and selective attention: Life Sci 25:1949–1956, 1979

47. Oades RD: The role of noradrenaline in tuning and dopamine in switching between signals in the CNS. Neurosci Biobehav Rev 9:261–282, 1985

48. Bever TG, Chiarello K: Cerebral dominance in musicians and non-musicians. Science 185:537–539, 1974

49. Johnson PR: Dichotically stimulated ear differences in musicians and non-musicians. Cortex 13:385–389, 1977

50. Marzi CA, Berlucchi G: Right visual field superiority of accuracy of recognition of famous faces in normals. Neuropsychologia 15:751–756, 1977

51. Papcun G, Krashen S, Terbeek D, et al: Is the left hemisphere specialized for speech, language and/or something else? J Acoust Soc Am 55:319–327, 1974

52. Barroso F: Hemispheric asymmetry of function in children, in The Neuropsychology of Language. Edited by Rieber RW. New York, Plenum, 1976, pp 157–180

53. Carmon A, Nachson I, Starinsky R: Developmental aspects of visual hemifield differences in perception of verbal material. Brain Lang 3:463–469, 1976

54. Miller LK, Turner S: Development of hemifield differences in word recognition. Journal of Educational Psychology 65:172–176, 1973

55. Miller LK, Turner S: Some boundary conditions for laterality effects in children. Dev Psychol 11:342–352, 1975

56. Porter RJ, Berlin CJ: On interpreting developmental changes in the dichotic right-ear advantage. Brain Lang 2:186–200, 1975

57. Gordon HW, Carmon A: Transfer of dominance in speed of verbal recognition to visually presented stimuli from right to left hemisphere. Percept Mot Skills 42:1091–1100, 1976

58. Kittler P, Turkewitz G, Goldberg E: Shifts in hemispheric advantage during familiarization with complex visual patterns. Cortex 25:27–32, 1989

59. Reynolds DM, Jevves MA: A developmental study of hemisphere specialization for recognition of faces in normal subjects. Cortex 14:511–520, 1978

60. Ross-Kossak P, Turkewitz G: Relationship between changes in hemispheric advantage during familiarization to faces and proficiency in facial recognition. Neuropsychologia 22:471–477, 1984

61. Voyer D, Bryden MP: Gender, level of spatial ability, and lateralization of mental rotation. Brain Cogn 13:18–29, 1990

62. Holtman AM: Manual reaction time to lateralized words, letters, faces, and symbols: structural and dynamic determination of hemispheric dominance. Unpublished doctoral dissertation, City University of New York, New York, 1978

63. Hellige JB: Changes in same-different laterality patterns as a function of practice and stimulus quality. Perception and Psychophysiology 20:273–276, 1976

64. Miller LK, Butler D: The effect of set size on hemifield asymmetries in letter recognition. Brain Lang 9:307–314, 1980

65. Basser LS: Hemiplegia of early onset and the faculty of speech with special reference to the effects of hemispherectomy. Brain 85:428–460, 1962

66. McFie J: The effects of hemispherectomy on intellectual functioning in cases of infantile hemiplegia. J Neurol Neurosurg Psychiatry 24:240–249, 1961

67. Grossberg S: Competitive learning: from interactive activation to adaptive resonance. Cognitive Science 11:23–63, 1987

68. Damasio AR: Prosopagnosia. Trends Neurosci 8:132–135, 1985

69. Galaburda AM, LeMay M, Kemper TL, et al: Right-left asymmetries in the brain. Science 199:852–856, 1978

70. LeMay M: Morphological cerebral asymmetries of modern man, fossil man, and nonhuman primate. Ann N Y Acad Sci 280:349–366, 1976

71. Hecaen H, Ruel J: Sièges lésionnels intrafrontaux et déficit au test de "fluence verbale." Rev Neurol (Paris) 137:277–284, 1981

72. Milner B: Some effects of frontal lobectomy in man, in The Frontal Granular Cortex and Behavior. Edited by Warren JM, Akert K. New York, McGraw-Hill, 1964, pp 313–334

73. Perret E: The left frontal lobe of man and the suppression of habitual responses in verbal categorical behavior. Neuropsychologia 12:323–330, 1974

74. Glosser G, Goodglass H: Disorders of executive control functions among aphasic and other brain-damaged patients. J Clin Exp Neuropsychol 12:485–501, 1990

75. Jones-Gottman M, Milner B: Design fluency: the invention of nonsense drawings after focal cortical lesions. Neuropsychologia 15:653–674, 1977

76. Fuster JM: The Prefrontal Cortex: Anatomy, Physiology, and Neuropsychology of the Frontal Lobe, 2nd Edition. New York, Raven, 1990

77. Goldman-Rakic PS: Circuitry of primate prefrontal cortex and representation of behavior by representational memory, in Handbook of Physiology—The Nervous System, Vol V. Edited by Plum F. Bethesda, MD, American Physiological Society, 1987, pp 373–417

78. Milner B: Effects of different brain lesions on card sorting. Arch Neurol 9:90–100, 1963

79. Larsen B, Skinhoj E, Lassen NA: Variations in regional cortical blood flow in the right and left hemispheres during automatic speech. Brain 101:193–209, 1978

80. Roland PE: Metabolic measurements of the working frontal cortex in man. Trends Neurosci 7:430–435, 1984

81. Roland PE, Larsen B: Focal increase of cerebral blood flow during stereognostic testing in man. Arch Neurol 33:557–558, 1976

82. Roland PE, Meyer E, Shibasaki T, et al: Regional cerebral blood flow changes in cortex and basal ganglia during voluntary movements in normal human voluntary movements in normal human volunteers. J Neurophysiol 48:467–480, 1982

83. Roland PE, Skinhoj E: Extrastriate cortical areas activated during visual discrimination in man. Brain Res 222:166–171, 1981

84. Roland PE, Skinhoj E, Lassen NA: Focal activations of human cerebral cortex during auditory discrimination. J Neurophysiol 45:1139–1151, 1981

85. Roland PE, Skinhoj E, Lassen NA, et al: Differential cortical areas in man in organization of voluntary movements in extrapersonal space. J Neurophysiol 43:137–150, 1980

86. Gevins AS: Distributed neuroelectric patterns of human neocortex during simple cognitive tasks, in The Prefrontal Cortex: Its Structure, Function, and Pathology (Progress in Brain Research, Vol 85). Edited by Uylings HBM, Van Eden CG, De Bruin JPC, et al. Amsterdam, The Netherlands, Elsevier Science, 1990, pp 337–355

87. Gevins AS, Cutillo BA, Bressler SL, et al: Event-related covariances during a bimanual visuomotor task, II: preparation and feedback. Electroencephalogr Clin Neurophysiol 74:147–160, 1989

88. Gevins AS, Morgan NH, Bressler SL, et al: Human neuroelectric patterns predict performance accuracy. Science 235:580–585, 1987

89. Ruchkin DS, Johnson R, Grafman J, et al: Distinctions and similarities among working memory processes: an event-related potential study. Cognitive Brain Research 1:53–66, 1992

90. Pardo JV, Fox PT, Raichle ME: Localization of a human system for sustained attention by positron emission tomography. Nature 349:61–64, 1991

91. Nishizawa Y, Olsen TS, Larsen B, et al: Left-right cortical asymmetries of regional blood flow during listening to words. J Neurophysiol 48:458–466, 1982

92. Roland PE: Cortical regulation of selective attention in man: a regional cerebral blood flow study. Neurophysiology 48:1059–1078, 1982

93. Knight RT, In S, Riggio PS, et al (eds): Epilepsy and the Functional Anatomy of the Frontal Lobes. New York, Raven, 1995

94. Andreasen NC, Rezai K, Alliger R, et al: Hypofrontality in neuroleptic-naive patients and in patients with chronic schizophrenia: assessment with xenon 133 single-photon emission computed tomography and the Tower of London. Arch Gen Psychiatry 49:943–958, 1992

95. Buchsbaum MS, Nuechterlein KH, Haier RJ, et al: Glucose metabolic rate in normals and schizophrenics during the Continuous Performance Test assessed by positron emission tomography. Br J Psychiatry 156:216–227, 1990

96. Rezai K, Andreasen NC, Alliger R, et al: The neuropsychology of the prefrontal cortex. Arch Neurol 50:636–642, 1993

97. Marenco S, Coppola R, Daniel DG, et al: Regional cerebral blood flow during the Wisconsin Card Sorting Test in normal subjects studied by xenon-133 dynamic SPECT: comparison of absolute values, percent distribution values, and covariance analysis. Psychiatry Res 50:177–192, 1993

98. Mazziotta JC, Phelps ME, Halgren E: Local cerebral glucose metabolic response to audiovisual stimulation and deprivation: studies in human subjects with positron CT. Human Neurobiology 2:11–23, 1983

99. Jones-Gotman M, Zatorre RJ: Odor recognition memory in humans: role of right temporal and orbitofrontal regions. Brain Cogn 22:182–198, 1993

100. Goldberg E, Costa LD: Qualitative indices in neuropsychological assessment: an extension of Luria's approach to executive deficit following prefrontal lesions, in Neuropsychological Assessment of Neuropsychiatric Disorders. Edited by Grant I, Adams KM. New York, Oxford University Press, 1986, pp 48–64

101. Lhermitte F: "Utilization behavior" and its relation to lesions of the frontal lobes. Brain 106:237–255, 1983

102. Lhermitte F, Pillion B, Sraru M: Human autonomy and the frontal lobes, part I: imitation and utilization behavior: a neuropsychological study of 75 patients. Ann Neurol 19:326–334, 1985

103. Drewe EA: The effect of type and area of brain lesion on Wisconsin Card Sorting Test performance. Cortex 10:159–170, 1974

104. Robinson AL, Heaton RK, Lehman RAW, et al: The utility of the Wisconsin Card Sorting Test in detecting and localizing frontal lobe lesions. J Consult Clin Psychol 48:605–614, 1980

105. Anderson SW, Damasio H, Jones RD, et al: Wisconsin Card Sorting Test performance as a measure of frontal lobe damage. J Clin Exp Neuropsychol 13:909–922, 1991

106. Podell K, Lovell M, Zimmerman M, et al: The cognitive bias task and lateralized frontal lobe functions in males. J Neuropsychiatry Clin Neurosci 4:491–501, 1995

107. Milner B: Cognitive effects of frontal lesions in man, in The Neuropsychology of Cognitive Function. Edited by Broadbent DE, Weiskrantz L. London, The Royal Society, 1982, pp 211–226

108. Milner B, Petrides M: Behavioural effects of frontal lobe lesions in man. Trends Neurosci 7:403–407, 1984

109. Petrides M, Milner B: Deficits on subject-ordered tasks after frontal- and temporal-lobe lesions in man. Neuropsychologia 20:249–262, 1982

110. McCarthy RA, Warrington EK: Cognitive Neuropsychology. New York, Academic Press, 1990

111. Goldberg E, Podell K, Harner R, et al: Cognitive bias, functional cortical geometry, and the frontal lobes: laterality, sex, and handedness. J Cogn Neurosci 6:274–294, 1994

112. Goldberg E, Podell K: Hemispheric specialization, cognitive novelty, and the frontal lobes, in Epilepsy and the Functional Anatomy of the Frontal Lobe (Advances in Neurology Series, Vol 66). Edited by Jasper H, Riggio S, Goldman-Rakic PS. New York, Raven, 1995, pp 85–96

113. Kimura D: Sex differences in cerebral organization for speech and praxic functions. Canadian Journal of Psychology 37:19–35, 1983

114. Kimura D: Are men's and women's brains really different? Canadian Journal of Psychology 28:133–147, 1987

115. Kimura D, Harshman RA: Sex differences in brain organization for verbal and non-verbal functions, in Sex Differences in the Brain (Progress in Brain Research, Vol 61). Edited by DeVries GJ, DeBruin JPC, Uylings HBM, et al. New York, Elsevier, 1984, pp 423–441

116. Shaywitz BA, Shaywitz SE, Pugh KR, et al: Sex differences in the functional organization of the brain for language. Nature 373:607–609, 1995

117. Goldberg E, Podell K: Lateralization in the frontal lobes: searching the right (and left) way. Biol Psychiatry 38:569–571, 1995

118. Goldberg E, Podell K: Adaptive versus veridical decision making and the frontal lobes. Conscious Cogn 8:364–377, 1999

119. Goldberg E, Podell K: Adaptive decision making, ecological validity and the frontal lobes. J Clin Exp Neuropsychol 22:56–68, 2000

120. McEwen BS: Steroid hormones are multifunctional messengers to the brain. Trends in Endocrinology and Metabolism 2:62–67, 1991

121. Geschwind N, Galaburda AM: Cerebral Lateralization: Biological Mechanisms, Associations and Pathology. Cambridge, MA, MIT Press, 1987

122. Geschwind N, Galaburda AM: Cerebral lateralization: biological mechanisms, associations, and pathology, I: a hypothesis and a program of research. Arch Neurol 42:428–459, 1985

123. Toran-Allerand CD: Gonadal hormones and brain development: cellular aspects of sexual differentiation. American Zoology 18:553–565, 1978

124. Dohler KD, Hancke JL, Srivastava SS, et al: Participation of estrogens in female sexual differentiation of the brain: neuroanatomical, neuroendocrine and behavioral evidence, in Sex Differences in the Brain (Progress in Brain Research, Vol 61). Edited by DeVries GJ, DeBruin JPC, Uylings HBM, et al. New York, Elsevier, 1984, pp 99–117

125. Goy RW, McEwen BS: Sexual Differentiation of the Brain. Cambridge, MA, MIT Press, 1980

126. Gerlach JL, McEwen BS, Toran-Allerand CD, et al: Perinatal development of estrogen receptors in mouse brain assessed by radioautography, nuclear isolation and receptor assay. Brain Res 11:7–18, 1983

127. Friedman WJ, McEwen BS, Toran-Allerand CD, et al: Perinatal development of hypothalamic and cortical estrogen receptors in mouse brain: methodological aspects. Brain Res 11:19–27, 1983

128. Sandu S, Cook P, Diamond MC: Rat cortical estrogen receptors: male-female, right-left. Exp Neurol 92:186–196, 1986

129. Sholl SA, Kim KL: Estrogen receptors in the rhesus monkey brain during fetal development. Brain Res 50:189–196, 1989

130. Ryan KJ, Naftolin F, Reddy V, et al: Estrogen formation in the brain. Am J Obstet Gynecol 114:454–460, 1972

131. Diamond MC: Rat forebrain morphology: right-left; male-female; young-old; enriched-impoverished, in Cerebral Laterality in Nonhuman Species. Edited by Glick SD. New York, Academic Press, 1985, pp 73–87

132. Diamond MC, Dowling GA, Johnson RE: Morphologic cerebral cortical asymmetry in male and female rats. Exp Neurol 71:261–268, 1981

133. Diamond MC, Johnson RE, Ingham CA: Morphological changes in young, adult and aging rat cerebral cortex, hippocampus, and diencephalon. Behavioral Biology 14:163–174, 1975

134. Diamond MC, Johnson RE, Young D, et al: Age-related morphologic differences in the rat cerebral cortex and hippocampus: male-female; right-left. Exp Neurol 81:1–13, 1983

135. Papas CTE, Diamond MC, Johnson RE: Morphological changes in the cerebral cortex of rats with altered levels of ovarian hormones. Behavioral and Neural Biology 26:298–310, 1979

136. Maggi A, Zucchi I: Sexual differentiation of mammalian frontal cortex. Life Sci 40:1155–1160, 1987

137. Sholl SA, Kim KL: Androgen receptors are differentially distributed between right and left cerebral hemispheres of the fetal male rhesus monkeys. Brain Res 516:122–126, 1990

138. Diamond MC: Asymmetry in the cerebral cortex: development, estrogen receptors, neuron/glial ratios, immune deficiency and enrichment/overcrowding, in Duality and Unity of the Brain: Unified Functioning and Specialization of the Hemispheres. Edited by Ottoson D. New York, Plenum, 1987, pp 37–52

139. Clark AS, Goldman-Rakic PS: Gonadal hormones influence the emergence of cortical functions in nonhuman primates. Behav Neurosci 103:1287–1295, 1989

140. Goldman PS, Crawford HT, Strokes LP, et al: Sex-dependent behavioral effects of cerebral cortical lesions in the developing rhesus monkey. Science 186:540–542, 1974

141. Goldman PS, MacBrown R: The influence of neonatal androgen on the development of cortical function in the rhesus monkey. Abstracts for Neuroscience 1:494, 1975

142. de Lacoste M-C, Horvath DS, Woodward DJ: Possible sex differences in the developing human fetal brain. J Clin Exp Neuropsychol 13:831–846, 1991

143. Robinson RG, Szetela B: Mood changes following left hemispheric brain injury. Ann Neurol 9:447–453, 1981

144. Robinson RG, Kubos KG, Starr LB, et al: Mood disorders in stroke patients: importance of lesion location. Brain 107:81–93, 1984

145. Starkstein SE, Robinson RG, Price TR: Comparison of cortical and subcortical lesions in the production of post-stroke mood disorders. Brain 110:1045–1059, 1987

146. Starkstein SE, Robinson RG: Affective disorders and cerebral vascular disease. Br J Psychiatry 154:170–182, 1989

147. Eastwood MR, Rifat SL, Nobbs H, et al: Mood disorder following cerebrovascular accident. Br J Psychiatry 154: 195–200, 1989

148. Sinyor D, Jacques P, Kaloupek DG, et al: Post-stroke depression and lesion location: an attempted replication. Brain 109:537–546, 1986

149. House A, Dennis M, Warlow C, et al: The relationship between intellectual impairment and mood disorder in the first year after stroke. Psychol Med 20:805–814, 1990

150. Starkstein SE, Robinson RG, Berthier ML, et al: Differential mood changes following basal ganglia versus thalamic lesions. Arch Neurol 45:725–730, 1988

151. Starkstein SE, Robinson RG, Price TR: Comparison of patients with and without post-stroke major depression matched for size and location of lesion. Arch Gen Psychiatry 45:247–252, 1988

152. Baxter LR, Schwartz JM, Phelps ME, et al: Reduction of prefrontal cortex glucose metabolism common to three types of depression. Arch Gen Psychiatry 46:243–250, 1989

153. Martinot JL, Hardy P, Feline A, et al: Left prefrontal glucose hypometabolism in the depressed state: a confirmation. Am J Psychiatry 147:1313–1317, 1990

154. Bench CJ, Friston KJ, Brown RG, et al: The anatomy of melancholia: focal abnormalities of cerebral blood flow in major depression. Psychol Med 22:607–615, 1992

155. Yazici KM, Kapucu O, Erbas B, et al: Assessment of changes in regional cerebral blood flow in patients with major depression using the ^{99m}Tc-HMPAO single photon emission tomography method. Eur J Nucl Med 19:1038–1043, 1992

156. Andreason PJ, Altemus M, Zametkin AJ, et al: Regional cerebral glucose metabolism in bulimia nervosa. Am J Psychiatry 149:1506–1513, 1993

157. Allen JJ, Iacono WG, Depue RA, et al: Regional EEG asymmetries in bipolar seasonal affective disorder before and after phototherapy. Biol Psychiatry 33:642–646, 1993

158. Davidson RJ, Schaffer CE, Saron C: Effects of lateralized presentations of faces on self-reports of emotion and EEG asymmetry in depressed and non-depressed subjects. Psychophysiology 22:353–364, 1985

159. Henriques JB, Davidson RJ: Left frontal hypoactivation in depression. J Abnorm Psychol 100:535–545, 1991

160. Schaffer CE, Davidson RJ, Saron C: Frontal and parietal electroencephalogram asymmetry in depressed and non-depressed subjects. Biol Psychiatry 18:753–762, 1983

161. Drevets WC, Raichle ME: Positron emission tomographic imaging studies of human emotional disorders, in The Cognitive Neuroscience. Edited by Gazzaniga MS. Cambridge, MA, MIT Press, 1995, pp 1153–1164

162. Silfverskiold P, Risberg J: Regional cerebral blood flow in depression and mania. Arch Gen Psychiatry 46:253–259, 1989

163. Henriques JB, Davidson RJ: Regional brain electrical asymmetries discriminate between previously depressed subjects and healthy controls. J Abnorm Psychol 99:22–31, 1990

164. Heller W: Neuropsychological mechanisms of individual differences in emotion, personality and arousal. Neuropsychology 7:476–489, 1993

165. Tomaraken AJ, Keener AD: Frontal brain asymmetry and depression: a self-regulatroy perspective. Cognition and Emotion 12:387–420, 1998

166. Dawson G, Klinger LG, Panagiotides H, et al: Infants of mothers with depressive symptoms: electroencephalographic and behavioral findings related to attachment status. Dev Psychopathol 4:67–80, 1992

167. Field T, Fox NA, Pickens J, et al: Relative right frontal EEG activation in 3- to 6-month old infants of "depressed" mothers. Dev Psychol 3:358–363, 1995

168. Dawson G, Frey K, Panagiotides H, et al: Infants of depressed mothers exhibit atypical frontal electrical brain activity during interactions with mother and with a familiar, non-depressed adult. Child Dev 70:1058–1066, 1999

169. Pardo JV, Pardo PJ, Raichle ME: Neural correlates of self-induced dysphoria. Am J Psychiatry 150:713–719, 1993

170. Tucker DM, Luu P, Pribram KH: Social and emotional self-regulation. Ann N Y Acad Sci 769:213–239, 1995

171. Liotti MD, Tucker DM: Right hemisphere sensitivity to arousal and depression. Brain Cogn 18:138–151, 1992

172. Tucker DM, Starslie CE, Roth RS, et al: Right frontal lobe activation and right hemisphere performance: decrement during a depressed mood. Arch Gen Psychiatry 38:169–174, 1981

173. Davidson RJ: Cerebral asymmetry, emotion and affective style, in Brain Asymmetry. Edited by Davidson RJ, Hugdahl K. Cambride, MA, MIT Press, 1995

174. Canli T, Desmond JE, Zhao Z, et al: Hemispheric asymmetry for emotional stimuli detected with fMRI. Neuroreport 9:3233–3239, 1998

175. Field T, Martinez A, Nawrocki T, et al: Music shifts frontal EEG in depressed adolescents. Adolescence 33:109–116, 1998

176. George MS, Lisanby SH, Sackiem HA: Transcranial magnetic stimulation: applications in neuropsychiatry. Arch Gen Psychiatry 56:300–311, 1999

177. Pascual-Leone A, Rubio B, Pallarado F, et al: Beneficial effects of rapid-rate transcranial magnetic stimulation of the left dorsolateral prefrontal cortex in drug-resistant depression. Lancet 348:233–237, 1996

178. George MS, Wassermann EM, Williams WE, et al: Mood improvements following daily left prefrontal repetitive transcranial magnetic stimulation in patients with depression: a placebo-controlled crossover trial. Am J Psychiatry 154:1752–1756, 1997

179. Menkes DL, Bodnar P, Ballesteros RA, et al: Right frontal lobe slow frequency repetitive transcranial magnetic stimulation is an effective treatment for depression: a case-control pilot study of safety and efficacy. J Neurol Neurosurg Psychiatry 67:113–115, 1999

180. Klien E, Kreinin I, Chistyakov A, et al: Therapeutic efficacy of right prefrontal slow repetitive transcranial magnetic stimulation in major depression: a double-blind study. Arch Gen Psychiatry 56:315–320, 1999

181. Triggs WJ, McCoy KJ, Greer R, et al: Effects of left frontal transcranial magnetic stimulation on depressed mood, cognition, and corticomotor threshold. Biol Psychiatry 45:1440–1446, 1999

182. Belmaker RH, Grisaru N: Does TMS have bipolar efficacy in both depression and mania (abstract)? Biol Psychiatry 43:755, 1998

183. Grisaru N, Cudakov B, Yaroslavsky Y, et al: TMS in mania: a controlled study. Am J Psychiatry 155:1608–1610, 1998

184. Rauch SL, Jenike MA, Alpert NM, et al: Regional cerebral blood flow measured during symptom provocation in obsessive-compulsive disorder using oxygen 15-labeled carbon dioxide and positron emission tomography. Arch Gen Psychiatry 51:62–70, 1994

185. Baxter LR, Schwartz JM, Guze BH, et al: PET imaging in obsessive compulsive disorder with and without depression. J Clin Psychiatry 51:61–69, 1990

186. Baxter LR, Schwartz JM, Mazziotta JC, et al: Cerebral glucose metabolic rates in nondepressed patients with obsessive-compulsive disorder. Am J Psychiatry 145:1560–1563, 1988

187. Baxter LR, Phelps ME, Mazziotta JC, et al: Local cerebral glucose metabolic rate in obsessive-compulsive disorder. Arch Gen Psychiatry 44:211–218, 1987

188. Benkalfat C, Nordahl TE, Semple WE, et al: Local cerebral glucose metabolic rates in obsessive-compulsive disorder: patients treated with clomipramine. Arch Gen Psychiatry 47:840–848, 1990

189. Flor-Henry P: The obsessive-compulsive syndrome: reflection of fronto-caudate dysregulation of the left hemisphere? Encephale 16:325–329, 1990

190. Swedo SE, Schapiro MB, Grady CL, et al: Cerebral glucose metabolism in childhood-onset obsessive-compulsive disorder. Arch Gen Psychiatry 46:518–523, 1989

191. Johanson AM, Risberg J, Silfverskiold P, et al: Regional changes of cerebral blood flow during anxiety in patients with anxiety neurosis, in The Roots of Perception. Edited by Hentschel U, Smith G, Draguns JG. Amsterdam, The Netherlands, North-Holland, 1986, pp 124–135

192. Insel TR: Toward a neuroanatomy of obsessive-compulsive disorder. Arch Gen Psychiatry 49:739–744, 1992

193. George MS, Trimble MR, Costa DC, et al: Elevated frontal cerebral blood flow in Gilles de la Tourette syndrome: a 99Tcm-HMPAO SPECT study. Psychiatry Res 45:143–151, 1992

194. Sacks OW: Neuropsychiatry and Tourette's, in Neurology and Psychiatry: A Meeting of Minds. Edited by Mueller J. Basel, Switzerland, S Karger, 1989

195. Rubin E, Sackheim HA, Prohovnik I, et al: Regional cerebral blood flow in mood disorders, IV: comparison of mania and depression. Psychiatry Res 61:1–10, 1995

196. Starkstein SE, Robinson RG: The role of the frontal lobes in affective disorders following stroke, in Frontal Lobe Function and Dysfunction. Edited by Levin HS, Eisenberg HM, Benton AL. New York, Oxford University Press, 1991, pp 288–303

7

Consciousness, Self-Awareness, and the Frontal Lobes

Donald T. Stuss, Ph.D., Terence W. Picton, M.D., Ph.D., Michael P. Alexander, M.D.

In this chapter, we present a biological view of human consciousness, highlighting the roles of the frontal lobes. Our understanding of the processes of consciousness emerges from analyzing the disorders of awareness that occur in patients with lesions of the brain. Our theory of consciousness has four distinct elements:

1. Awareness results from cerebral processes that construct models of the world.
2. These model-making processes of the brain are arranged hierarchically.
3. Within any one level of the hierarchy, the processes operate in a modular manner.
4. The frontal lobes play a particularly important role at the highest levels of conscious processing, with the right frontal lobe being particularly important for self-awareness.

Our understanding of consciousness proposes that the brain generates a model to fit the information that it receives and experiences the model rather than the information. Similar concepts have been proposed in philosophy,[1] in cognitive psychology,[2,3] and in artificial intelligence.[4] In terms of the brain, the modeling process is most evident in the cerebral cortex.[5] The modeling process underlying consciousness requires interactions between different sets of neurons (Figure 7–1). Some neurons spontaneously generate patterns of activity to balance incoming activity; others compare how well the generated activity fits with the input. Our general view is that each level of the brain's hierarchy functions much as diagrammed in Figure 7–1.

The hierarchy is set up such that higher levels use the modeling capabilities of lower levels (Figure 7–2). A model active at one level of the hierarchy can control the modeling at lower levels in two ways: 1) it can activate the lower generator neurons to model incoming information more intensively, or 2) it can either accentuate or attenuate the comparison process so that the modeling is more or less accurate. These processes allow top-down control of lower levels of processing according to the needs of the modeling at higher levels. Also, a bottom-up flow of sensory information and arousal signals activates generator neurons at higher levels (particularly when modeling at the lower levels does not successfully fit the input).

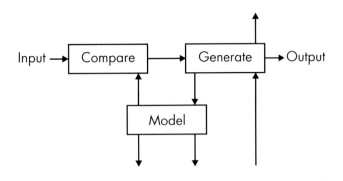

FIGURE 7–1.   The modeling process.

The crucial part of this process is a set of cortical neurons that "generate" patterns of activity that serve as a model for incoming information. These cells can be active spontaneously or in response to signals from higher or lower levels within the nervous system. Most commonly, they are excited by incoming information from the "input" pathways, particularly if such input is not appropriately modeled. Once active, they initiate the firing of "model" cells that encode both a perceptual model and a model for action. The modeling process continues until the model "compares" well with the input. A lack of fit of the model to the input brings about further generator activity. Once set up, the activity patterns of the model cells can become dormant until initiated again by the generator cells (following renewed input).

We conceive of four main levels to the hierarchy. At the lowest level, there is no internal modeling of incoming information. This level makes simple behavioral responses to incoming stimuli and activates higher levels of the nervous system. Feedback at this level of the system occurs not between a model and incoming information but between motor responses and sensory input. This level mainly involves the brain stem reticular system and mediates the arousal aspects of consciousness. The second level, involving the sensory and motor regions of the neocortex, provides the basic analysis of incoming sensory information and the construction of complex motor activity. A third level, probably involving the frontal lobes, mediates the executive functions that integrate the information provided by the sensory systems and organizes goal-directed behavior. A final level considers information from the viewpoint of a personal history, remembered from the past and projected to the future. This level of self-awareness is related to the frontal lobe and its limbic connections, with the right frontal lobe playing a crucial role. Consciousness occurs at the level of the highest active generator system, and the contents of consciousness are the model at that particular level.

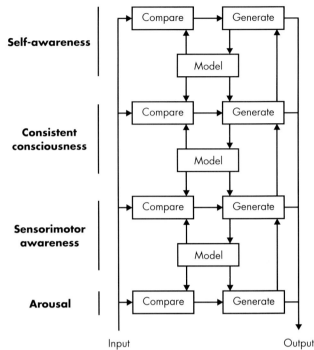

FIGURE 7–2.   Hierarchies of processing.

This figure shows how the modeling processes can be set up in hierarchies. Four different levels are portrayed. The bottom level does not involve any internal models and is concerned with making simple responses and arousing higher levels to consider new information. The highest level deals with self-awareness. The generator neurons at any one level can activate the generator neurons at higher levels to take care of information that cannot be fully modeled at their level. The models at one level can control the generator neurons and the comparison processes at lower levels.

In addition to being arranged in a hierarchical manner, many parts of the nervous system function in a self-contained or modular manner. At any one level, information is handled by multiple independent processors (Figure 7–3). The outputs from such processors are then integrated at higher levels. Modularity allows for the rapid and efficient processing of information. Modularity is most evident at the level of sensorimotor processing. Efficient cortical systems process the various visual characteristics of a scene, the meanings of heard words, and the joint movements necessary for skilled motor performance. However, modularity also may be present at higher levels. We have begun to fractionate different executive functions and relate them to different areas of the frontal lobes.[6,7] Self-awareness also may be modular to some extent. An individual wears many hats. In different contexts, a person perceives and acts using different memories, styles, and goals.

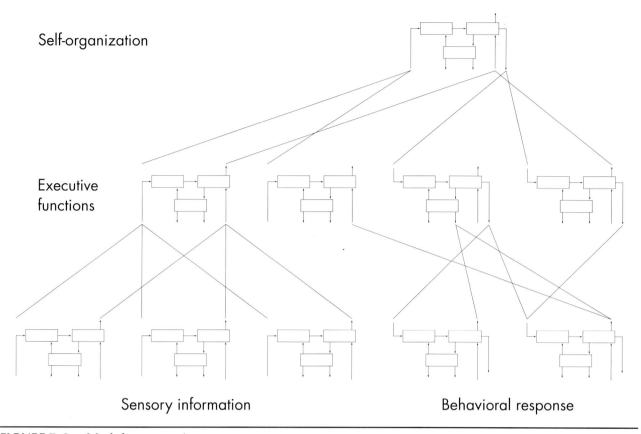

Self-organization

Executive functions

Sensory information   Behavioral response

FIGURE 7–3. Modular processing.

At any level of processing, many different modeling processes can be performed independently of others. A major difference is between sensory modules (*left side*) that transmit information toward higher levels and motor modules (*right side*) that organize output down through the lower levels. Integration of sensory modeling and organization of behavioral modeling occur at higher levels. Only some of the many connections between levels are shown.

This approach to consciousness[5,8–11] combines ideas of modeling, hierarchy, and modularity. It derives from neuropsychology and neurobiology but has many components in common with theories of self in social psychology.[12] The hierarchy reflects the different levels of model-making of the human brain and relates to different levels of experienced consciousness. The afferent component at the different levels ranges from simple sensory information, such as the color of an object, to the experience of oneself as a distinct sentient entity. The efferent component ranges from simple reflex movements to self-directed volitional actions.

The approach has many features in common with modern theories of memory.[13] Memory consists of several systems, each characterized by a specific relation to consciousness.[14] Simple memories such as conditioned reflexes and perceptual priming occur without direct awareness (*anoetic*) and are highly modular. Semantic memories involve the experience of know-

ing or *noetic* consciousness. These memories are modular in the sense of different domains of knowledge. Episodic memory is the remembering of personal experiences and is characterized by an *autonoetic* consciousness that involves the self. Tulving,[14] based on Ingvar's[15] blood flow work, postulated that this autonoetic consciousness would depend on the integrity of the frontal lobes. Thus, the neural organization of memory illuminates both the hierarchies of modeling within the human brain and the modular structures within each level of the hierarchy.

AROUSAL AND ACTIVATION

Disorders of consciousness resulting from damage at the lowest levels of the hierarchy result in diminished general arousal. The neural bases for the processes of arousal and general responsiveness are the brain stem reticular formation and the specific brain stem nuclei and their projection to the thalamus and cortex. These systems not only initiate simple behavioral responses but also arouse the cortex to consider other aspects of the sensory input than the requirement for immediate response.

Coma is the most extreme deficit of consciousness. In coma, an individual is completely unresponsive except for simple spinal or bulbar reflexes. Coma differs from other states of unconsciousness such as sleep, from which the individual can be aroused by stimulation, and anesthetic unconsciousness, from which the individual can be aroused by withdrawal of the anesthetic medication. Coma is associated with either widespread damage or dysfunction in the cerebral cortex or lesions to the mesencephalic reticular formation.[16]

From coma to normal wakefulness, a continuum of disorders exists. Coma is associated with no response, stupor is characterized by cortical activity that is elicited only by intense stimuli and not sustained for any time, and obtundation (or torpor) is evidenced by a slow and poorly integrated responsiveness.[16] These presumably represent different degrees of damage to the brain stem arousal systems.

With focal pathology in the brain stem reticular activating system, a patient can only pay attention transiently (phasic attention) but rapidly reverts to a somnolent state because of a disorder in ongoing alertness (tonic attention).[17] In certain disorders, a patient may have wandering attention, in which tonic attention is relatively intact but phasic attention is impaired, resulting in distractibility. The pathology, if found, involves the diffuse thalamic projection system. Delirium also has been used to describe a state like wandering attention. Lipowski[18] used the terms *hypoactive* and *hyperactive delirium* to encompass the range of disturbed consciousness from drifting (stupor) to wandering (delirium) attention.

Another condition of pathological unconsciousness is the persistent vegetative state. This differs from coma in that the brain stem arousal systems operate relatively normally. The patient cycles through different levels of arousal, similar to the normal changes between sleep and wakefulness. The eyes may open, and nonpurposeful roving eye movements may occur. These are often quite disconcerting because the patient appears to be looking at things. However, the patient is completely unconscious. The cortex is so profoundly damaged that no normal cortical activity can be elicited: arousal is present, but consciousness is empty of any content.

Damage to one specific brain stem area—the dopaminergic ventral tegmental area or its projection to frontal cortex via the medial forebrain bundle—produces impaired general responsiveness despite normal arousal and intact cortical functioning. This condition of "akinetic mutism" is characterized by an inability to activate mental operations. Some degree of voluntary responsiveness may be seen when cognitively undemanding requests are made or when emotionally potent stimuli are presented. However, purposeful integrated cortical function does not occur. Unlike patients in a coma or persistent vegetative state, patients with akinetic mutism have purposeful eye movements, and fixation is normal. In this condition, arousal is present and cortical function is possible, but there is little activation of these functions.

Coma, the persistent vegetative state, and akinetic mutism must be distinguished from the unresponsiveness that occurs in the "locked-in" syndrome. This lack of responsiveness is not caused by unconsciousness but by the patient being disconnected from any output. Consciousness is normal, but damage to all efferent motor systems precludes any volitional action.

The states of disturbed consciousness that relate to the lower levels of the brain's hierarchy are characterized by a general decrease in or absence of responsiveness. Two basic patterns of lesion are found. In the first (akinetic mutism, brain stem coma), the cortex is relatively spared but is not sufficiently activated to function normally. The lesion may be in the lower levels (the brain stem reticular formation)[19] or in bilateral anterior cingulate regions affecting limbic drive and activation.[20,21] In the second (persistent vegetative state, cortical coma), the cortex is extensively damaged and cannot function normally despite incoming activation. The lower levels of the brain's hierarchy provide an ongoing activation for higher levels of consciousness and awareness. In terms of the modeling processes, they provide the activation for the generative activity that permits the models to develop. If the cortex does not function normally because of damage or a lack of activation, modeling cannot occur, and consciousness is absent.

CONTENT OF ACTIVATED CONSCIOUSNESS

The next level of the brain's hierarchical organization provides the processing that underlies the simple awareness of the sensory world and one's bodily responses. At the previous level, we were concerned with responsiveness and arousal and not with awareness. After brain stem projections sufficiently arouse and activate the cortex, modeling of incoming afferent information is possible, and awareness can occur. Disorders of consciousness at this level are characterized by specific disturbances in the content of consciousness that depend on which module of the cortex is injured.

Fodor[22] proposed a theory of modularity in cognitive operations. The brain processes information with multiple separate modules, each working on specific aspects of information. Modules are domain-specific and process information automatically. They are determined by inherited neural structures that, through development and experience, gradually create models of their domain to guide interpretation and response. The operations of the modules are impenetrable (i.e., they are not accessible to awareness and are not influenced by intention). However, the results of these operations reach conscious awareness when some higher cognitive processors direct attention to them. Because disturbances at this level are domain-specific, impaired awareness reveals itself as an actual absence of the created models within the damaged domain, a disturbance of knowledge, or an agnosia.

The classical clinical neurology of focal brain lesions delineates many different types of domain-specific disturbed awareness. For example, a lesion in the left posterior temporal lobe typically produces Wernicke's aphasia, characterized by an inability to understand language and a fluent speech with specific substantive words replaced by neologisms.[23] In addition, however, the patient is unaware of either the failure to comprehend or the abnormal speech. Indeed, as the patient recovers and becomes more aware of the problem, a significant psychological reaction often occurs. Another example is the neglect of the left side that occurs with right parietal lesions. Patients with this lesion may be completely unaware of any perceptual disability. The general term *anosognosia* was coined by Babinski[24] to describe patients who are unaware of their deficits.

The posterior cerebral hemispheres model many different aspects of incoming sensory information. Focal damage to these areas produces not only an inability to process information in a particular way but also a domain-specific unawareness of the deficit. In terms of modeling processes, arousal and activation are normal, but domain-specific modeling systems at the sensorimotor levels are not able to function. Higher mod-

eling processes can occur but cannot use the lower damaged modeling processes. The patient's awareness therefore does not include either information from the domain of the damaged module or the fact that this information is missing.

FRONTAL LOBES AND CONTROL OF CONSCIOUSNESS

Both experimental and clinical evidence indicate the preeminence of the frontal lobes in the higher levels of awareness. Monkeys with frontal lesions are indifferent to their surroundings and to their own actions.[25] From the earliest clinical reports of human patients with frontal damage, a similar indifference was noted, and, when probed, introspection and self-awareness were deficient. Patients showed a dissociation between knowledge (the content of consciousness) and the use of this knowledge to control their own behavior. Freeman and Watts[26] evaluated patients who had undergone frontal lobectomies and observed impairments in two levels of self-awareness: a visceral consciousness of one's own identity and a more abstract and reflective consciousness of the self. The more abstract self-consciousness seemed dependent on more anterior frontal structures. That there are levels of self-awareness is apparent in neuroethnology. Gallup[27] used the "mirror test" and found no evidence that a monkey can recognize its reflection as an image of itself. However, chimpanzees, orangutans, and human children after a certain age easily perform this act of visceral consciousness. Only humans, among primates, appear to have a reflective consciousness of the self as an entity across time.

The frontal lobes probably play a role at two distinct levels of consciousness. One level involves making sense of all the sensory information that has been evaluated in the posterior areas of the brain and putting together an appropriate set of behavioral responses to this information. At this level, we are dealing with the executive functions of the brain,[7] the functions that select which information to attend to, that activate or inhibit the patterns of voluntary behavior, and that resolve discrepancies between various sources of information. The modeling system at this level acts to construct a world model from the models of specific aspects of the world that are formed at the lower levels of processing. A model of the world that is consistent with reality can then control behavior. A second level of frontal processing concerns self-awareness. This is highly developed in human primates, in whom actions are governed by the goals of a self that exists from past to future.

Impairments in the higher-level reflective consciousness or in self-awareness may take several forms. Patients never complain of these disorders, and families and clinicians generally will not see the patient's problems in terms of reflective consciousness or self-awareness. Two case histories will illustrate the key role of frontal lobe damage in producing abnormalities of reflectiveness and of self-awareness.

Executive Functions—Forming a Consistent World Model

Mr. A[28] had a severe traumatic brain injury with prolonged coma, then prolonged amnesia before finally showing slowly improving cognition and memory. Computed tomography scan indicated bilateral frontal damage that was very extensive on the right, with right frontal and anterior temporal damage.

Several months after the injury, Mr. A began to report that he had a "new" second family virtually identical to his first family. In the psychiatric literature, this behavior is labeled Capgras' syndrome. In the neurological literature, the term *reduplicative paramnesia* may be used, but this often is reserved for duplication of place. Even as he improved over the next months, he maintained that he had two families. Neuropsychological testing demonstrated high to average intelligence, normal facial recognition, and normal memory. Impairments were seen only on executive function tests. He was able to judge that the story of two identical families was "unbelievable" when it was presented as a hypothetical story involving someone else. He regrettably insisted that he "wouldn't believe it," but he would then immediately assert that his story was nonetheless a true experience.

Years later, when Mr. A knew that his continued assertion of the two families was the only obstacle to his going home, he would still insist that the story was true.

William James[29] claimed that the experience of an integrated self required strong feelings of personal unity and continuity. These feelings emerge from seamless, warm, and salient memories. When we scrutinized the time course of Mr. A's reduplication, we could see how his world became discontinuous. As his confusion and amnesia were clearing, months after the accident, he had his first home visit. In that intervening time, his wife had purchased a new car, his teenage children were almost 1 year older, and in his

honor, his wife had a new hairstyle. He experienced a family, almost identical to the one he remembered, in a warm and familiar environment at a time of significant problems in judgment (caused by the frontal damage) and still recovering memory. He had two separate but similar experiences, both of which became part of his consciousness. His significant executive dysfunction, even when other faculties had recovered, left him with deficits in planning, judgment, and monitoring of his own situation. Most critically, however, these deficits left him unable to create a mental model of his own situation that would reconcile the two experiences (of his family and home) into one.

This case represents a disorder of model construction and monitoring at a high level, distinct from the focal deficiencies of awareness in patients with posterior lesions. The patient has a model of the world, but it is inconsistent and unreal.

Self-Awareness and the Right Frontal Lobe

Growing evidence indicates that if the frontal lobes are involved in self-awareness, then the most important region may be the right frontal lobes. Mr. A had maximum right frontal pathology. In the literature on neurological cases of reduplicative paramnesia and/or Capgras' syndrome, the preponderance of cases have right frontal damage.[30,31] Positron-emission tomography activation studies of episodic memory have shown a "hemispheric encoding-retrieval asymmetry," with preferential right prefrontal cortical involvement in episodic retrieval tasks.[32,33] Wheeler and colleagues[34] summarized the literature on self-awareness and episodic memory and suggested that autonoetic consciousness (the experience of personal memories) depends on the right frontal lobe.

Mr. B[11] underwent a resection of a right frontal astrocytoma. Although his intelligence remained superior and performance on standard frontal lobe tests (of executive functions) was normal on postoperative testing, he could not maintain the high level of productivity required for the position that he held. Although his knowledge of his workplace difficulties was precise, he steadfastly blamed the problems on others. For example, Mr. B personally often could not complete tasks in a timely manner (a problem that he acknowledged and that was addressed in weekly rehabilitation sessions), but he blamed his problems on subordinates. He was clearly concerned about his difficulties, as shown by his desire to continue regular rehabilitation/therapy sessions. In role-playing procedures with Mr. B as the employer, he had no difficulty identifying appropriate corrections to the problems (e.g., early retirement, financial and personal counseling). However, he would not or could not act accordingly. He showed two characteristics of this level of disturbed consciousness: an unawareness of the implications of his disorder and an inability to use intact semantic knowledge to guide personal decisions.

Mr. B knows what he should do, but he does not act in his own self-interest. He lacks a mental model of his own self, which leaves him without any clear purpose to organize his perceptions and actions. We believe that this impairment of self-awareness is due to right prefrontal pathology.

CONSCIOUSNESS AND TIME

Self-awareness then is the highest level of consciousness. A model of the self is generated through experience and used to analyze incoming information and direct behavior. Monitoring the present state of the self is necessary for a full human life. In addition, however, this chapter has hinted at another important principle—the interpretation of experience (the construction of the model) must be monitored across time. This temporal integration varies with the hierarchical level. At the domain-specific level, the subunit operations of even complex operations are overlearned or routinized—the time scale is very brief. The temporal order at this lower level relates to immediate actions and reactions, wherein "the brain follows, rather than prescribes, that order."[35]

At the level of awareness associated with executive functioning, the model construction and monitoring are slow and deliberate—"conscious effort" is required. At this level, we sculpt a view of the world that is realistic and consistent. The processing involves more than direct experiences. These are modified by intentional decisions. We may discount sensory input as illusory and attempt to interpret causes and effects. The timing is what we perceive as the present.

The highest level of self-awareness involves a longer subjective time, a reflectiveness of past and future events. Ingvar[15] connected the frontal lobes with "memories of the future." Wheeler and colleagues[34] proposed that the prefrontal regions transform episodic memory—the recall of personal past with its subjective time and its reconstructed emotional associations—into autonoetic or self-reflective consciousness. This highly personal consciousness, shared by

no one else, generates and executes plans for the future. James[29] expressed the temporal aspects of self-awareness clearly, dissociating the consciousness of the immediate present from the longer-lasting consciousness that enables a personal history and an anticipatory vision of the future.

> In short, the practically cognised present is no knife-edge, but a saddle-back, with a certain breadth of its own on which we sit perched, and from which we look in two directions into time. The unit of composition of our perception of time is a duration, with a bow and a stern, as it were—a rearward and a forward looking end.[29] (p. 399)

For James, time and self are intimately connected, each hierarchically. The highest level of self-awareness emerges from the perception of the self from the past into the future. When the anterior frontal lobes are damaged, only the perceptual present remains,[36] but abstract models of the self in other times—past or present, real or imagined—are deficient.

PSYCHIATRIC IMPLICATIONS

Many psychiatric problems can be viewed from the principle of modeling the external world.[37] Depressed individuals may have faulty mental models of self or defective models of the world's expectations of them. The inability to reconcile these abstract models generates the depressed mood. Cognitive therapy focuses on remodeling belief systems and self-perceptions.[38]

Delusional states in affective disorder or in schizophrenia may be generated by the same inability to integrate experience with mental models, as shown by our patient with reduplication. Delusions in brain diseases are common after frontal lobe damage, and perhaps neurochemical disturbances of frontal functions in psychiatric disease produce equivalent executive impairments and self-awareness.

Confabulations may indicate a lack of ability to compare the model with incoming information. The model generator therefore creates explanations for this information without any regard for the actual external reality. Confabulations have been related to impaired frontal lobe control functions, particularly of the fantastic kind.[39,40] The model-building concept might explain confabulation in split-brain patients.[41] Once the right hemisphere makes a response based on information it received, the disconnected left hemisphere attempts to explain itself by inventing a plausible but incorrect reason for the response. Schizophrenic patients have clear abnormalities in self-awareness. The patient has difficulty maintaining a self who is able to understand incoming information and who is in control of action.

CONCLUSIONS

Conscious experience does not come from a passive reception of incoming information but involves the active construction of mental models of the world. We remember, we think, and we plan by using mental models. We are not so much conscious of the world as conscious of our models thereof. Consciousness is hierarchical, with self-awareness occurring at the highest levels. Caution is essential when speculating about the cerebral localization of such complex processes. Nevertheless, the frontal lobes and their connections are clearly critical for self-awareness. In the frontal lobes, affect and cognition have the maximum opportunity for integration.[42,43] The right frontal lobe, once considered a functionally silent cerebral zone, may be particularly important.

REFERENCES

1. Craik K: The Nature of Explanation. Cambridge, MA, Cambridge University Press, 1943

2. Miller GA, Galanter EH, Pribram KH: Plans and the Structure of Behavior. New York, Holt, Rinehart & Winston, 1960

3. Yates J: The content of awareness is a model of the world. Psychol Rev 92:249–284, 1985

4. Johnson-Laird PN: Mental Models: Towards a Cognitive Science of Language, Inference, and Consciousness. Cambridge, MA, Harvard University Press, 1983

5. Picton TW, Stuss DT: Consciousness, in Principles of Medical Biology. Edited by Bittar EE, Bittar N. JAI Press (in press)

6. Stuss DT, Alexander MP, Palumbo CL, et al: Organizational strategies of patients with unilateral or bilateral frontal lobe injury in word list learning tasks. Neuropsychology 8:355–373, 1994

7. Stuss DT, Shallice T, Alexander MP, et al: A multidisciplinary approach to anterior attentional functions. Ann N Y Acad Sci 769:191–212, 1995

8. Picton TW, Stuss DT: Neurobiology of conscious experience. Curr Opin Neurobiol 4:256–265, 1994

9. Stuss DT, Benson DF: The Frontal Lobes. New York, Raven, 1986

10. Stuss DT: Disturbance of self-awareness after frontal system damage, in Awareness of Deficit After Brain Injury: Clinical and Theoretical Issues. Edited by Prigatano GP, Schacter DL. New York, Oxford University Press, 1991, pp 63–83

11. Stuss DT: Self, awareness, and the frontal lobes: a neuropsychological perspective, in The Self: Interdisciplinary Approaches. Edited by Strauss J, Goethals GR. New York, Springer-Verlag, 1991, pp 255–278

12. Carver CS, Scheier MF: Self-regulation and the self, in The Self: Interdisciplinary Approaches. Edited by Strauss J, Goethals GR. New York, Springer-Verlag, 1991, pp 168–207

13. Challis BH, Velichkovsky BM, Craik FIM: Levels of processing effects on a variety of memory tasks: new findings and theoretical implications. Conscious Cogn 5:142–164, 1996

14. Tulving E: Memory and consciousness. Canadian Journal of Psychology 26:1–10, 1985

15. Ingvar DH: "Memory of the future": an essay on the temporal organization of conscious awareness. Human Neurobiology 4:127–136, 1985

16. Plum F, Posner JB: The Diagnosis of Stupor and Coma, 3rd Edition. Philadelphia, PA, FA Davis, 1980

17. Benson DF, Geschwind N: Psychiatric conditions associated with focal lesions of the central nervous system, in American Handbook of Psychiatry, 2nd Edition, Vol 4: Organic Disorders and Psychomatic Medicine. Edited by Arieti S, Reiser M. New York, Basic Books, 1975, pp 208–243

18. Lipowski ZJ: Delirium: Acute Confusional States. New York, Oxford University Press, 1990

19. Ross EO, Stewart RM: Akinetic mutism from hypothalomic damage: successful treatment with dopamine antagonists. Neurology 32:1435–1439, 1981

20. Damasio AR, Van Hoesen GW: Emotional disturbances associated with focal lesions of the limbic frontal lobe, in Neuropsychology of Human Emotion. Edited by Heilman KM, Satz P. New York, Guilford, 1983, pp 83–110

21. Devinsky O, Morrell M, Vogt BA: Contributions of anterior cingulate cortex to behavior. Brain 118:279–306, 1995

22. Fodor JA: The Modularity of Mind. Cambridge, MA, MIT Press, 1983

23. Benson DF: Aphasia, Alexia, and Agraphia. New York, Churchill Livingstone, 1979

24. Babinski J: Contribution a l'étude des troubles mentaux dans l'hémiplegie organique cérébrale (anosognosie). Rev Neurol (Paris) 27:845–848, 1914

25. Bianchi L: The Mechanism of the Brain and the Functions of the Frontal Lobes. New York, William Wood, 1922

26. Freeman W, Watts JW: Frontal lobe functions as revealed by psychosurgery. Digest of Neurology and Psychiatry, Institute of Living 16:62–68, 1948

27. Gallup GG Jr: Do minds exist in species other than our own? Neurosci Biobehav Rev 9:631–641, 1985

28. Alexander MP, Stuss DT, Benson DF: Capgras syndrome: a reduplicative phenomenon. Neurology 29:334–339, 1979

29. James W: The Principles of Psychology (1890). Chicago, IL, Encyclopaedia Britannica, 1952

30. Malloy P, Duffy J: The frontal lobes in neuropsychiatric disorders, in Handbook of Neuropsychology, Vol 9. Amsterdam, The Netherlands, Elsevier, 1994, pp 203–232

31. Malloy PF, Richardson ED: The frontal lobes and content-specific delusions. J Neuropsychiatry Clin Neurosci 6:455–466, 1994

32. Tulving E, Kapur S, Craik FIM, et al: Hemispheric encoding retrieval asymmetry in episodic memory: positron emission tomography findings. Proc Natl Acad Sci U S A 91:2016–2020, 1994

33. Nyberg L, Cabeza R, Tulving E: PET studies of encoding and retrieval: the HERA model. Psychonomic Bulletin and Review 3:135–148, 1996

34. Wheeler MA, Stuss DT, Tulving E: Toward a theory of episodic memory: the frontal lobes and autonoetic consciousness. Psychol Bull 121:331–354, 1997

35. Fuster JM: Temporal organization of behavior. Human Neurobiology 4:57–60, 1985

36. Hutton EL, Lond BS: The investigation of personality in patients treated by prefrontal leucotomy. Journal of Mental Science 371:275–281, 1942

37. Benson DF, Stuss DT: Frontal lobe influences on delusions: a clinical perspective. Schizophr Bull 16:403–411, 1990

38. Beck AT: Cognitive Theory and the Emotional Disorders. New York, International Universities Press, 1976

39. Stuss DT, Alexander MP, Lieberman A, et al: An extraordinary form of confabulation. Neurology 28:1166–1172, 1978

40. Shapiro BE, Alexander MP, Gardner H, et al: Mechanisms of confabulation. Neurology 31:1070–1076, 1981

41. Gazzaniga MS: Brain mechanisms and conscious experience, in Experimental and Theoretical Studies of Consciousness (Ciba Foundation Symposium 174). Chichester, UK, Wiley, 1993, pp 43–60

42. Nauta WJH: Connections of the frontal lobe with the limbic system, in Surgical Approaches in Psychiatry. Edited by Laitinen SV, Livingston KE. Baltimore, MD, University Park Press, 1973, pp 303–314

43. Pandya DN, Barnes CL: Architecture and connections of the frontal lobe, in The Frontal Lobes Revisited. Edited by Pereceman E. New York, IRBN Press, 1987, pp 41–72

PART 3

Prefrontal Syndromes in Clinical Practice

8

Regional Prefrontal Syndromes

A Theoretical and Clinical Overview

James D. Duffy, M.B., Ch.B., John J. Campbell III, M.D.

The term *frontal lobe syndrome* has become entrenched in the language of neuropsychiatry; however, its genesis and validity warrant further inspection. The term appears to denote a constellation of clinical signs and symptoms that are referable to a specific neuroanatomical focus, the frontal lobe. However, the persistence of this anatomically based descriptive term is an anachronism that draws support from a strict localizationalist approach to brain-behavior relationships. Although there is no doubt that focal lesions involving the prefrontal cortex produce a predictable constellation of executive cognitive deficits, there is equally robust evidence that lesions distant from the anterior cortical mantle may produce a similar constellation of behavioral abnormalities.[1–4] Because a syndrome comprises a cluster of signs and symptoms rather than an anatomical location, it is more appropriate to describe a "dysexecutive syndrome" rather than a "frontal lobe syndrome" when describing patients who manifest abnormalities in executive cognition. This nomenclature is more consistent with current theories that describe large-scale distributed neuronal networks subserving behavior.[5] It also pro-

vides a more rational template for evaluating patients who show deficits in the complex behavior subserved by executive cognition.

HISTORICAL PERSPECTIVES

A brief review of the historical antecedents to the emergence of the frontal lobe syndrome will clarify the genesis of the term. Although a vague association between the frontal areas of the brain and higher intellect was hinted at throughout the Greek and Roman eras,[6,7] Guido Lanfranchi[8] was probably the first clinician to describe the typical clinical sequelae of frontal lobe damage. In the fourteenth century, he described two soldiers who became "dull witted" following damage to the anterior cortex. Almost three centuries later, in 1614, Felix Platter[9] provided a detailed clinical description of a patient demonstrating apathy and "dementia" that he argued was a direct consequence of a large encapsulated frontal tumor. Although Emanuel Swedenborg[10] (1688–1772) wrote that the frontal lobes were intimately involved in the generation of higher cognitive processes as the "highest court of the cerebrum," his manuscripts were not publicly dispersed during his lifetime. It was therefore not until the emergence of phrenology (as the progenitor of localization theory) that the role of the frontal lobe in higher cognition was firmly established. In France, Jean Cruvelhier[11] provided a detailed description of the behavioral sequelae of frontal lobe damage in his classic text *L'Anatomie Pathologique du Corps Humain* (1842). Meanwhile, in America, John Harlow's[12] presentation of Phineas Gage to the Boston Neurologic and Psychiatric Society (1868) provided the early impetus for the study of the neurological underpinnings of higher cognitive function. These early clinical observations were soon supported by the elegant experiments of David Ferrier[13] (1843–1928) and Leonardo Bianchi[14] (1848–1927), who described qualitative alterations in the behavior of laboratory animals who had undergone surgical ablation of the prefrontal lobes.

The precise origin of the term *frontal lobe syndrome* remains obscure, but it probably arose from the increasing conviction of early neurologists that, in accordance with the findings of Broca and Wernicke, the site of all sensorimotor and cognitive functions could be localized in the cerebrum. Building on this theoretical foundation, the late nineteenth century witnessed the publication of a flurry of case studies that described a remarkably consistent constellation of clinical characteristics referable to frontal lobe damage.[15] The elaboration of the syndrome and its widespread acceptance were facilitated by two world wars that resulted in large cohorts of patients with focal frontal injuries.

Unfortunately, through the brief but rampant popularization of prefrontal lobotomy, the mid-twentieth century witnessed a "medical assault" on the frontal lobes. Although thousands of psychiatric patients underwent psychosurgical procedures involving the prefrontal lobes, virtually no attempt was made to scientifically evaluate the behavioral and cognitive consequences of such lesions. Despite the lack of any scientific monitoring, the devastating clinical effects of frontal lobotomy in producing "demented imbeciles"[16] were soon recognized, and this particular form of psychosurgery was abandoned in favor of less destructive procedures.[17]

Recent advances in neuroimaging and in our understanding of the distributed neural networks subserving complex behavior have reconfirmed that many patients with executive cognitive deficits have neuropathological changes distant from the prefrontal cortex. It is clearly a misnomer to describe these patients as having a frontal lobe syndrome. We would argue that the descriptive term *dysexecutive syndrome* provides a more valid and clinically useful description of the particular neural system dysfunction underlying such behavioral alterations.

DEFINING EXECUTIVE COGNITION

The qualitative nature of executive cognition makes it difficult to define. Rather than being limited to any particular cognitive or functional domain, *executive cognition* refers to the qualitative organizing principles necessary to navigate the fluctuating and ambiguous challenges confronted in autonomous social behavior. These "metacognitive" functions are necessary to produce context-appropriate, goal-oriented behavior, including motivation, planning, self-regulation, and self-monitoring.[18] A deficit in any of these supervisory mental processes will result in a breakdown in appropriate autonomous behavior and will render the individual incapable of generating self-determined rather than environmentally determined (i.e., stimulus-bound) behavior.

Although the behavioral consequences of executive dysfunction are well recognized (see Table 8–1), the overarching and fundamental processes involved in the generation of executive cognition remain uncertain. Several theoretical models capable of explaining the organizing principles of executive cognition have been proposed. A brief review of these models is helpful to appreciate the fundamental dysfunction experienced by patients with deficits in executive cognition.

Working Memory

Baddeley[19] has described "working memory" as a "neural scratch-pad" that provides the real-time neural cognitive representation necessary for executive decision making.

Fuster[20] extended the working memory model and proposed that the overarching function of the prefrontal cortex (and the core characteristic of executive cognition) is "the integration of sensory information and motor acts into novel, complex and purposive behavioral sequences." He suggested that the prefrontal cortex accomplishes this "synthetic" function through its coordination of three fundamental executive cognitive functions: 1) providing the template for provisional short-term memory, 2) developing response strategies, and 3) suppressing internal and external stimuli that might disrupt the enactment of the prioritized behavioral strategy.

Modulation of Large-Scale Neurocognitive Networks

Mesulam[21] suggested that the widespread corticocortical and cortical-subcortical connections of the prefrontal lobes enable them to assume an organizing (executive) role in behavior by appropriately activating, inhibiting, and integrating widely distributed ideomotor and sensorimotor neural networks. The individual is able to respond to a particular stimulus on the basis of a distillate of previous experience and current environmental stimuli; for example, "Although I'm tired, I must continue studying if I want to pass the exam tomorrow." Mesulam[21] highlighted two important computational characteristics of the prefrontal lobe's role in executive cognitive function: 1) a high density of connections with other networks and 2) relative autonomy from sensorimotor activities.

The clinical ramification of this theoretical framework of large distributed neuronal networks is that lesions anywhere within the extended neuronal network will produce a similar functional deficit.

The Somatic Marker Hypothesis

Damasio[22] postulated that portions of the ventromedial prefrontal cortex provide a repository for the linkage of current contingencies with the individual's previous emotional experience of similar situations. Damasio postulated that the orbitofrontal cortex does not contain factual information pertinent to the current contingency but provides "somatic markers" that enable the individual to "learn by experience" whether a particular behavior will produce positive or negative bioregulatory states (interpreted by the individual as emotions). This linkage of factual sets (held in the appropriate association cortices) and emotional sets (held in the ventromedial frontal cortex) is thought to modify the response of the individual to environmental stimuli and to facilitate logical reasoning. According to this hypothesis, individuals who fail to develop context-appropriate somatic markers (either through a "sociopathic temperament" or through injury to the ventromedial frontal cortex) will have inappropriate stimulus-bound behavior typical of sociopathy.

FRONTAL LOBE ANATOMY

An understanding of prefrontal neuroanatomy and connectivity is a prerequisite to appreciating the complex nature and multiple etiologies of these syndromes.

The prefrontal cortex is histologically heterogeneous. Furthermore, extensive and discrete connections exist with multiple cortical, subcortical, and brain stem sites. The elucidation of these connections provides a framework within which to infer the contributions of the prefrontal cortex to human behavior.

Precise identification of the frontal lobe is difficult and varies depending on the particular gross histological or connectionist system used. On a gross level, the frontal lobe approximates the configuration of four interconnected triangular surfaces with a posterior white matter "wall" composed of massive afferent and efferent tracts, a medial gray matter surface abutting the falx, a basal gray matter floor resting on the bony roof of the orbits, and a convex lateral cortical surface. An anterior pole is formed by the convergence of the medial, basal, and anterior surfaces posterior to the frontal bone.

The posterolateral margin is the central sulcus of Rolando. The posteromedial margin is an imaginary line dropped from the superomedial aspect of the central sulcus to the corpus callosum. The posterobasal margin runs laterally from the optic chiasm to the temporal poles.

Cytoarchitectonic differentiation of the frontal cortex was accomplished by Brodmann and von Economo. Brodmann's areas 4, 6, 8–12, and 43–47 are located on the lateral convexity. The medial surface is composed of areas 6, 8–12, 24, 25, 32, and 33. The basal surface contains areas 10–15, 25, and 27. von Economo[23] used a different approach and identified two primary types of cortex in the frontal lobes. Heterotypic frontal agranular cortex subserves motor function and includes Brodmann's area 4 and the primary motor strip or precentral gyrus, along with premotor areas 6, 8, and 43–45. Homotypic frontal granular cortex is nonmotor and includes areas 9–15, 46, and 47. Area 8, the frontal eye fields, represents a transition between these cortices.

Frontal thalamocortical afferent connections respect the neuroanatomical boundaries described by von Economo.[23] The ventral anterior and ventral lateral thalamic nuclei synapse with the primary motor and premotor heterotypic agranular cortex, respectively. The dorsomedial thalamic nucleus is exclusively linked to the homotypic granular cortex in the frontal lobes. This serves as one means of defining the nonmotor or prefrontal cortex, with *prefrontal* referring to its location anterior to the premotor gyrus.

The regional heterogeneity within the prefrontal cortex is reflected by topographic organization within the dorsomedial nucleus.[23] The lateral parvocellular region of the dorsomedial nucleus projects to areas 9 and 10 on the lateral convexity but not to the basal orbitofrontal cortex. The medial magnocellular region provides efferent connections to the mesial and orbitofrontal cortices. These thalamocortical projections constitute the final linkage in a series of parallel cortical-striatal-pallidal-thalamic-cortical loops influencing motor and nonmotor frontal functions.[24] Despite their close proximity, it appears that very little cross-communication occurs among these circuits and that the loops remain segregated. Two nonmotor loops channel information processed through the ventral or limbic striatum, with a third nonmotor loop connecting the dorsolateral frontal cortex to the head of the caudate nucleus, lateral globus pallidus, and parvocellular thalamus.[25] This circuitry may form the anatomical basis for "frontal" dysfunction observed in the context of subcortical injury, as is seen with stroke[26–29] or basal ganglia pathology.[30–36] The neuropsychiatry of these frontal subcortical loops has been reviewed by Cummings.[37]

Massive white matter tracts subserve frontocortical connections. Prefrontal cortex is unique in that it is the sole cortical area receiving highly processed sensory information of all modalities. The frontal lobes also participate in multiple distributed neurocognitive networks mediating attention, language, and memory.[38,39] The superior longitudinal fasciculus channels reciprocal information between prefrontal and parietal heteromodal cortices. Information from temporal heteromodal association cortex arrives through the uncinate bundle.

The granular prefrontal cortex has rich connections with the limbic system, particularly the posterior orbitofrontal cortex. Limbic connections contribute emotional and motivational relevance to incoming sensory information.[40] Livingston and Escobar[41] defined two frontolimbic circuits: 1) a medial system described by Papez[42] that includes brain stem reticular and hypothalamic information concerning the internal milieu and 2) a basolateral circuit, involving orbitofrontal cortex, dorsomedial thalamus, anterior temporal heteromodal association cortex, and amygdala, that processes sensory data concerning the external milieu.

Brain stem input to the prefrontal cortex involves primarily the reticular core via the thalamic reticular nucleus. This modulates the level of arousal for the entire cortex, providing a matrix for complex behavior.[43] Cortical tone is further modulated by the biogenic amine nuclei of the brain stem that project to the cortex via the median longitudinal fasciculus. The locus coeruleus and dorsal raphe nuclei provide noradrenergic and serotonergic input, respectively. A dopaminergic system involving the ventral tegmental area and substantia nigra provides input to the neostriatum, medial prefrontal area, cingulum, entorhinal areas and septum, olfactory tubercle, nucleus accumbens, amygdala, and piriform cortex. These constitute the mesocortical and mesolimbic systems.[44] Reciprocal corticofugal fibers modulate the firing patterns of these nuclei and serve to finely tune the regulation of arousal and cortical tone, possibly influencing the efficiency of all cortical functional systems.[45]

Finally, there is an extensive reciprocal innervation between the cerebellum and the cortical association areas, particularly the prefrontal and parietal heteromodal cortex.[46] Cortical neurons synapse in the basis pontis and then pass through the contralateral middle cerebellar peduncle to terminate in the cerebellar cortex.[47] The contribution of this corticopontine cerebellar system to executive cognition remains uncertain.[48]

The intricate and extensive connectivity of the prefrontal cortex establishes an anatomical basis for ongoing, goal-directed behavior. Highly processed sensory information arrives infused with emotional relevance, and the state of the internal milieu is constantly represented. Fine adjustments to the response threshold are possible. The groundwork is laid for a weighing of external demands and internal impulses in the service of the organism. Functionally, the frontal lobes cannot be considered as autonomous structures but must be conceived as one aspect of an executive system involving many structures of the central nervous system.

CLINICAL CHARACTERISTICS OF THE PREFRONTAL SYNDROMES

Although functional divisions within the prefrontal system (and its extensive connectivity) have been identified, in clinical practice, lesions are seldom confined to any one of these systems. Patients are therefore likely to manifest the clinical features of more than one of the symptom clusters described below. With this caveat in mind, three distinct prefrontal syndromes have been identified (Table 8–1).

Dorsal Convexity Dysexecutive Syndrome

The high-level cognitive functions mediated by the dorsolateral prefrontal lobe and its connections, which have been summarized by Milner and Petrides,[49]

TABLE 8–1.   Core characteristics of the regional prefrontal syndromes

Dysexecutive type (dorsal convexity system)	Disinhibited type (orbitofrontal system)	Apathetic type (mesial frontal system)
Diminished judgment, planning, insight, and temporal organization	Stimulus-driven behavior	Diminished spontaneity
Cognitive impersistence	Diminished social insight	Diminished verbal output (including mutism)
Motor programming deficits (may include aphasia and apraxia)	Distractibility	Diminished motor behavior (including akinesis)
Diminished self-care	Emotional lability	Urinary incontinence
		Lower extremity weakness and sensory loss
		Diminished spontaneous prosody
		Increased response latency

include cognitive flexibility, temporal ordering of recent events, planning, regulating actions based on environmental stimuli, and learning from experience. Patients with dysfunction in these cognitive domains are concrete and perseverative and show impairment in reasoning and mental flexibility.[50–52] In addition, such patients are characterized by a profound paucity in spontaneous behavior and will act only if acted upon. They therefore appear apathetic and are usually irritable when attempts are made to rouse them from their inertia. Although they may be able to perform within normal limits on tests that are designed to assess learned knowledge or sensorimotor skills (such as the Mini-Mental State Exam and the Wechsler intelligence and memory scales), they have difficulty on tests designed to assess their problem-solving skills (such as the Wisconsin Card Sorting Test and the Tower of London).[53] Their inability to appropriately maintain, prioritize, and redirect their attention results in the classic signs of distractibility, perseveration, and impersistence. Without the constant direction and structure of the interviewer (or their environment), they rapidly "lose set" and exhibit purposeless, disorganized behavior. Their difficulty in sequencing tasks is reflected in an inability to perform novel motor sequences such as those originally devised by Luria (such as three-step hand sequences and rhythm tapping).[54]

One such patient in our clinic who had experienced a severe closed head injury "solved" a Porteus Mazes Test by "making her own exit" and drawing a straight line out of the maze. This response was a dramatic metaphor for the numerous problems she experienced in daily life. She would do her laundry by placing the box of detergent in the washing machine with her clothes. She would occasionally wear her undergarments over her clothes if they had been laid out in the wrong order. She deduced that "money trees" exist because "money is green and so are leaves, so money

must grow on trees." In cold weather, she would wear a hat, scarf, sweater, and gloves and dress her dog similarly before walking it. She was formerly a hospital dietitian, but her cognitive processes had degenerated to Piaget's[55] preoperational subperiod, normally noted between ages 2 and 7 years. The apathy, environmental disregard, and personal disrepair of patients with dorsal convexity syndrome are frequently misinterpreted by clinicians as depression or as passive-aggressive and avoidant personality traits.[56]

The common denominator for the signs and symptoms found in this behavioral syndrome appears to be metacognitive disorganization. It may therefore be appropriate to name this symptom cluster the "prefrontal syndrome–dysexecutive type."

Orbitofrontal Disinhibition Syndrome

The orbitofrontal cortex rests on the coarse, bony orbital roof and is commonly subjected to contusion during acceleration/deceleration injury. The orbitofrontal cortex has discrete connections with the paralimbic cortex and thus plays a role in the elaboration and integration of limbic drives.[57] This area receives highly processed information about the individual's experience of an environmental stimulus and the anticipated consequences of various behavioral responses to it.[58] This process allows a person to maintain consistent behavior in keeping with his or her self-concept.

Patients with orbitofrontal damage have poor impulse control, explosive aggressive outbursts, inappropriate verbal lewdness, jocularity, and a lack of interpersonal sensitivity.[58] One such patient, who had a history of closed head injury, was evaluated after psychiatric admission for an impulsive drug overdose. Her conduct was inappropriate and her manner facetious. She undressed in front of the examiner and propositioned him, finding his discomfort humorous.

Perhaps the classic description of orbitofrontal disinhibition was published by Harlow[12] in 1868 following an evaluation of Phineas Gage, a construction foreman who blasted an iron tamping rod through his left frontal lobe:

> He is fitful, irreverent, indulging at times in the grossest profanity (which was not previously his custom), manifesting but little deference for his fellows, impatient of restraint or advice when it conflicts with his desires, at times pertinaciously obstinate, yet capricious and vacillating, devising many plans of future operation which are no sooner arranged than they are abandoned in turn for others appearing more feasible.

Such patients are often given diagnoses of mania or antisocial personality disorder despite the absence of neurovegetative signs of primary mood disorder or of a history of conduct disorder. These "pseudopsychopathic" behaviors inevitably result in a life characterized by downward social mobility and sporadic "crimes of passion," with numerous encounters with the legal system.

Because this syndrome is characterized primarily by impulse dyscontrol, it would be appropriate to describe it as the "prefrontal syndrome–disinhibited type."

Mesial Frontal Apathetic Syndrome

Mesial frontal pathology generally affects the functional balance between the cingulum and the supplementary motor area. These structures appear to participate in an exploratory system involving motivation and action.[59] Electrical stimulation of the cingulum induces wakefulness and arousal,[59] whereas stimulation of the supplementary motor area produces cessation of volitional activity, with a subjective sense of absence of the will to move.[60] Disconnection of cingulum input to the supplementary motor area may result in varying degrees of "release" of supplementary motor area activity, leading to a dysmotivational picture ranging from apathy to akinetic mutism. When present, an abulic syndrome will dominate a "mixed" type of dysexecutive syndrome (J. Cummings, personal communication, 1993).

These patients often appear depressed, yet they lack the dysphoria, negative cognitions, and neurovegetative signs of a major depression. Their indifference may be misconstrued as willful behavior, resulting in strained relationships. One patient, after a gunshot wound to both frontal lobes, was essentially inert when left alone. When questioned, he related an awareness of a personality change. He denied boredom and described it as a "loss of motivation" in that he entertained numerous ideas for activities but felt no impetus to act on them. His facial expression was one of casual indifference, and he would often respond with simple gestures instead of speaking.

Considering that the predominant characteristic of this syndrome is hypokinesis, it would be appropriate to describe it as the "prefrontal syndrome–apathetic type."

ETIOLOGY OF THE DYSEXECUTIVE SYNDROMES

The syndromes described above may be produced by lesions occurring anywhere within the extended neuronal network subserving executive cognition. Injuries to the different structures within this complex system produce various degrees of behavioral dysfunction. For example, even small lesions in the head of the caudate are likely to produce marked deficits in executive cognition. Conversely, relatively large areas of frontal ablation may result in relatively minor behavioral deficits.

An understanding of the anatomical hierarchical system subserving executive cognition is helpful when attempting to determine the etiology of a patient's regional prefrontal syndrome. Table 8–2 provides an anatomically based outline of the multiple causes of the different regional prefrontal syndromes.

An extensive discussion of the multiple causes of a dysexecutive syndrome is beyond the scope of this chapter. However, a brief discussion of the clinical disorders associated with lesions at different levels of the hierarchy will be helpful to the clinician.

Cortical

The vast expanse of the prefrontal cortex is particularly vulnerable to trauma. In particular, the orbitomediofrontal cortex is vulnerable to damage during a closed head injury. It is unusual, however, for injury to be localized to this region of the prefrontal cortex, and most significant prefrontal injury also will involve the dorsal convexity regions. In addition, severe trauma also may produce diffuse axonal injury that disrupts frontosubcortical connections and further compounds the severity of the dysexecutive syndrome.

The frontotemporal dementias are a heterogeneous group of neurodegenerative disorders characterized

TABLE 8–2. Etiology of the dysexecutive syndromes

Pathology	Cortical	White matter	Neuroanatomical site Thalamic	Striatal	Other
Degenerative	Frontotemporal dementias Pick's disease Advanced Alzheimer's disease FLD/motor neuron disease	Progressive subcortical gliosis	Primary degenerative syndromes	Huntington's disease Parkinson's disease Progressive supranuclear palsy Neuroacanthocytosis	
Traumatic	Focal Closed head injury Iatrogenic	Closed head injury		Dementia pugilistica	
Cerebrovascular	CVA Ruptured ACA aneurysm	Subcortical encephalomalacia	CVA (anterior and medial dorsal nuclei)	Lacunar state	? Pontine lesions Ventral tegmental lesions ? Cerebellar lesions
Toxic/other	Alcoholic dementia Anoxia Tumor Hydrocephalus	Demyelinating diseases (e.g., MS, infectious, diffuse axonal injury, radiation, methotrexate) AIDS-related dementia Hydrocephalus Toluene	Wernicke-Korsakoff syndrome	Wilson's disease Carbon monoxide and manganese poisoning (globus pallidus)	Disruption of the medial longitudinal fasciculus (e.g., craniopharyngioma)

Note. FLD=frontal lobe dementia; CVA=cerebral vascular accident; ACA=anterior communicating artery; MS=multiple sclerosis.

clinically by a progressive decline in executive cognition. The clinical and neuropsychological features of these dementing disorders are therefore distinct from Alzheimer's disease.[61] Although Pick's disease is the most commonly known (and therefore most often clinically diagnosed) type of frontotemporal dementia, neuropathological studies suggest that it is an unusual cause of this type of dementia.[61] Various terms have been used to describe this "non-Pick's" dementing illness, including *frontal lobe dementia*,[61] *dementia of the frontal lobe type*,[62] and *dementia lacking distinctive neuropathological features*.[63] The disease has a nonspecific pathological picture consisting of neuronal loss, gliosis, and superficial cortical spongy degeneration.[62] As one would expect, patients with frontal lobe dementia typically have disorders in executive functioning, personality change, apathy, and irritability. Unfortunately, this constellation of signs and symptoms is frequently misinterpreted as indicating a primary psychiatric disorder such as depression or sociopathy.

Chronic and significant alcohol abuse may produce prominent executive deficits and diminished prefrontal metabolism.[64] Fortunately, subsequent abstinence from alcohol is likely to be associated with a prompt improvement in cognition.[64] Although Alzheimer's disease predominantly affects the temporoparietal cortex, histopathological, neuropsychological, and functional imaging studies found that the frontal lobe is also frequently included in the pathophysiology of this disease process.[65]

Cerebrovascular lesions involving the prefrontal cortex may produce secondary mood disorders. Lesions close to the left prefrontal pole are likely to produce a secondary depressive disorder, whereas right anterior lesions may produce anosognosia. Secondary mania has most often been reported with right frontotemporal lesions.[58] Rupture of an anterior communicating artery aneurysm will likely produce orbitomesiofrontal deficits, with a behavioral disorder characterized by apathy and disinhibition.[66]

White Matter

The disruption of ascending and descending projections to and from the prefrontal cortex will result in a functional disconnection of the distributed neural system subserving executive cognition. Any subcortical white matter disease (such as multiple sclerosis, HIV encephalopathy, or diffuse axonal injury) may produce a constellation of varied cognitive deficits, including but not limited to the executive cognitive system. The neuropsychological significance of subcortical microvascular disease remains controversial, but it does appear that severe disease is likely to produce a dysexecutive syndrome.[67]

Thalamic

The mediodorsal and anterior nuclei of the thalamus are the thalamic members of the frontosubcortical circuitry.[24] Vascular or degenerative disorders involving these thalamic nuclei are likely to result in typical dysexecutive syndromes. The most common etiology of thalamic injury is Wernicke-Korsakoff syndrome, which is characterized by periventricular hemorrhagic microinfarcts that frequently affect the dorsomedial nucleus of the thalamus.[68] The diencephalic and mediothalamic distribution of these lesions explains the classic amnesia, confabulation, and dysexecutive syndrome that characterize this disorder.[68] Finally, craniopharyngiomas, obstructive hydrocephalus, and tumors in the region of the third ventricle may cause destruction to the medial thalamus, globus pallidus, and ventral striatum.[69]

Subcortical

Each of the five parallel circuits that constitute the frontal subcortical pathways includes the frontal lobes, neostriatum, globus pallidus, substantia nigra, and thalamus.[37] Projections are progressively focused onto fewer and fewer neurons as they pass from cortical to subcortical sites.[37] The dorsolateral prefrontal cortex projects to the dorsolateral caudate, the orbitofrontal cortex projects to the ventromedial region of the caudate, and the anterior cingulate gyrus projects to the ventral striatum and nucleus accumbens.[37] Although focal lesions are very rarely restricted to just one part of the striatum, Mendez et al.[29] described patients whose disorganized or disinhibited clinical syndromes correlated with dorsal and ventral lesions, respectively. The most common neurological disorder affecting the caudate is Huntington's disease, in which the patient's cognitive and behavioral abnormalities correspond to dysfunction in corticostriatal connections.[37] Lacunar infarcts occasionally may produce focal striatal lesions. Many patients with Parkinson's disease are likely to show dysexecutive symptoms, primarily of the disorganized type, secondary to a reduction in the dopamine input to this prefrontal cortical system.[70] Finally, the rare neurodegenerative syndrome neuroacanthocytosis primarily involves the caudate nucleus and produces a classic dysexecutive syndrome.[71]

Although relatively rare, focal lesions of the globus pallidus have been reported following carbon monoxide poisoning, manganese intoxication, and vascular insult.[72,73] Patients with globus pallidus lesions may have any of the typical dysexecutive syndromes.

Cerebellar Lesions

The cerebellum's contribution to executive cognition is the focus of recent research. As described earlier in this chapter, there are considerable corticopontocerebellar connections linking the parietal, temporal, and prefrontal association cortices. Lesions of the cerebellar hemispheres reportedly result in executive cognitive defects characterized by diminished insight, planning, and associative learning. Focal pontine lesions that disconnect cortical and cerebellar structures may theoretically produce a dysexecutive syndrome.[74–76]

Ventral Tegmentum

Although the disruption of mesocortical projections has long been considered an important contributor to the dysexecutive clinical features of Parkinson's disease, the widespread nature of neuropathological changes in this disorder has made it difficult to assign these clinical features to any one site. Recently, however, Adair et al.[77] reported on a patient who had apathy and executive cognitive deficits following a ventral tegmental lesion.

CONCLUSIONS

We have attempted to outline a theoretical approach to executive cognition that has clinical utility. An understanding of the distributed neuronal networks subserving executive cognition enables the clinician to develop a reasoned approach to the evaluation and treatment of the dysexecutive disorders. In this regard, a clinical nosology that distinguishes among three different regional prefrontal syndromes will facilitate the more effective diagnosis and management of these common disorders.

REFERENCES

1. Barris RW, Schuman HR: Bilateral anterior cingulate gyrus lesions. Neurology 3:44–52, 1953
2. Gentilini M, De Renzi E, Crisi G: Bilateral paramedian thalamic artery infarcts: report of eight cases. J Neurol Neurosurg Psychiatry 50:900–909, 1987
3. Ross ED, Stewart RM: Akinetic mutism from hypothalamic damage: successful treatment with dopamine agonists. Neurology 31:1435–1439, 1981
4. Moossy J, Martinez J, Hamin I, et al: Thalamic and subcortical gliosis with dementia. Arch Neurol 44:510–513, 1987
5. Goldman-Rakic PS: Topography of cognition: parallel distributed networks in primate association cortex. Annu Rev Neurosci 11:137–156, 1988
6. Finger S: Origins of Neuroscience. New York, Oxford University Press, 1994
7. Clarke E, Dewhurst K: An Illustrated History of Brain Function. Berkeley, CA, University of California Press, 1968
8. Lanfranchi G: Chirurgia Magna (c. 1300). London, Marsh, 1565
9. Platter F: Observatinum…Libri Tres. Basel, Switzerland, König, 1614
10. Swedenborg E: The Brain, Considered Anatomically, Physiologically, and Philosophically. London, Speirs, 1882–1887
11. Cruvelhier J: L'Anatomie Pathologique du Corps Humain. Paris, France, J B Balliere, 1829–1842
12. Harlow JM: Recovery after severe injury to the head. Publication of the Massachusetts Medical Society 2:327–346, 1868
13. Ferrier D: The Gulstonian lectures of localization of cerebral disease. BMJ 1:397–402, 1878
14. Bianchi L: The functions of the frontal lobes. Brain 18:497–530, 1895
15. Starr MA: Cortical lesions of the brain: a collection and analysis of the American cases of localized cerebral disease. Am J Med Sci 88:114–141, 1884
16. Sullivan HS. Editorial. Am J Psychiatry 100:228–229, 1949
17. Duffy JD: A means to an end—a history of psychosurgery, in The Search for the Magic Bullet. Edited by Duffy JD. Unpublished manuscript
18. Goldman-Rakic PS: Specification of higher cortical functions. J Head Trauma Rehabil 8:15–23, 1993
19. Baddeley AD: Working memory. Proceedings of the Royal Society of London 302:311–324, 1983
20. Fuster JM: The prefrontal cortex, mediator of cross-temporal contingencies. Human Neurobiology 4:169–179, 1985
21. Mesulam M: Large scale neurocognitive networks and distributed processing for attention, language, and memory. Ann Neurol 28:597–613, 1990
22. Damasio AR: The somatic marker hypothesis and the possible functions of the prefrontal cortex. Philos Trans R Soc Lond B Biol Sci 351:1413–1420, 1996
23. von Economo C: The Cytoarchitectonics of the Human Cerebral Cortex. New York, Oxford University Press, 1929
24. Alexander GE, Crutcher MD: Functional architecture of basal ganglia circuits: neural substrates of parallel processing. Trends Neurosci 13:266–271, 1990

25. Gerfen CR: The neostriatal mosaic: multiple levels of compartmental organization. Trends Neurosci 15:133–138, 1992

26. Sandson TA, Daffner KR, Carvalho PA, et al: Frontal lobe dysfunction following infarction of the left sided medial thalamus. Arch Neurol 48:1300–1303, 1991

27. Eslinger PJ, Warner GC, Grattan LM, et al: "Frontal lobe" utilization behavior associated with paramedian thalamic infarction. Neurology 41:450–452, 1991

28. Caselli RJ, Graff-Radford NR, Rezai K: Thalamocortical diaschisis: single photon emission tomographic study of cortical blood flow changes after focal thalamic infarction. Neuropsychiatry Neuropsychol Behav Neurol 4:193–214, 1991

29. Mendez MF, Adams NL, Lewandowski KS: Neurobehavioral changes associated with caudal lesions. Neurology 39:349–354, 1989

30. Flowers KA, Robertson C: The effect of Parkinson's disease on the ability to maintain a mental set. J Neurol Neurosurg Neuropsychiatry 48:517–529, 1985

31. Perlmutter JS, Raichle ME: Regional blood flow in hemiparkinsonism. Neurology 55:1127–1134, 1985

32. Wolfson LI, Leenders KL, Brown LL, et al: Alterations of regional cerebral blood flow and oxygen metabolism in Parkinson's disease. Neurology 35:1399–1405, 1985

33. Kuhl DE, Phelps ME, Markham CH, et al: Cerebral metabolism and atrophy in Huntington's disease determined by 18F-FDG and computed tomographic scan. Ann Neurol 12:425–434, 1982

34. Weinberger DR, Berman KF, Iadarda M, et al: Prefrontal cortical blood flow and cognitive function in Huntington's disease. J Neurol Neurosurg Psychiatry 51:94–104, 1988

35. DeVolder AG, Francart J, Dooms G, et al: Decreased glucose utilization in the striatum and frontal lobe in probable striatonigral degeneration. Arch Neurol 26:239–247, 1989

36. Blin J, Baron JC, Dubois B, et al: Positron emission tomography study in progressive supranuclear palsy: brain hypometabolic pattern and clinicometabolic correlations. Arch Neurol 47:747–752, 1990

37. Cummings SJ: Frontal subcortical circuits and human behavior. Arch Neurol 50:873–880, 1993

38. Mesulam M-M: A cortical network for directed attention and unilateral neglect. Ann Neurol 10:309–325, 1981

39. Morecraft RJ, Guela C, Mesulam M: Architecture of connectivity within a cingulo-frontal-parietal neurocognitive network for directed attention. Arch Neurol 50:279–284, 1993

40. Mesulam M-M: Frontal cortex and behavior. Ann Neurol 19:320–324, 1986

41. Livingston KE, Escobar A: Tentative limbic system models for certain patterns of psychiatric disorders, in Surgical Approaches in Psychiatry. Edited by Laitenen VL, Livingston LE. Baltimore, MD, University Park Press, 1973

42. Papez JW: A proposed mechanism of emotion. Archives of Neurology and Psychiatry 38:725–743, 1937

43. Moruzzi G, Magoun HW: Brainstem reticular formation and activation of the EEG. Electroencephalogr Clin Neurophysiol 1:459–473, 1949

44. Bjorkland A, Lindvall O: Dopamine containing systems in the CNS, in Handbook of Clinical Neuroanatomy, Vol 2: Classical Transmitters in the CNS, Part I. Edited by Bjorkland A, Hokfelt T. Amsterdam, The Netherlands, Elsevier, 1984

45. Mesulam M-M: Principles of Behavioral Neurology. Philadelphia, PA, FA Davis, 1985

46. Schmahmann JD: An emerging concept: the cerebellar contribution to higher cognition. Arch Neurol 48:1178–1187, 1991

47. Allen GI, Tsukuhara N: Cerebrocerebellar communication systems. Physiol Rev 54:957–1008, 1974

48. Leiner HC, Leiner AL, Dow RS: Reappraising the cerebellum: what does the hindbrain contribute to the forebrain? Behav Neurosci 103:998–1008, 1989

49. Milner B, Petrides M: Behavioral effects of frontal-lobe lesions in man. Trends Neurosci 7:403–407, 1984

50. Benton AL: Differential behavioral effects in frontal lobe disease. Neuropsychologia 6:53–60, 1986

51. Paradiso S, Chemerinski E, Yazici KM, et al: Frontal lobe syndrome reassessed: comparison of patients with lateral or medial frontal brain damage. J Neurol Neurosurg Psychiatry 67:664–667, 1999

52. Filley CM, Young DA, Reardon MS, et al: Frontal lobe lesions and executive dysfunction in children. Neuropsychiatry Neuropsychol Behav Neurol 12:156–160, 1999

53. Shallice T, Burger PW: Deficits in strategy application following frontal lobe damage in man. Brain 114:727–741, 1991

54. Luria AR: Human Brain and Psychological Processes. New York, Harper & Row, 1966

55. Piaget J: The Early Growth of Logic in the Child. New York, WW Norton, 1969

56. Grace J, Stout JC, Malloy PF: Assessing frontal lobe behavioral syndromes with the frontal lobe personality scale. Assessment 6:269–284, 1999

57. Gallagher M, McMahan RW, Schoenbaum G: Orbitofrontal cortex and representation of incentive value in associative learning. J Neurosci 19:6610–6614, 1999

58. Malloy PF, Duffy JD: The frontal lobes in neuropsychiatric disorders, in Handbook of Neuropsychology, Vol 8. Edited by Boller F, Spinnler H. New York, Elsevier, 1992, pp 203–232

59. Parent A: Extrinsic connections of the basal ganglia. Trends Neurosci 13:254–258, 1990

60. Penfield W, Welch K: Supplementary motor area of cortex; clinical and experimental study. Archives of Neurology and Psychiatry 66:289–317, 1951

61. Brun A: Frontal lobe degeneration of the non-Alzheimer type, I: neuropathology. Archives of Gerontology and Geriatrics 6:193–208, 1987

62. Neary D, Snowden JS, Northen B, et al: Dementia of the frontal lobe type. J Neurol Neurosurg Psychiatry 51: 353–361, 1988

63. Knopman DS, Mastri AR, Frey WH, et al: Dementia lacking distinctive histologic features: a common non-Alzheimer type degenerative dementia. Neurology 40:251–260, 1990

64. Lishman WA: Alcohol and the brain. Br J Psychiatry 156:635–644, 1990

65. Kemper T: Neuroanatomical and neuropathological changes in normal aging and dementia, in Clinical Neurology of Aging. Edited by Albert ML. New York, Oxford University Press, 1984

66. Freedman M, Oscar-Berman M: Bilateral frontal lobe disease and selective delayed-response deficits in humans. Behav Neurosci 100:337–342, 1986

67. Salloway S, Malloy P, Kohn R, et al: MRI and neuropsychological diferences in early- and late-life onset geriatric depression. Neurology 6:157–174, 1996

68. Victor M, Adama RD, Collins GH: The Wernicke-Korsakoff syndrome. Philadelphia, PA, FA Davis, 1989

69. Lavy S: Akinetic mutism in a case of craniopharyngioma. Psychiatric Neurology 138:369–374, 1959

70. Litvan I, Mohr E, Williams J, et al: Differential memory and executive functions in demented patients with Parkinson's disease and Alzheimer's disease. J Neurol Neurosurg Psychiatry 54:25–29, 1991

71. Wyszynski B, Merriam A, Medalia A, et al: Choreoacanthocytosis: report of a case with psychiatric features. Neuropsychiatry Neuropsychol Behav Neurol 2:137–144, 1989

72. LaPlane D, Baulac M, Wildacher D, et al: Pure psychic akinesia with bilateral lesions of the basal ganglia. J Neurol Neurosurg Psychiatry 47:377–385, 1984

73. Mena I, Marin O, Fuenzalida S, et al: Chronic manganese poisoning. Neurology 17:128–136, 1967

74. Duffy JD, Johnson J, Richardson E: Postulating a cortico-ponto-cerebellar disconnection syndrome. Poster presented at the annual meeting of the American Neuropsychiatric Association, Newport, RI, July 1994

75. Schmahmann JD, Sherman J: The cerebellar cognitive affective syndrome. Brain 121:561–579, 1998

76. Winn P: Frontal syndrome as a consequence of lesions in the pedunculopontine tegmental nucleus: a short theoretical review. Brain Res Bull 47:561–563, 1998

77. Adair JC, Williamson DJ, Schwartz RL, et al: Ventral tegmental area injury and frontal lobe disorder. Neurology 46:842–843, 1996

9

Assessment of Frontal Lobe Functions

Paul F. Malloy, Ph.D., Emily D. Richardson, Ph.D.

In this chapter, we describe methods for conducting a thorough assessment of functions subserved by frontal lobe systems. In all evaluations of neuropsychological functioning, the skilled practitioner must be guided by a theoretical model of brain systems and their characteristic disturbances by various diseases. In no area is this more important than in assessment of frontal lobe functions, given their highly complex nature. To set the stage for discussion of assessment techniques, this chapter therefore begins with a brief discussion of frontal lobe subsystems (this topic is covered in detail by the other contributors to this section) and the effects of lesions on these subsystems. We then describe both bedside and psychometric methods of assessing these deficits.

OVERVIEW OF FRONTAL LOBE SYSTEMS

Historically, frontal lobe functions have been poorly understood by many clinicians. Past clinical descriptions of behavior consequent to frontal lesions have been dramatic and evocative but have generally lacked the anatomical-clinical correlations necessary for complete understanding of these syndromes. The historical use of the generic term *frontal lobe syndrome,*

for example, fails to account for the diversity of frontal lobe functions.

Situated as they are at the pinnacle of human brain-behavior relationships, frontal functions are complex and difficult to describe, and only recently have researchers clearly elucidated frontal subsystems. Through the efforts of both animal and human researchers over the past three decades,[1,2] our understanding of frontal lobe functions has improved dramatically. Several functional subdivisions now have been identified: the *primary motor* area, the *premotor* area, the *frontal eye fields,* the *dorsolateral prefrontal* area, the *orbital prefrontal* area, and a medial area composed of the *supplementary motor area* and *anterior cingulate gyrus.*

Each of these frontal zones has extensive connections with posterior cortical and subcortical structures (particularly certain thalamic nuclei and the basal ganglia). As Mega and Cummings have illustrated in Chapter 3 in this volume, frontal cortical zones act in concert with these other structures to form frontal lobe subsystems. Lesions at any level of these subsystems can disrupt the functioning of the frontal system to which it contributes. In the remaining sections of this chapter, we describe the functions of each frontal subsystem, the effects of lesions on complex behavior, and both informal clinical and formal psychometric methods of assessing dysfunction in each subsystem.

MOTOR SUBSYSTEM

The motor area (Brodmann's area 4) is critical to pyramidal motor functions, that is, control of fine motor movement. The motor area receives projections from posterior cortical areas (especially in the primary tactile area of the parietal lobe) involved in somatosensory perception, as well as subcortical input from the ventral lateral thalamic nucleus. Primary motor output travels via the internal capsule to the pyramidal tracts.

Large lesions to the motor area result in flaccid hemiplegia in the contralateral side of the body, which typically resolves into spastic hemiplegia. Less severe lesions to the primary motor area or its connections may result in weakness (hemiparesis) and incoordination rather than frank paralysis.

The clinician can test basic motor functions at the bedside via the familiar maneuvers of the elementary neurological examination. Of course, motor deficits also may be a result of lesions to the cerebellum, extrapyramidal system, or descending white matter tracts, and the clinician must interpret results from the tests that follow in the context of the entire examination. Motor strength can be tested by having the patient squeeze the examiner's fingers and then attempting to extricate them. This allows the comparison of the relative strengths of the two hands, which should be approximately equal (i.e., it should be difficult or impossible to remove the fingers from the grasp of either hand of most healthy adults). Motor speed and dexterity can be assessed by having the patient perform rapid movements with the hands and feet.

Neuropsychological tests of motor abilities often consist of standardization of the neurological examination maneuvers. For example, the Reitan Grip Strength test[3] uses a dynamometer to assess the strength of each hand precisely. Similarly, fine motor speed can be measured precisely with the Finger Tapping Test,[3] which counts the average number of taps made with the index finger during several 10-second trials. As with all standardized neuropsychological tests, the availability of norms allows the neuropsychologist to detect subtle asymmetries that may elude the bedside examiner and to correct for handedness, sex, and age. This can be very important in that most women have significantly lower grip strength than men,[4,5] and motor speed declines with age.[6,7]

PREMOTOR SUBSYSTEM

The premotor area (Brodmann's area 6) is involved in sensorimotor integration and in complex volitional movement or praxis. The premotor area has connections with secondary somatosensory areas in the parietal lobe and (to a lesser extent) with primary somatosensory areas.[8] It has connections with the ventral anterior nucleus of the thalamus, with extrapyramidal motor structures (especially the caudate nucleus), and with the primary motor area. Hence, it is well positioned to modify motor plans in a dynamic way on the basis of changing sensory, motor tone, and postural feedback.

Lesions in the premotor area result in 1) the inability to use sensory feedback to modify movements smoothly and 2) apraxia. Sensorimotor abilities can be tested at the bedside by having the patient touch each finger to the thumb sequentially and observing for clumsiness, slowing, or inaccuracies. The test can be made more sensitive by requiring the patient to close his or her eyes, emphasizing the use of somatosensory rather than visual information to guide the movements. Luria[9] also has described a set of bedside assessment tasks that elegantly dissociate motor, sensory, and interhemispheric (or collosal) aspects of sensorimotor abilities. Luria's kinesthetic motor tasks involve the reproduction of finger positions, first with eyes open (to demonstrate intact unilateral motor abilities), then unilaterally with eyes closed (to demonstrate unilateral sensorimotor loops), and finally with eyes closed with the patient attempting to reproduce the passive position of one hand with the opposite hand (to demonstrate callosal transfer of sensory information from one hemisphere to the other).

Apraxia, in its strictest sense, is defined as the inability to carry out a motor movement or gesture to command. Apraxia is commonly found in association with left hemisphere lesions,[10] with frontal as well as nonfrontal localization.[11] Thus, the presence of apraxia should not be viewed as pathognomonic of frontal dysfunction, but praxis should be included in any comprehensive assessment of frontal abilities. The clinician can test praxis at the bedside by requiring the patient to perform single and serial limb, whole body, and facial movements. Movements should include transitive ("Show me how you use scissors"), intransitive symbolic ("Show me how you salute"), and nonsymbolic movements. To document the presence of an apraxia, the examiner must prove that the patient has the basic motor abilities to perform the movement. This can be done by requiring use of the same muscle groups in simpler movements during the formal examination and by observing the incidental movements of the patient on the unit (e.g., the patient spontaneously scratches an itch in the right eye but cannot point to the eye on command). Evidence suggests that the specialized motor system subserving praxis shares much cerebral territory with the language system; hence, apraxias are often found in combination with aphasia. The examiner therefore also must show that the patient understands the instruction for the movement in order to document an apraxia. Often, the patient will attempt a partial or distorted variant of the required movement. Requiring the patient to imitate gestures after failing to perform a command also can be useful in this regard, although this removes many of the ideational aspects of praxis from the task.

Clinicians unfamiliar with the assessment of praxis may wish to consult the Boston Diagnostic Aphasia Examination,[12] which includes a comprehensive set of maneuvers for assessing praxis among other supplementary, nonlanguage tests. Although several other apraxia examinations have been developed for experimental and clinical purposes,[10,13] none has truly psychometric properties or adequate norms. This is not crucial for most clinical applications because persons without apraxia can be expected to perform all common movements to command without error. Of course, the tasks may be failed for multiple reasons, such as disturbed attention in the delirious patient or failure of the aphasic patient to understand the command. The astute clinician must be prepared to devise tasks at the bedside to discriminate these deficits.

Various neuropsychological tests are available for studying other aspects of complex movement and its disturbances. The Purdue Pegboard[14] and the Grooved Pegboard[15] require the patient to place as many pegs into holes on a board as possible within a time limit. Both tests assess visuomotor coordination and speed, with the Grooved Pegboard adding the visuospatial demand of orienting the grooved pegs correctly in space so that they fit in the holes. The Motor Steadiness Battery is useful in patients with frontal subcortical systems disturbances such as Parkinson's disease. These tests permit the quantification of tremor in static postures and during intentional movement by counting the number of times an electrically wired stylus touches the sides of progressively smaller holes or grooves.

FRONTAL EYE FIELDS

The frontal eye fields (Brodmann's area 8) are necessary for voluntary gaze and visual search. The frontal eye fields permit volitional eye movements in the contralateral visual field, but as with other frontal subsystems, this function is complex and involves integration with other brain regions. Crowne[16] argued that the frontal eye fields may play a role in directing complex attention, particularly during defensive maneuvers or pursuit of a target. Fuster[17] has similarly suggested that the frontal eye fields integrate "a running blend of current sensory input with prospective information by which the eye field continuously adjusts the motor apparatus and sensory mechanisms in order to ensure coherence in both perception and movement" (p. 93). Studies also have suggested that the frontal eye fields act in concert with dorsolateral frontal zones in guiding eye movements during goal-directed behavior, especially when memory is involved.[18]

Lesions in the frontal eye fields result in transient ipsilateral eye deviation and more persistent contralateral gaze paresis. The patient may be capable of passively following the examiner's finger throughout both right and left hemispace (hence demonstrating that there is no neglect) but cannot move the eyes to the contralateral side to command or when engaged in active visual search. Secondary to these deficits in eye movement, the patient will be unable to efficiently pursue a target or actively search visual space.

The clinician also can test these functions with visual search stimuli consisting of a page of randomly arranged letters or symbols; the patient is required to find all occurrences of a target letter or symbol. Patients with frontal eye field lesions will be unable to actively search the side of the page contralateral to their lesion, although they will be capable of passive eye movements in the same visual field. The intactness of passive gaze distinguishes such patients from those with hemispatial neglect.

A patient's description of a complex figure such as the well-known "Cookie Theft" picture[12] can be revealing in regard to ability to organize a search of an entire stimulus. More complex search instruments with psychometric norms also have been developed. For example, in the Visual Search Test by Lewis and collaborators,[19] the patient is required to match a checkerboard pattern presented in the center of a page with its twin from a set of patterns around the page.

DORSOLATERAL PREFRONTAL SUBSYSTEM

The dorsolateral subsystem is responsible for executive functions. The dorsolateral area has extensive connections with the posterior tertiary association cortex and hence is the recipient of highly processed sensory information in all modalities. For example, the dorsolateral area receives extensive input from angular and supramarginal gyri, association areas involved in multimodal processing. Executive functions include integration of multimodal sensory input, generation of multiple response alternatives, maintenance of set and goal-directedness, modification of behavior as conditions change, and self-evaluation.

Lesions of the dorsolateral area result in 1) the inability to effortfully integrate disparate sensory elements into a coherent whole, 2) a stereotyped or limited response repertoire, 3) easy loss of task set, 4) perseveration and inflexibility, and 5) a lack of self-monitoring of errors. These executive functions have been the object of the most extensive study of all frontal lobe functions, and consequently there is a large armamentarium from which the neuropsychiatrist or neuropsychologist can draw for the psychometric assessment of executive abilities.

Royall et al.[20] developed a brief bedside test for measuring a variety of frontal lobe functions—the Executive Interview (EXIT). The EXIT includes tasks derived from several sources, including so-called frontal release signs from the neurological examination, abbreviated versions of neuropsychological tests such as word fluency, and Luria's techniques. Many of the tasks are cleverly arranged to elicit frontal executive dysfunction. For example, the patient is first asked to describe a picture of a cat climbing a tree and then asked to memorize the words "book, tree, house." The patient is next required to spell "cat" as a distraction task and finally to recall the three words after this brief delay. The recent exposure to the "tree-cat" picture and the interpolation of the word "cat" during the delay makes perseverative error of "cat" on recall likely. Validation of the EXIT to date has been limited largely to demonstrations that it is sensitive to cognitive changes in dementia[21] and the discrimination of cortical from subcortical dementias when used with other brief screening instruments.[22] Richardson et al.[23] provided preliminary evidence that individuals with chronic surgical frontal lesions perform in the more pathological range on the EXIT when compared with either Alzheimer-type dementia patients or psychiatric patients. However, these investigators suggested that these findings may have been confounded by level of care. In fact, Royall and colleagues[21] have shown that the EXIT is a good predictor of level of care required, independent of the neuroanatomical location of the pathology. Thus, the specificity of the EXIT in regard to frontal lesions remains to be demonstrated.

Poor integration of disparate pieces of sensory input can be measured by tests such as the Hooper Visual Organization Test[24] (HVOT). The HVOT presents the patient with pictures of common objects, such as a dog, that have been cut apart and rearranged on the page like a puzzle. The patient is required to put the pieces together mentally and determine what the object is. The patient with frontal lesions will be unable to initiate the active processing necessary to identify the complete object and will erroneously extrapolate from detail. Thus, one patient with a frontal convexity lesion identified the shape shown in Figure 9–1 from the HVOT as "Benjamin Franklin" because he fixated on the part of the figure on the lower left and failed to integrate the whole.

Similarly, Luria described a set of incomplete pictures[25] that are fragmented or out of focus, so that the patient must "fill in the blanks" to determine the identity of the object. Luria[9] also demonstrated that dorsolateral frontal lesions can result in visual search deficits of quite a different sort from those resulting from frontal eye field lesions. By actually measuring eye movements with a mechanical apparatus, he showed that patients with frontal lesions failed to formulate an effective plan for scanning a narrative picture, adopting instead one of two maladaptive strategies: 1) randomly searching all of the picture or 2) getting "stuck" on one salient aspect and making inappropriate extrapolations. For example, one of our patients viewed a picture of a man in a horse-drawn sleigh and exclaimed, "Oh, there is snow—that must be my uncle's farm in New Hampshire." He failed to actively search the remainder of the picture to confirm or disconfirm his idea.

Generation of multiple response alternatives can be measured by word and figure fluency tasks. The most widely used word fluency task is the Controlled Oral Word Association Test[26] (COWA). Ruff and his colleagues[27] showed that word fluency performance can be affected by nonfrontal deficits, such as auditory attention and word knowledge, but that prefrontal functions also can contribute to poor performance. This test requires the patient to produce as many words as possible in 1 minute beginning with F, then A, then S, while simultaneously maintaining a complex instruc-

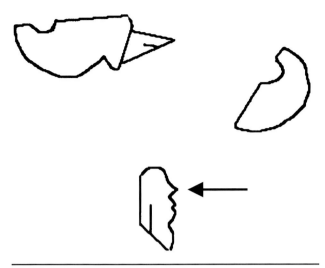

FIGURE 9–1. Stimulus from the Hooper Visual Organization Test.

Arrow indicates feature identified as "Benjamin Franklin" by a patient with a frontal lobe lesion.

tional set. Other categorical fluency tasks (i.e., naming animals, fruits, and vegetables) have been shown to be more sensitive and specific in detecting dementia,[28] but they may not tap executive functions to the same extent as the COWA. The COWA requires not only multiple response generation but also maintenance of a complex task set—-the words must not include proper names and must not consist of previously used words with a suffix. Second, the test presents the opportunity to observe perseverative and intrusion errors. A within-task perseveration consists of repeating a previous word on the same letter list without awareness or self-correction. Between-task perseverations consist of repeating words beginning with a previous letter. Intrusions consist of words that do not begin with any of the letters, usually caused by disinhibited associations (e.g., "at, after, apple, peaches, oranges,…"). In addition, the letters *F, A,* and *S* seem to "pull" for vulgar or socially inappropriate words used by frontal patients with disinhibitory deficits. We therefore routinely record not only the number of words produced but also the number of incorrect words according to the complex rules, number of perseverations, and number of socially inappropriate words.

A nonverbal or figural fluency task was developed by Jones-Gotman and Milner,[29] who reported that left frontal patients failed verbal fluency, but right frontal patients differentially failed figural fluency. Their version of the figural fluency task involves having the pa-

tient produce as many nonrepresentational drawings as possible in 5 minutes and then produce as many figures with four parts as possible in 4 minutes. However, clinicians have encountered some difficulty with reliable scoring of this test because of difficulty in determining whether a design is "different" or perseverative, and normative data have not been gathered to date. Ruff[30] therefore developed a figural fluency task incorporating some constraints to enhance reliability. In the Ruff Figural Fluency Test, the patient is required to draw a figure within a grid of lines, enhancing the examiner's ability to discern different and perseverative shapes. The Ruff Figural Fluency Test has been shown to be sensitive to right versus left frontal lesions,[31] and large-scale norms are available for adults.[32]

Lezak[33] developed another task that assesses generation of multiple response alternatives in a clever manner. In her Tinkertoy Test, the patient is presented with several pieces from the child's construction toy and instructed in a deliberately vague manner to make whatever he or she likes from the pieces. Subjects without frontal lesions or patients with posterior lesions typically will produce a reasonably complex, representational object such as a car, whereas the frontal syndrome patient will be able to produce only simple, unimaginative, and unnameable objects. Unstructured tests like the Tinkertoy Test can be useful in distinguishing patients with multiinfarct dementia from patients with Alzheimer's dementia, presumably because of the greater disruption of frontal systems in the patients with multiinfarct dementia.[34] Performance on the Tinkertoy Test also predicts ability to return to work in patients with head injury.[35]

Luria[9] has described several bilateral hand movements and alternating graphic sequences that theoretically require intact motor, premotor, and executive functions, particularly the ability to produce alternating response sets. Versions of these tasks are included in the Luria-Nebraska Neuropsychological Battery[25] and some other neuropsychological instruments such as the Dementia Rating Scale[36] and the Behavioral Dyscontrol Scale.[37]

Malloy and colleagues[38] reported that these tasks are performed more poorly by patients with focal frontal lesions than by patients with comparably sized posterior lesions. The technique that we use ensures that a response set is established and then changed and also that the task is sustained long enough to observe subtle executive dysfunction. On the reciprocal hand movements, the patient first must place one hand up and one hand down and then must reverse the hand positions, moving both hands simultaneously in a coordinated effort. Next, the patient must place one hand in an extended position and the other in a clenched position and then reverse the positions repeatedly. Finally, the patient must tap asymmetrical rhythms, twice with one hand and once with the other. The examiner notes how quickly and smoothly the patient performs the motions and observes certain pathognomonic errors: within-task perseverations (e.g., tapping three times rather than twice), cross-task perseverations (e.g., thrusting the hands as on the previous task rather than tapping with clenched fists), and oversimplifications (e.g., tapping twice with each hand rather than the required asymmetrical two-to-one pattern).

On alternating graphic sequences, we first require the patient to copy a pattern of two crosses and a circle repeatedly. After the patient completes one line of this pattern, the model is removed and the patient is asked to continue the pattern, increasing the demands of the task in regard to maintenance of set. Next, the patient is required to copy a more difficult pattern of alternating peaks and plateaus. Typical frontal errors include within-task perseverations (repeating too many crosses), cross-task perseverations (inserting crosses into the peaks and plateaus), oversimplifications (simply drawing a series of peaks rather than the alternating pattern), and intrusions of habitual responses (writing letters rather than the required pattern of shapes).

Figure 9–2 presents examples of typical errors by a patient with dementia of the frontal type[39,40] on these tasks. Note that the patient understands the task demands, and she is initially able to reproduce the figure correctly. Hence, her eventual failure is not due to language or basic construction deficits. After moving beyond the first model, however, she begins to oversimplify the figure from the asymmetrical ++0++0 to the simpler +0+0. Similarly, she begins to copy the second model correctly but then displays within-task perseverative errors (multiple peaks rather than alternating peaks and plateaus) as well as cross-task perseverations (crosses from the first task). Note also that her pattern is stimulus bound, gradually moving up to overlap the model.

The Wisconsin Card Sorting Test[41] (WCST) has been considered the premiere test of executive functions for many years. It taps a variety of executive abilities, including maintenance of task set, flexibility in response to feedback or changing circumstances, and perseverative tendencies. The WCST requires the patient to sort cards into piles under four sample cards that differ in color, form (shapes on the card), and number of shapes. The patient is not provided with these categories but must discern them based on feedback from the examiner. The "correct" category varies throughout the test, and measures are derived of ability to stick with the currently correct category and shift to the new category when appropriate. The WCST has been shown to be sensitive to effects of frontal lobe lesions in several studies.[42,43] Subjects without frontal lobe lesions have increased dorsolateral frontal metabolism/activation during WCST performance on quantified electroencephalogram, single photon emission computed tomography,[44,45] and functional magnetic resonance imaging.[46] However, negative findings also have been reported regarding the frontal specificity of the test.[47–49]

In his seminal book *Brain and Intelligence: A Quantitative Study of the Frontal Lobes*, Halstead[50] developed many of the tests that would come to constitute the Halstead-Reitan Neuropsychological Battery (HRNB). As the title of Halstead's book indicates, the frontal lobes were thought to provide the essential biological basis for intellectual activity. Although this would now be considered an oversimplification, many of the tests in the HRNB continue to be used as putative tests of frontal lobe functioning. The Category Test and Trail Making Test have generally been considered measures of abstraction, set maintenance, and cognitive flexibility. Hence, clinicians frequently use these tests as measures of dorsolateral frontal functions. However, research has indicated that these tests are multidimensional[51,52] and are failed by patients with nonfrontal as well as frontal lesions.[53–56]

Model   ++0++0

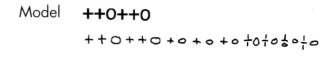

Model

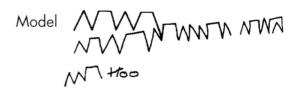

FIGURE 9–2.   Performance of a patient with dementia of the frontal type on Luria's Alternating Figures.

ORBITAL PREFRONTAL SUBSYSTEM

Few measures of orbitofrontal functions in humans exist. Clinicians may therefore have difficulty detecting common behavioral sequelae of orbitofrontal damage. However, review of the literature suggests that anosmia, disinhibited personality change, and failure on neuropsychological tests of inhibition are reliable signs of orbitofrontal dysfunction. Although these signs can occur with lesions of other brain areas, their presence together is highly suggestive of orbitofrontal damage.[57]

Smell discrimination is often omitted from the routine neurological examination, but the presence of anosmia in a variety of disorders with effects on frontal functions makes this a cardinal error. For example, anosmia, often an early sign of degenerative dementia, is common in Korsakoff's syndrome[58] and is seen in nearly 90% of the patients who have undergone repair of anterior cerebral aneurysms.[59] Loss of smell abilities is frequently seen in frontal traumatic insult,[60,61] particularly right orbitofrontal damage.[62] Assessment of smell by clinicians is also important in that orbitofrontal dysfunction has dire prognostic implications. For example, head-injured patients with anosmia have poorer social and vocational outcomes than patients without this evidence of orbital damage.[63]

Anosmia can be assessed clinically by having the patient identify common aromatic substances such as coffee, tobacco, or cocoa. Volatile or irritating substances should be avoided so that the anosmic patient cannot identify them based on trigeminal stimulation. Psychometric assessment of smell discrimination is possible with the University of Pennsylvania Smell Identification Test,[64] which provides 40 "scratch-and-sniff" items with age-corrected norms. Norms are essential in smell assessment when the patient is not completely anosmic because major declines in smell thresholds occur with normal aging.[64–66] The examiner also must keep in mind the myriad medical causes of reduced smell discrimination, such as infections of the nasal passages, smoking, and medication use.[66]

Disinhibited or socially inappropriate behavior can be observed informally on the treatment unit, and family reports always should be sought. Orbitofrontal patients may show behaviors such as facetious humor, inappropriate sexual behavior (e.g., open masturbation, sexual overtures to strangers), and labile emotionality. Disinhibited and socially problematic behaviors may reach proportions resembling antisocial personality disorder in some patients with orbital lesions.[67] We

have developed a psychometric instrument for assessing changes in behavior due to frontal dysfunction—the Frontal Lobe Personality Scale (FLOPS). Patient, staff and family versions of the instrument have been developed, with the expectation that frontal patients will be unaware of deficits that are readily apparent to their caregivers. Studies to date have found that the FLOPS can differentiate frontal lesions from posterior lesions,[68] subtypes of dementia with distinct behavioral features,[69] and behavioral changes after traumatic brain injury[70] and pallidotomy.[71]

Rosenkilde[72] reviewed animal research on frontal lobe function and concluded that animals with orbitofrontal lesions perform more poorly than animals with other lesions on go/no-go tasks. Go/no-go tasks require the subject to make a response to a *go* signal and withhold or inhibit the response to the *no-go* signal. The task can be made more difficult by changing the habitual meaning of the signals (e.g., *go* to a red light, *no-go* to a green light). A bedside example of this task can involve asking the patient to tap his or her fist when the examiner says "stop" and not tap when the examiner says "go." We have shown that healthy subjects display activation of the orbital cortex on topographic electroencephalogram during the inhibitory portion of a go/no-go task.[73] In that same study, patients with obsessive-compulsive disorder failed to show the same orbital activation, a finding that is consistent with functional neuroimaging studies showing orbital dysfunction in obsessive-compulsive disorder.[74,75]

SUPPLEMENTARY MOTOR AREA AND ANTERIOR CINGULATE GYRUS

Goldberg and Bloom[76] have argued that the supplementary motor area and anterior cingulate gyrus form a reciprocal system responsible for environmental search and inhibition of exploratory behavior. The cingulate gyrus appears to supply the drive for this environmental exploration, and the supplementary motor area appears to supply the inhibitory component. Hence, lesions to the anterior cingulate gyrus can result in akinetic mutism, in which the patient fails to respond to environmental stimuli and remains inert. Unilateral lesions usually result in transient akinesia, whereas bilateral lesions result in more permanent deficits.[77] Conversely, lesions to the supplementary motor area and corpus callosum result in the fascinating disorder known as "alien hand syndrome."[76] The patient with "alien hand" may grab objects, throw things, and otherwise explore the environment in a disinhibited manner. The patient feels as though he or she has no control over these movements, whereas in reality they are probably due to the actions of the right hemisphere in initiating actions while disconnected from the verbal left hemisphere. The dramatic syndromes of akinetic mutism and alien hand obviously require no special assessment techniques beyond the ability of the examiner to make the appropriate anatomical-clinical correlations.

The Stroop Test[78] is another task that places demands on inhibitory abilities as well as on sustained and directed attention. The published version of this test consists of three stimulus arrays. On the first page, the patient is required to read the words "red," "green," and "blue" printed in black ink in randomly ordered columns. On the second page, the patient must state the color of X's printed in red, green, or blue ink. The third page provides the critical interference trial: The patient is required to state the color of the ink, ignoring the word printed in that color. For example, the patient sees the word "red" printed in blue ink and must say "blue." Because the printed word is more salient than the color, the patient has to inhibit the tendency to say the word. Recent research has shown that both orbitofrontal and anterior cingulate frontal zones are activated in healthy subjects during the Stroop Test.[79–81]

"FRONTAL" ERRORS ON TESTS OF OTHER COGNITIVE FUNCTIONS

As Kaplan[82] has eloquently argued, how a patient approaches a task is frequently more informative than whether he or she fails the task. Hence, a "process approach" to test analysis can detect patterns of deficits not apparent in total scores. This is nowhere more true than in deficits due to frontal dysfunction, which impair higher order mental processes or "metacognition."

On memory testing, for example, the frontal patient often will show impoverished learning strategies, intrusions and perseverations,[83] poor retrieval strategies,[84] and difficulty with temporal tagging of learned information.[85] The California Verbal Learning Test (CVLT) provides an excellent tool for examining these process dimensions.[86] The CVLT involves the presentation of a 16-word list over five learning trials, with free, cued, and recognition recall of the original list after an interpolated interference list. Indices are provid-

ed for a number of learning and memory processes typically disturbed by frontal dysfunction. Hence, it is possible to observe the frontal patient producing a shallow learning curve across the five trials (due to inefficient encoding strategies), mixing up the first and second lists (due to problems in temporal tagging), showing inordinate gains from cued or recognition recall in comparison to free recall (due to inability to formulate a retrieval strategy), and producing large numbers of perseverations and intrusions. This is a markedly different pattern from the patient with Alzheimer's disease, for example, who typically will not benefit from cueing or recognition to any significant degree.

Delis and his collaborators[87] also developed a variation of the card-sorting technique, which allows the examiner to analyze qualitative or process aspects of problem-solving abilities. In its initial validation trial, the test was administered to four subject groups: 1) patients with focal frontal lobe lesions, 2) patients with both frontal dysfunction and amnesia (Korsakoff's syndrome), 3) patients with circumscribed (non-Korsakoff) amnesia, and 4) control subjects without dysfunction. The patients with frontal lobe lesions and patients with Korsakoff's syndrome were impaired on eight of the nine process components of the task. Qualitative analysis showed a wide spectrum of deficits in abstract thinking, cognitive flexibility, and use of knowledge to regulate behavior, all of which contributed to the problem-solving impairment in these patients.

Frontal patients often perform well on simple attentional tasks such as digits forward but make characteristic errors on complex attentional tasks requiring active manipulation of information. This deficit is often most apparent when the patient is required to overcome overlearned or habitual behavior patterns. For example, when asked to recite the days of the week backward, the frontal patient has difficulty reorganizing the information and returns to the habitual pattern in which the material is usually used: "Sunday, Saturday...Friday...Thursday...Friday, Saturday, Sunday."

This process approach can be applied to discriminating the effects of lesions to frontal subsystems. For example, Crowe[88] reported that qualitative analysis of errors on fluency tasks can be useful in discriminating orbital from other frontal lesions. Patients with orbitofrontal lesions produced more disinhibited responses on word fluency than did patients with dorsolateral frontal lesions. We commonly observe that patients with closed head injury and orbital damage produce vulgar or sexually oriented responses on the COWA, whereas patients with posterior lesions or psychiatric disorders do not.

GENERAL GUIDELINES FOR BEDSIDE ASSESSMENT

Although formal neuropsychological testing is a valuable diagnostic resource, the clinician must have some practical clinical tools that allow the sensitive evaluation of frontal functions at the bedside. It could be argued that the only truly valid assessment of executive functions can be obtained through the observation of an individual's behavioral response to the ambiguous and shifting challenges encountered in autonomous social behavior. Bearing this in mind, the clinician should seize every opportunity to observe the patient's ability to show insight, plan ahead, and execute effective strategies to different environmental challenges. For example, is the patient able to efficiently schedule an appointment and arrive at the clinician's office on time? Typically, the patient with executive deficits will require a third party to identify the necessity for the psychiatric intervention and plan his or her schedule. Similarly, the task of understanding one's medical insurance policy represents a considerable test of executive skills!

The physical appearance of the patient also may provide valuable clues. In extreme cases, frontal patients neglect personal hygiene, presenting with soiled clothes, unshaven face, and even incontinence about which they show no concern. In less severe cases, the observant examiner will note inappropriate attire such as a heavy jacket in summer, an unzipped fly, or a mismatched outfit.

The social demeanor of the patient is often revealing in regard to the disinhibited personality change discussed earlier in relation to the orbitofrontal subsystem. Such patients may become overly familiar with the examiner, asking inappropriately personal questions, making comments about the examiner's appearance, offering sexual overtures, or engaging in rude or embarrassing behavior. Emotional overreaction is also seen and often has a rapid on/off quality.

It is particularly important that the clinician appreciate his or her role in shaping the patient's behavior. For example, the interviewer may unconsciously compensate for a patient's apathy and cognitive disorganization, assuming a directive and paternal role and us-

ing only closed-ended questions. In other words, the examiner may "act as the patient's frontal lobes" and thereby miss important clues. The apparently simple task of describing one's presenting complaint in a cohesive and pertinent fashion places considerable demands on frontal functions such as insight, judgment, social sensitivity, and self-reflection. Indeed, patients with frontal lesions have been shown to be remarkably poor at providing coherent autobiographical information.[89] A detailed history that includes work, hobbies, daily routine, and interpersonal relationships will provide valuable information about the patient's ability to orchestrate his or her life. But the examiner must question family or caregivers as well because a discrepancy between patient and family report of problems is a hallmark of frontal lobe dysfunction.

Although the examiner must refrain from providing too much structure during the early stages of the examination, it can be equally useful to deliberately provide additional structure once it is established that frontal deficits exist. In this way, the clinician can show that the reason for failure lies in a dysexecutive syndrome rather than in more basic cognitive functions. For example, if one observes that the patient fails a complex construction task such as copying the Rey-Osterreith figure, it is often useful to provide a strategy to the patient ("Start with this big rectangle, and then draw these diagonal lines...") to see if performance then improves markedly.

From this discussion, it should be clear that the evaluation of frontal lobe functions should not be limited to the formal mental status examination. Executive functions provide an overarching or superordinate qualitative influence on the performance of virtually all mental processes. By the time the examiner begins the formal cognitive examination, he or she should have already obtained significant indications of the patient's capacities. All components of the mental status examination will then provide data about the patient's ability to effectively strategize, monitor, and adapt his or her cognitive behavior to changing circumstance and to evaluate his or her own performance.

EFFECTS OF AGE ON FRONTAL LOBE FUNCTIONS

Clinicians should be particularly cautious in assessing frontal lobe functions in children and the elderly. Evidence indicates that the frontal lobes do not fully mature until adolescence[90,91] and that children perform much more poorly than adults on most frontal lobe tests[92] (if indeed they are capable of understanding instructions). Conversely, research has clearly shown that loss of neurons is greater in the frontal lobes than in posterior areas with normal aging,[93] and frontal lobe functioning changes more than other abilities.[94] For example, performance on the WCST markedly declines with age[41]: the average 30-year-old produces only 10 perseverative errors on this task, whereas the average 70-year-old produces more than 20. In contrast, confrontational naming performance, dependent mainly on the posterior left hemisphere, appears to change little with age.[95] Even primitive behaviors such as so-called frontal release signs (glabellar, grasp, palmomental, snout, suck, root, and jaw jerk reflexes) are strongly affected by aging, with 40% of healthy individuals showing some of these signs after age 60.[96] Neuropsychological assessment is therefore extremely useful in children and the elderly because availability of norms allows age corrections.

LIMITATIONS TO LOCALIZATION OF FRONTAL FUNCTIONS

We have taken a highly localizational approach to frontal systems, which at minimum should provide a useful resource for clinicians to organize their thinking. However, it is important to recognize the limitations of any localizational model.

First, the examiner must remember that most complex behaviors require that various frontal subsystems act in concert to produce adaptive functioning. Sustained and directed attention is an example of an ability involving multiple frontal zones (including dorsolateral, orbital, and cingulate areas).[79,97] Utilization behavior is another example. In this condition, the patient automatically uses objects in his or her environment in a habitual way, regardless of whether this use is appropriate at the time. Lhermitte et al.[98] described a former nurse with frontal damage who spied a syringe in the examining room and attempted to inject the examiner with it. This emergence of habitual or high probability behavior in response to environmental stimuli has been reported with large bilateral frontal lesions,[99] mesial frontal lesions,[100] caudate infarction,[101] and thalamic infarction.[102] Thus, utilization behavior probably represents dysfunction in multiple frontal subsystems.

Second, many patients will show combinations of the frontal syndromes described above because natu-

rally occurring lesions damage multiple subsystems. This situation is found in most areas of neuropsychology, yet a theoretical schema remains essential in organizing the clinical examination. In aphasia, for example, an understanding of the localization and connections of the language system and aphasia subtypes is crucial, even though most patients have mixed aphasias rather than pure subtypes. This knowledge ensures that the examiner comprehensively assesses language abilities (fluency, comprehension, repetition, naming, reading, and writing), allows the examiner to make sense of the findings, and often yields behavioral data that can be correlated with neuroimaging.

Third, some deficits may be the result of either frontal or nonfrontal lesions. For example, abstract reasoning can be viewed as a measure of ability to shift mental set from the specific (i.e., more concrete or tangible) to the general (i.e., abstract) principle. It is often measured at the bedside via proverb interpretation or similarities. However, abstract reasoning is strongly dependent on innate intelligence and education, and most such complex abilities cannot be highly localized. Thus, although abstraction is very susceptible to the effects of injury involving frontal systems, poor ability to abstract is not specific to frontal injury.

In summary, the skilled clinician must be knowledgeable about frontal lobe subsystems and their roles in determining specific types of abnormal behavior. Bedside maneuvers can then be designed to discriminate dysfunction, and the clinician will be alerted to changes in incidental behavior that indicate frontal impairment. Neuropsychological assessment is an invaluable tool for testing frontal lobe functions because of the complexity of these behaviors and the profound effects of maturation and aging on frontal functions.

REFERENCES

1. Goldman-Rakic PS: Circuitry of the primate prefrontal cortex and regulation of behavior by representational memory, in Handbook of Physiology: the Nervous System: Higher Functions of the Brain, Vol 5, Sect 1. Edited by Plum F, Mountcastle V. Bethesda, MD, American Physiological Society, 1987, pp 373–417
2. Cummings JL: Frontal-subcortical circuits and human behavior. Arch Neurol 50:873–880, 1993
3. Reitan RM, Wolfson D: The Halstead-Reitan Neuropsychological Test Battery. Tucson, AZ, Neuropsychology Press, 1985

4. Kupke T, Lewis R, Rennick P: Sex differences in the neuropsychological functioning of epileptics. J Consult Clin Psychol 47:1128–1130, 1979

5. Fromm-Auch D, Yeudall LT: Normative data for the Halstead-Reitan Neuropsychological Tests. J Clin Exp Neuropsychol 5:221–238, 1983

6. Ernst J, Warner MH, Townes BD, et al: Age group differences on neuropsychological battery performance in a neuropsychiatric population: international descriptive study with replications. Archives of Clinical Neuropsychology 2:1–12, 1987

7. Villardita C, Cultrera S, Cupone V, et al: Neuropsychological test performances and normal aging. Archives of Gerontology and Geriatrics 4:311–319, 1985

8. Pandya DN, Barnes CL: Architecture and connections of the frontal lobe, in The Frontal Lobes Revisited. Edited by Perecman E. New York, IRBN Press, 1987, pp 41–72.

9. Luria AR: Higher Cortical Functions in Man. New York, Basic Books, 1980

10. DeRenzi E, Motti F, Nichelli P: Imitating gestures: a quantitative approach to ideomotor apraxia. Arch Neurol 37:6–10, 1980

11. Kolb B, Milner B: Performance of complex arm and facial movements after focal brain lesions. Neuropsychologia 19:491–503, 1981

12. Goodglass H, Kaplan E: The Assessment of Aphasia and Related Disorders. Philadelphia, PA, Lea & Febiger, 1972

13. Kertesz A: The Western Aphasia Battery. London, ON, Canada, University of Western Ontario, 1980

14. Foundation PR: Examiner's Manual for the Purdue Pegboard. Chicago, IL, Science Research Associates, 1948

15. Lafayette Instrument Company: Instructions for the Grooved Pegboard. Lafayette, IN, Lafayette Instrument Company

16. Crowne DP: The frontal eye fields and attention. Psychol Bull 93:232–260, 1983

17. Fuster JM: The Prefrontal Cortex: Anatomy, Physiology, and Neuropsychology of the Frontal Lobe. New York, Raven, 1980

18. Pierrot DC, Israel I, Berthoz A, et al: Role of the different frontal lobe areas in the control of the horizontal component of memory-guided saccades in man. Exp Brain Res 95:166–171, 1993

19. Lewis RF, Rennick PM: Manual for the Repeatable Cognitive-Perceptual-Motor Battery. Grosse Pointe Park, MI, Axon Publishing, 1979

20. Royall DR, Mahurin RK, Gray KF: Bedside assessment of executive cognitive impairment: the executive interview [see comments]. J Am Geriatr Soc 40:1221–1226, 1992

21. Royall DR, Mahurin RK, True JE, et al: Executive impairment among the functionally dependent: comparisons between schizophrenic and elderly subjects. Am J Psychiatry 150:1813–1819, 1993

22. Royall DR, Mahurin RK, Cornell J, et al: Bedside assessment of dementia type using the Qualitative Evaluation of Dementia. Neuropsychiatry Neuropsychol Behav Neurol 6:235–244, 1993

23. Richardson ED, Duffy J, Royall DR: Examination of a new bedside measure for assessment of executive dysfunction (abstract). J Neuropsychiatry Clin Neurosci 5:452–453, 1993

24. Hooper HE: The Hooper Visual Organization Test Manual. Beverly Hills, CA, Western Psychological Services, 1958

25. Golden CJ, Hammeke TA, Purisch AD: Manual for the Luria-Nebraska Neuropsychological Battery. Los Angeles, CA, Western Psychological Services, 1980

26. Benton AL: Differential behavioral effects in frontal lobe disease. Neuropsychologia 6:53–60, 1968

27. Ruff RM, Light RH, Parker SB, et al: The psychological construct of word fluency. Brain Lang 57:394–405, 1997

28. Monsch AU, Bondi MW, Butters N, et al: Comparisons of verbal fluency tasks in detection of dementia of the Alzheimer type. Arch Neurol 49:1253–1258, 1992

29. Jones-Gotman M, Milner B: Design fluency: the invention of nonsense drawings after focal cortical lesions. Neuropsychologia 15:653–674, 1977

30. Ruff RM: Ruff Figural Fluency Test Administration Manual. San Diego, CA, Neuropsychological Resources, 1988

31. Ruff RM, Allen CC, Farrow CE, et al: Figural fluency: differential impairment in patients with left versus right frontal lobe lesions. Archives of Clinical Neuropsychology 9:41–55, 1994

32. Ruff RM, Light R, Evans R: The Ruff Figural Fluency Test: a normative study with adults. Developmental Neuropsychology 3:37–51, 1987

33. Lezak M: Neuropsychological Assessment, 2nd Edition. New York, Oxford University Press, 1983

34. Mendez MF, Ashla-Mendez M: Differences between multi-infarct dementia and Alzheimer's disease on unstructured neuropsychological tasks. J Clin Exp Neuropsychol 13:923–932, 1991

35. Bayless JD, Varney NR, Roberts RJ: Tinker toy test performance and vocational outcome in patients with closed-head injuries. J Clin Exp Neuropsychol 11:913–917, 1989

36. Mattis S: Dementia Rating Scale Professional Manual. Odessa, FL, Psychological Assessment Resources, 1973

37. Grigsby J, Kaye K, Robbins LJ: Reliabilities, norms and factor structure of the Behavioral Dyscontrol Scale. Percept Mot Skills 74:883–892, 1992

38. Malloy PF, Webster JS, Russell W: Tests of Luria's frontal lobe syndrome. International Journal of Clinical Neuropsychology 7:88–94, 1985

39. Neary D, Snowden JS, Northen B, et al: Dementia of frontal lobe type. J Neurol Neurosurg Psychiatry 51:353–361, 1988

40. Rahman S, Sahakian BJ, Hodges JR, et al: Specific cognitive deficits in mild frontal variant frontotemporal dementia. Brain 122:1469–1493, 1999

41. Heaton RK, Chelune GJ, Talley JL, et al: Wisconsin Card Sorting Test Manual: Revised and Expanded. Odessa, FL, Psychological Assessment Resources, 1993

42. Milner B: Effects of different brain lesions on card sorting. Arch Neurol 9:90–100, 1963

43. Drewe EA: The effect of type and area of brain lesion on Wisconsin Card Sorting Test performance. Cortex 10:159–170, 1974

44. Tien AY, Schlaepfer TE, Orr W, et al: SPECT brain blood flow changes with continuous ligand infusion during previously learned WCST performance. Psychiatry Res 82:47–52, 1998

45. Marenco S, Coppola R, Daniel DG, et al: Regional cerebral blood flow during the Wisconsin Card Sorting Test in normal subjects studied by xenon-133 dynamic SPECT: comparison of absolute values, percent distribution values, and covariance analysis. Psychiatry Res 50:177–192, 1993

46. Volz HP, Gaser C, Hager F, et al: Brain activation during cognitive stimulation with the Wisconsin Card Sorting Test—a functional MRI study on healthy volunteers and schizophrenics. Psychiatry Res 75:145–157, 1997

47. van den Broek MD, Bradshaw CM, Szabadi E: Utility of the Modified Wisconsin Card Sorting Test in neuropsychological assessment. Br J Clin Psychol 32:333–343, 1993

48. Heck ET, Bryer JB: Superior sorting and categorizing ability in a case of bilateral frontal atrophy: an exception to the rule. J Clin Exp Neuropsychol 8:313–316, 1986

49. Axelrod BN, Goldman RS, Heaton RK, et al: Discriminability of the Wisconsin Card Sorting Test using the standardization sample. J Clin Exp Neuropsychol 18:338–342, 1996

50. Halstead WC: Brain and Intelligence: A Quantitative Study of the Frontal Lobes. Chicago, IL, University of Chicago Press, 1947

51. Golden CJ, Kushner T, Lee B, et al: Searching for the meaning of the Category Test and the Wisconsin Card Sort Test: a comparative analysis. Int J Neurosci 93:141–150, 1998

52. Allen DN, Goldstein G, Mariano E: Is the Halstead Category Test a multidimensional instrument? J Clin Exp Neuropsychol 21:237–244, 1999

53. Reitan RM: An investigation of the validity of Halstead's measures of biological intelligence. Archives of Neurology and Psychiatry 73:28–35, 1955

54. Reitan RM: Impairment of abstraction ability in brain damage: quantitative versus qualitative changes. J Psychol 9:211–215, 1959

55. Pendleton MG, Heaton RK: A comparison of the Wisconsin Card Sorting Test and the Category Test. J Clin Psychol 38:392–396, 1982

56. Klove H: Validation studies in adult clinical neuropsychology, in Clinical Neuropsychology: Current Status and Applications. Edited by Reitan RM, Davison LA. Washington, DC, VH Winston & Sons, 1974, pp 211–227

57. Malloy PF, Bihrle A, Duffy J, et al: The orbitomedial frontal syndrome. Archives of Clinical Neuropsychology 8:185–202, 1993

58. Jones BP, Butters NM, Moskowitz HR, et al: Olfactory and gustatory capacities of alcoholic Korsakoff patients. Neuropsychologia 16:323–338, 1978

59. Eriksen KD, Boge RT, Kruse LC: Anosmia following operation for cerebral aneurysms in the anterior circulation. J Neurosurg 72:864–865, 1990

60. Potter H, Butters N: An assessment of olfactory deficits in patients with damage to prefrontal cortex. Neuropsychologia 18:621–628, 1980

61. Yousem DM, Geckle RJ, Bilker WB, et al: Posttraumatic smell loss: relationship of psychophysical tests and volumes of the olfactory bulbs and tracts and the temporal lobes. Acad Radiol 6:264–272, 1999

62. Zatorre RJ, Jones-Gotman M: Human olfactory discrimination after unilateral frontal or temporal lobectomy. Brain 114 (pt 1A):71–84, 1991

63. Varney N: Prognostic significance of anosmia in patients with closed head trauma. J Clin Exp Neuropsychol 10:250–254, 1988

64. Doty RL: The University of Pennsylvania Smell Identification Test Administration Manual. Philadelphia, PA, Sensonics, 1983

65. Cain WS, Gent JF: Olfactory sensitivity: reliability, generality, and association with aging. J Exp Psychol Hum Percept Perform 17:382–391, 1991

66. Ship JA, Weiffenbach JM: Age, gender, medical treatment, and medication effects on smell identification. J Gerontol 48:26–32, 1993

67. Meyers CA, Berman SA, Scheibel RS, et al: Case report: acquired antisocial personality disorder associated with unilateral left orbital frontal lobe damage. J Psychiatry Neurosci 17:121–125, 1992

68. Grace J, Stout JC, Malloy PF: Assessing frontal lobe behavioral syndromes with the Frontal Lobe Personality Scale. Assessment 6:269–284, 1999

69. Paulsen JS, Stout JC, DelaPena J, et al: Frontal behavioral syndromes in cortical and subcortical dementia. Assessment 3:327–337, 1996

70. Cicerone K, Tanenbaum LN: Disturbance of social cognition after traumatic orbitofrontal brain injury. Archives of Clinical Neuropsychology 12:173–188, 1997

71. Trepanier LL, Saint-Cyr JA, Lozano AM, et al: Neuropsychological consequences of posteroventral pallidotomy for the treatment of Parkinson's disease. Neurology 51:207–215, 1998

72. Rosenkilde CE: Functional heterogeneity of the prefrontal cortex in the monkey: a review. Behavioral and Neural Biology 25:301–345, 1979

73. Malloy P, Rasmussen S, Braden W, et al: Topographic evoked potential mapping in obsessive-compulsive disorder: evidence of frontal lobe dysfunction. Psychiatry Res 28:63–71, 1989

74. Baxter LJ, Phelps ME, Mazziotta JC, et al: Local cerebral glucose metabolic rates in obsessive-compulsive disorder: a comparison with rates in unipolar depression and in normal controls. Arch Gen Psychiatry 44:211–218, 1987

75. Saxena S, Brody AL, Schwartz JM, et al: Neuroimaging and frontal-subcortical circuitry in obsessive-compulsive disorder. Br J Psychiatry 35 (suppl):26–37, 1998

76. Goldberg G, Bloom KK: The alien hand sign: localization, lateralization and recovery. Am J Phys Med Rehabil 69:228–238, 1990

77. Damasio AR, Van Hoesen GW: Emotional disturbances associated with focal lesions of the limbic frontal lobe, in Neuropsychology of Human Emotion. Edited by Heilman KM, Satz P. New York, Guilford, 1983, pp 85–110

78. Stroop JR: Studies of interference in serial verbal reactions. J Exp Psychol 18:643–662, 1935

79. Bench CJ, Frith CD, Grasby PM, et al: Investigations of the functional anatomy of attention using the Stroop test. Neuropsychologia 31:907–922, 1993

80. Peterson BS, Skudlarski P, Gatenby JC, et al: An fMRI study of Stroop word-color interference: evidence for cingulate subregions subserving multiple distributed attentional systems. Biol Psychiatry 45:1237–1258, 1999

81. Brown GG, Kindermann SS, Siegle GJ, et al: Brain activation and pupil response during covert performance of the Stroop Color Word Task. J Int Neuropsychol Soc 5:308–319, 1999

82. Kaplan E: The process approach to neuropsychological assessment of psychiatric patients. J Neuropsychiatry Clin Neurosci 2:72–87, 1990

83. Vilkki J: Perseveration in memory for figures after frontal lobe lesion. Neuropsychologia 27:1101–1104, 1989

84. Kopelman MD: Frontal dysfunction and memory deficits in the alcoholic Korsakoff syndrome and Alzheimer-type dementia. Brain 114:117–137, 1991

85. Shimamura AP, Janowsky JS, Squire LR: Memory for the temporal order of events in patients with frontal lobe lesions and amnesic patients. Neuropsychologia 28:803–813, 1990

86. Delis DC, Kramer JH, Kaplan E, et al: The California Verbal Learning Test: Research Edition. New York, Psychological Corporation, 1987

87. Delis DC, Squire LR, Bihrle A, et al: Componential analysis of problem-solving ability: performance of patients with frontal lobe damage and amnesic patients on a new sorting test. Neuropsychologia 30:683–697, 1992

88. Crowe SF: Dissociation of two frontal lobe syndromes by a test of verbal fluency. J Clin Exp Neuropsychol 14:327–339, 1992

89. Della SS, Laiacona M, Spinnler H, et al: Autobiographical recollection and frontal damage. Neuropsychologia 31:823–839, 1993

90. Yakolev PI, Lecours AR: The myelogenetic cycles of regional maturation of the brain, in Regional Development of the Brain. Edited by Minkowski A. Philadelphia, PA, FA Davis, 1967, pp 3–70

91. Passler MA, Isaac W, Hynd GW: Neuropsychological development of behavior attributed to frontal lobe functioning in children. Developmental Neuropsychology 1:349–370, 1985

92. Levin HS, Colhane KA, Hartmann J, et al: Developmental changes in performance on tests of purported frontal lobe functioning. Developmental Neuropsychology 7:277–396, 1991

93. Coffey CE, Wilkinson WE, Parashos IA, et al: Quantitative cerebral anatomy of the aging human brain: a cross-sectional study using magnetic resonance imaging. Neurology 42:527–536, 1992

94. Boone KB, Miller BL, Lesser IM: Frontal lobe cognitive functions in aging: methodologic considerations. Dementia 4:232–236, 1993

95. Van Gorp WG, Satz P, Kiersch ME, et al: Normative data on the Boston Naming Test for a group of normal older adults. J Clin Exp Neuropsychol 6:702–705, 1986

96. Jacobs L, Gossman MD: Three primitive reflexes in normal adults. Neurology 30:184–188, 1980

97. Bianchi A, Zolo P, Salmaso D: Effects of frontal lesions on a selective attention task. Ital J Neurol Sci 14:355–359, 1993

98. Lhermitte F, Pillon B, Serdaru M: Human autonomy and the frontal lobes, part I: imitation and utilization behavior: a neuropsychological study of 75 patients. Ann Neurol 19:326–334, 1986

99. Hoffmann MW, Bill PL: The environmental dependency syndrome, imitation behaviour and utilisation behaviour as presenting symptoms of bilateral frontal lobe infarction due to moyamoya disease. S Afr Med J 81:271–273, 1992

100. Shallice T, Burgess PW, Schon F, et al: The origins of utilization behaviour. Brain 112:1587–1598, 1989

101. Degos JD, da Fonseca N, Gray F, et al: Severe frontal syndrome associated with infarcts of the left anterior cingulate gyrus and the head of the right caudate nucleus: a clinico-pathological case. Brain 116:1541–1548, 1993

102. Eslinger PJ, Warner GC, Grattan LM, et al: "Frontal lobe" utilization behavior associated with paramedian thalamic infarction. Neurology 41:450–452, 1991

10

Diagnosis and Treatment of "Frontal Lobe" Syndromes

Stephen P. Salloway, M.D., M.S.

Impairment of frontal lobe functions is a common reason for admission to an inpatient neuropsychiatry service. A wide variety of clinical syndromes is seen, and many cases are difficult to diagnose and treat. Three common subtypes of frontal systems impairment seen in clinical practice can be defined in terms of the functional organization of the prefrontal cortex. In Chapter 8 in this volume, Duffy and Campbell divide frontal system dysfunction into a disorganized type, a disinhibited type, and an apathetic type. It is common for patients to present with a mixture of symptoms from each subtype, but one symptom cluster often dominates the clinical presentation. "Frontal lobe" symptoms may arise from a lesion anywhere in the frontal-striatal-thalamic circuit.[1]

Differentiating depression from apathy and frontal lobe epilepsy from symptoms of conversion is a substantial clinical challenge, and a comprehensive history and examination are essential for accurate diagnosis. A complete history can rarely be obtained from the patient alone; information also must be sought from family members and other informants. In addition, structural brain imaging, especially magnetic resonance imaging (MRI), and neuropsychological testing

are key parts of the diagnostic workup. Electroencephalography (EEG), simultaneous videotaping and EEG, and functional brain imaging can sometimes be helpful in arriving at a clinical diagnosis.

Assessing the effect of the patient's illness on family functioning is integral to the neuropsychiatric evaluation of patients with frontal systems impairment. Treatment is directed at educating both the patient and the family about the illness and helping them to understand and modulate the environmental factors that influence the patient's behavior. Carefully structuring the home environment can make a major difference in the patient's functional status and can improve the family's level of comfort.[2]

The judicious use of psychoactive medication may be quite helpful, but adverse effects are common. Few controlled medication trials have been carried out to guide clinicians in the treatment of apathetic, disinhibited, and disorganized behavior.

In this chapter, I describe nine representative cases of patients with frontal systems dysfunction seen on an inpatient neuropsychiatry service during a 24-month period. The cases represent apathetic, disinhibited, and disorganized syndromes as well as cases of late-life depression and frontal lobe epilepsy that do not fit neatly into the diagnostic subtypes. I discuss the clinical features, diagnostic evaluation, and treatment of each case.

APATHETIC SYNDROMES

Case 1: Apathy

A 56-year-old right-handed man was admitted from a rest home because of apathy and intermittent episodes of mildly destructive behavior. At age 46, he had developed a confusional episode after a period of binge drinking. He may have had several partial complex seizures at the onset of his illness. He suddenly left his job as the bartender and proprietor of a successful cocktail lounge and moved to Florida with one of the barmaids. Over 9 months, he depleted the family savings and then called his wife to pick him up. When he returned to Rhode Island, his wife noted that he had changed. He had become jocular, impulsive, shallow, and disinterested in his financial and personal affairs. Neuropsychological testing at that time revealed an extensive retrograde memory loss and extreme difficulty in learning new material, consistent with a diagnosis of Korsakoff's amnesia. He eventually had an MRI scan, which showed bilateral increased signal in the anteromedial thalamus, increased signal in the right putamen, and minimal cortical atrophy, probably reflecting subcortical midline necrosis caused by thiamine deficiency (Figure 10–1). The differential diagnosis also includes infarction of a single bilateral thalamic polar artery. The signal abnormalities have not changed in size on repeated scans.

Over the past 10 years, he developed a behavioral pattern of profound apathy alternating with intermittent disinhibition. His wife was unable to care for him at home, and he was placed in a rest home. There he sat contentedly for hours at a time, taking no interest in work or leisure-time activities. Occasionally, he stuffed toilets, peeled wallpaper, and dismantled window blinds for no apparent reason and without any malicious intent. He also had a voracious appetite and ate indiscriminately. At one point, the nursing home had him work in the vegetable garden; unfortunately, he ate all the fruits and the vegetables off the vine, leaving nothing for the other residents. His voracious appetite caused his weight to increase to more than 350 pounds at one stage and necessitated the institution of a very strict diet. Psychotic symptoms and aggression toward others were never noted. He had been treated with a number of neuroleptics, anxiolytics, anticonvulsants, and antidepressants to try to curb these acts of minor property destruction, without success. The rest home staff felt that

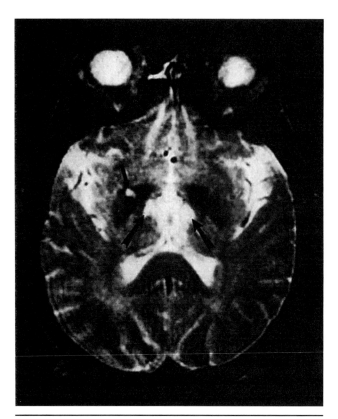

FIGURE 10–1. Case 1, a 56-year-old right-handed man with amnesia, apathy, and disinhibition.

T_2-weighted axial magnetic resonance imaging scan at the level of the thalami reveals increased signal in the anteromedial thalamus bilaterally (long arrows) and a small area of increased signal in the right putamen–globus pallidus (short arrow). The thalamic lesions are most likely caused by paramedian thalamic artery infarction.

these destructive episodes were increasing and asked for help from the neuropsychiatry service.

On examination, we found him to be in good general health. At the time of admission, he was taking carbamazepine, 300 mg three times a day; fluphenazine, 5 mg three times a day; benztropine, 0.5 mg twice a day; clomipramine, 25 mg three times a day; thiamine; and aspirin. He was apathetic and initiated no activities on his own. He was not distressed by his lack of drive, and he denied feeling depressed. His speech was fluent, although the amount of spontaneous speech was limited. He could register three objects but recalled zero of three at 5 minutes. Cueing did not help with recall. He was disoriented to time: he thought the year was 1963 and that Kennedy was president. He did not know why he was in the hospital. Remote memories of events before he became ill were generally intact. He recalled owning a bar and being a bartender and remembered a time when he was very busy and liked going out. He was able to name seven animals in 1 minute. Neuropsychological testing showed amnesia for all material once a delay or interference was introduced. However, some preservation of procedural learning was noted. Sensorimotor examination results were normal except for mild dysarthria and mild incoordination of the left arm and leg.

His MRI was unchanged. A brain single photon emission computed tomography (SPECT) ^{99m}Tc-hexamethylpropyleneamine oxime (HMPAO) scan showed minimal evidence of punctate areas of subcortical hypoperfusion but normal perfusion to the cortex. Quantitative measurement did not indicate decreased flow to the frontal lobes.

The fluphenazine, benztropine, and clomipramine were discontinued in an effort to streamline his medication regimen and eliminate agents that might be depressing his cognitive status without clearly improving his behavioral control. He made no attempt to damage property during a 2-week stay. His food and cigarette intake had to be carefully monitored. Without careful supervision, he would eat all of the desserts on the tray for the entire ward. Apathy was the most striking feature of his behavior. No change in his behavior was noted after discontinuation of the neuroleptics and clomipramine.

Bromocriptine was added and gradually increased to a dose of 30 mg three times a day on an outpatient basis after he returned to the rest home. No significant change was noted in his apathy or destructive behaviors. However, follow-up cognitive testing showed surprising improvement in attention and orientation. He gave the year as 1992 and said that Bush was the president (Clinton had just been elected). He could recall two of three objects at 5 minutes and could produce a word list of 14 animals in 1 minute.

Comment: This case shows that a dramatic prefrontal syndrome can follow a strategically placed subcortical lesion. This patient presented with executive dysfunction caused by bilateral medial thalamic lesions. The dorsomedial nucleus of the thalamus is a key relay in several prefrontal subcortical circuits.[1] His most prominent symptom was apathy, most likely due to interruption of connections from the anterior cingulate gyrus to the damaged thalamus. The Korsakoff's amnesia was probably related to injury to the anterior thalamic nuclei, disrupting diencephalic-limbic memory circuits. In addition, he had cognitive impairment related to the dorsolateral prefrontal cortex–subcortical circuit, intermittent dyscontrol related to the orbitofrontal subcortical dysfunction, and weight gain and loss of satiety secondary to hypothalamic dysfunction. This syndrome of paramedian thalamic artery infarction has been described.[3–5]

The MRI was helpful in detecting the thalamic injury. The perfusion pattern to the frontal lobes on ^{99m}Tc-HMPAO SPECT was normal despite his dramatic symptoms. The patient showed enhanced cognitive performance but lack of improvement in apathy after treatment with bromocriptine.

In anecdotal case reports, dopamine agonists have been shown to be beneficial in treating apathy.[6,7] Bromocriptine was chosen in this case because the apathy could have been related to disruption of presynaptic dopaminergic fibers. Postsynaptic dopamine augmentation would probably have the greatest likelihood of success in this case because the forebrain postsynaptic neurons should still be reasonably intact. Bromocriptine did not increase the patient's level of drive, but it did have a modest effect on memory, attention, verbal fluency, and cognitive speed. There are prominent dopaminergic inputs to the prefrontal cortex and the medial temporal lobe,[8] and dopamine has been shown to play a role in cognition.[9]

An alternative explanation for his cognitive improvement is that withdrawal of neuroleptics resulted in improved intellectual function. Against this explanation are the observations that the cognitive deficits were present before the neuroleptics were begun and that a trial of discontinuation of bromocriptine caused his cognitive status to deteriorate to his pretreatment baseline. This case example provides further clinical evidence that dopamine plays a role in cognition. Caution is recommended, however, in generalizing from an uncontrolled case report.

Although his cognition improved somewhat, the change did not have a significant effect on the patient's overall clinical status. His ability to control his impulsive behavior was limited because motivation, self-monitoring, and other key elements of executive function were still markedly deficient. It is not uncommon for patients with problems of behavioral control to be asymptomatic when observed in a structured clinical setting. He engaged in occasional destructive pranks after his return to the rest home. Rest home personnel tried to monitor his behavior more closely, but he returned to the neuropsychiatry service twice since his last admission for a brief stay to provide respite for the rest home staff.

Apathy is a common symptom in patients with neuropsychiatric illness. Symptoms of apathy usually can be differentiated from symptoms of depression by careful examination and observation.

Case 2: Differentiating Apathy From Depression

A 70-year-old right-handed man had presented to several different physicians with muscle stiffness, frequent crying, and decreased interest in his usual activities. He had no history of neurological or psychiatric illness, and no major life stressors could be identified. He was thought to have major depression. Antidepressants were prescribed, but they were not beneficial. The family sought another opinion.

On examination, he had paucity of speech and prominent psychomotor retardation. He was apathetic and had pathological affect, with brief bursts of tearfulness during the examination. He denied depressed mood but complained of muscle stiffness. Cognition was mildly impaired, particularly psychomotor speed. He could recall three of three words at 5 minutes. Cranial nerve testing showed decreased vertical gaze, with upgaze more impaired than downgaze. Oculocephalic reflexes were normal. Saccadic eye movements were slow. The gag reflex was hyperactive bilaterally. His neck was stiff, and tone in his extremities was mildly increased. No tremor was noted. He had mild difficulty in initiating gait and had moderate retropulsion.

Computed tomography (CT) and MRI of the brain showed normal findings. He was given the diagnosis of progressive supranuclear palsy (PSP). Treatment with carbidopa/levodopa led to a resolution of his pathological affect and improvement in his muscle stiffness and gait. Over the next year, apathy became his most prominent symptom. He denied feeling depressed. He did not initiate any activities and was content to do chores around the house when directed by his wife. He depended on others to oversee his self-care.

During the second year, bradykinesia and gait disturbance became more problematic. The levodopa was increased and bromocriptine added. Daytime sleepiness increased, and low doses of methylphenidate were added with a good response.

Comment: PSP was diagnosed by paying careful attention to the motor examination. Structural imaging studies were not helpful. Before the diagnosis of PSP, the patient's wife had been quite angry with him for not carrying his weight at home. Establishing the diagnosis and educating the family about the illness helped them learn to understand and anticipate problems. Seeing the patient and family together periodically during office visits was helpful in discussing the symptoms and in forming realistic expectations for his daily activities.

Apathy and pathological affect are common features of PSP, which was one of the first syndromes reported to be associated with subcortical dementia.[10]

PSP is a progressive neurodegenerative disorder caused by the widespread deposition of tangles in the superior colliculus, substantia nigra, striatum, and limbic system. The apathy may be caused by subcortical disconnection of cingulate circuits by the diencephalic pathology. Motor symptoms usually respond partially to dopamine replacement early in the illness. No treatment substantially alters the natural course of PSP.

This patient was thought to have major depression because he had lost interest in normal activities, had hypersomnia and somatic complaints, and was tearful at times, even though he did not report depressed mood. Standard antidepressant treatment was not helpful. In this case, motor symptoms and pathological affect responded to dopamine replacement but apathy did not.

THREE EXAMPLES OF DISINHIBITION

Disinhibition and aggression frequently lead to psychiatric admission and nursing home placement. In 1986, Lhermitte and colleagues[11,12] presented a large series of cases that they described as "utilization behavior" because they are stimulus bound and make use of whatever objects are in the room. This was thought to be a form of environmental dependency most often associated with lesions in the orbital aspects of the frontal lobe.

Case 3: Utilization Behavior and Environmental Dependency

A 78-year-old right-handed woman was admitted from a nursing home because of manic-type behavior. Her behavior and memory had been declining over the past few years. She wandered from room to room picking up and using a wide variety of objects without any apparent purpose. If there was a scale in the room, she had to weigh herself.

On examination, she had a bright affect, and she was restless and energetic. She had clanging, rhyming, pressured speech. Her manner was carefree, disinhibited, and jocular. She mimicked the examiner's movements without being asked, tried to auscultate the examiner with a stethoscope, and attempted to give herself an injection with a plastic syringe (fortunately, the needle was not attached). She registered three words but recalled zero of three words at 5 minutes. Naming also was impaired. Sensorimotor examination results were normal except for exaggerated deep tendon reflexes and positive grasp, glabellar, snout, and palmomental reflexes. Formal neuropsychological testing was difficult to complete, but her findings were most consistent with Alzheimer's disease.

CT of the brain without contrast revealed generalized atrophy, with prominent midline frontal atrophy (Figure 10–2). In addition, a watershed infarct was seen over the left parieto-occipital junction.

Comment: Utilization behavior can be caused by a wide variety of syndromes producing orbitofrontal dysfunction and can be associated with an activated or an apathetic state, depending on the posterior extent of the lesion.[13] Alzheimer's disease is a common cause of disinhibition and utilization behavior because of frontal lobe atrophy as the disease progresses. This patient's behavior had a disinhibited, pseudopsychopathic, maniclike quality often seen in patients with orbitofrontal dysfunction. She was environmentally dependent and stimulus bound.

Treatment with low-dose neuroleptics and carbamazepine provided partial improvement in behavioral control. Structuring the environment and redirecting her behavior were the most useful interventions.

During the last year of her life, her cognitive decline progressed, and behavioral problems abated as she became more listless and apathetic.

Case 4: Frontal Lobe Dementia

A 56-year-old right-handed man presented with violent aggressive outbursts. Three years before, he had developed obsessive-compulsive symptoms. After a year, he had become more vulgar in his speech, and his behavior had become more disinhibited. During the past year, he had struck out at family and attendants without clear provocation, at times causing others physical injury. He had become disheveled and was no longer able to carry out his activities of daily living (ADLs). He was transferred to a nursing home. His speech had become slurred, and his memory had begun to deteriorate. He continued to make aggressive outbursts despite high doses of haloperidol. He spent his days in a geriatric chair with a locking top to prevent wandering and aggressive behavior.

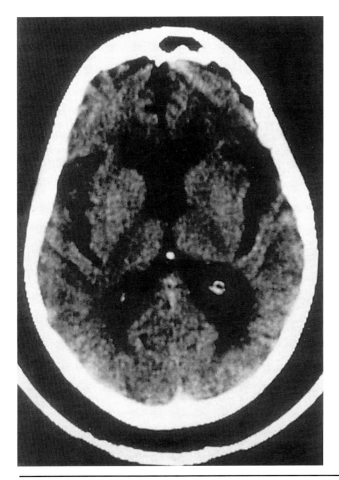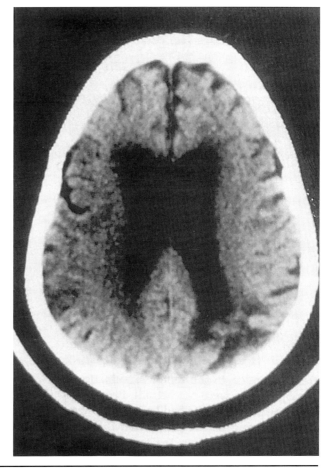

FIGURE 10–2.   Case 3, a 78-year-old woman with dementia and dramatic utilization behavior.
Noncontrast computed tomography scan at the level of the lateral ventricles shows generalized atrophy, ventricular enlargement, and prominent midline frontal and sylvian fissure atrophy. A left parieto-occipital watershed infarct can be seen (*right*).

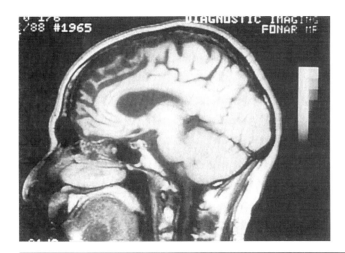 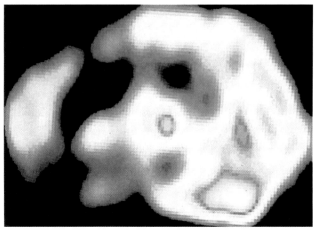

FIGURE 10–3.   Case 4, a 56-year-old man with disinhibition and violent outbursts.
Left: T_1-weighted midline sagittal magnetic resonance imaging scan shows marked segmental atrophy of the frontal lobe.
Right: Single photon emission computed tomography (SPECT) [^{99m}Tc]hexamethylpropyleneamine oxime (HMPAO) scan at the same level shows severe hypoperfusion to the frontal regions. The neuroimaging findings are consistent with frontal lobe dementia.

MRI of the brain revealed extensive frontal lobe atrophy with midline predominance, and a ^{99m}Tc-HMPAO SPECT scan showed marked frontal hypoperfusion (Figure 10–3). The behavior change and imaging studies were consistent with frontal lobe dementia, most likely Pick's disease.

Comment: The patient's self-monitoring functions were almost nonexistent. Once regulatory systems in the orbitomedial area are severely impaired, it is difficult to achieve satisfactory control of aggressive behavior with medication or behavior modification techniques. Controlled clinical trials for treatment of aggressive, disinhibited behavior in this population have not been pursued, although controlled trials[13A–13D] are in progress to evaluate the treatment of psychosis and agitation in Alzheimer's disease.

A consensus conference on frontal lobe dementia recently published its findings.[14] Three clinical syndromes related to frontal lobe dementia were identified—frontotemporal dementia, progressive nonfluent aphasia, and semantic dementia. Frontotemporal dementia is most relevant to this case. Frontotemporal dementia is a syndrome of focal lobar atrophy involving the frontal and temporal lobes. Pick's disease is the most common form, although other causes have been reported. The disease is usually sporadic, although a gene has recently been identified in families with frontotemporal dementia.[15] Clinically, changes in behavior and comportment are more striking than amnesia. Onset is usually insidious, before age 65, with gradual progression. Emotional blunting and loss of insight occur early. Hygiene and grooming are impaired early, and the patient may resist bathing. Hyperorality, stereotyped behavior, and utilization behavior may occur. Impulse-control problems are common and disturbing, as in this case. Stuttering speech, echolalia, and dysarthria may be present.

Case 5: Intermittent Explosive Disorder

A 40-year-old right-handed man had a 5-year history of multiple sclerosis that began with plaques in the brain stem causing mild hemisensory loss and hemiparesis. In the ensuing years, he experienced exacerbations and remissions. Fatigue was his most plaguing problem. He was admitted to the neuropsychiatry service because of aggressive outbursts directed toward his family.

The patient was the father of five children. In the past, he had been very even tempered and could handle family conflicts without difficulty. Lately, he had been coming home from work fatigued and confused, which caused him to misinterpret family arguments. He became prone to angry outbursts with limited provocation. During these episodes, he was likely to swear at the children or break things around the house. He always recalled what had happened and was remorseful after these events.

On examination, his mood was normal, but he was discouraged about his poor control of his behavior. Intelligence tested in the superior range without significant cognitive deficits. Neurological evaluation revealed mild bilateral intranuclear ophthalmoplegia and right lateral gaze diplopia. Hyperreflexia was present in the lower extremities, and mild proximal right leg weakness was present.

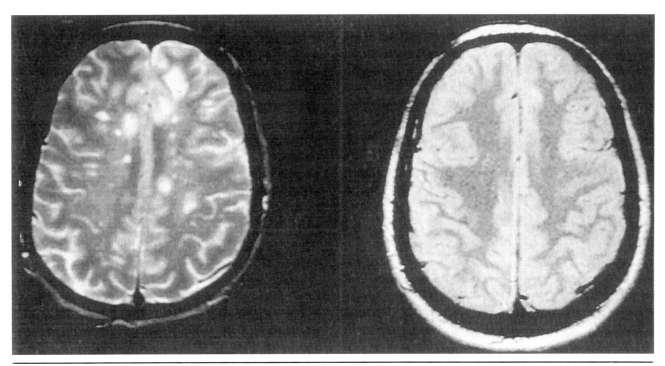

FIGURE 10–4. Case 5, a man with multiple sclerosis.
Right: At age 36, before the onset of intermittent explosive disorder, an axial proton density magnetic resonance imaging (MRI) scan at the level of the centrum semiovale is normal. **Left:** At age 40, a T_2-weighted MRI scan at the same level shows multiple plaques in the anterior subfrontal white matter.

MRI of the brain (Figure 10–4) showed many plaques in the midline subfrontal matter and periventricular region as well as in the brain stem. Administration of gadolinium contrast showed multiple small areas of uptake consistent with active plaques.

A 5-day course of intravenous methylprednisolone was administered. The right leg weakness, urinary urgency, and diplopia resolved. Symptoms of fatigue temporarily improved. Ten days after receiving methylprednisolone, he was readmitted to the hospital with a diagnosis of intermittent explosive disorder, exacerbated by the steroids, after he tried to hit his son with his car during an intense family argument. His behavior returned to normal without pharmacological treatment over 5 days in a structured setting.

Meetings were held with the patient and his family to educate them about multiple sclerosis and the effect it can have on behavior as well as to explore the family patterns that are likely to cause loss of control. The patient eventually had to give up his job because of fatigue. Fatigue was helped initially by bupropion. Later, the bupropion was discontinued, and sertraline was begun. Sertraline improved his alertness, mood, and sense of well-being. The patient has been taking interferon-β for the past year and has had no major flare-ups of multiple sclerosis. He has also had no more aggres-

sive outbursts. Further steroid treatment has been avoided.

Comment: This patient was at risk for episodes of dyscontrol when he was fatigued, confused, and overstimulated. The midline subfrontal plaques caused damage to orbitofrontal centers that normally monitor and regulate aggressive impulses. His tendency toward aggressive behavior was further brought out by treatment with corticosteroids, which can promote disinhibition.

Family counseling helped identify and limit factors that tended to promote the aggressive outbursts. Treating the underlying multiple sclerosis with interferon-β decreased the frequency and severity of flare-ups. Confusion and fatigue improved during the time he was taking interferon-β. The serotonin agonist sertraline helped him feel calmer.

DYSEXECUTIVE SYNDROME

Case 6: Traumatic Brain Injury

A 25-year-old right-handed woman with a history of depression was involved in a major motor vehicle accident, in which she experienced a loss of consciousness lasting 24 hours, left hemiparesis, and decreased coordination in her left hand, 3 years prior to assessment. For the past 2½ years, she had carried out her ADLs in a disorganized manner. She often did her laundry by placing the box of detergent in the washing machine with her clothes. She occasionally wore her undergarments over her clothes if they had been laid out in the wrong order. She wandered at night and would sometimes get lost, did not know how to ask for help, and could not remember her telephone number. She had great difficulty in organizing her living area and carrying out multiple-step tasks. She was admitted to the neuropsychiatry service because of disorganized behavior, mood swings, and decreased self-care.

On examination, her thinking was concrete and disorganized. She had trouble understanding common idioms (e.g., "What kind of things cause you to blow up?" "Blow up—you mean like dynamite?"). Her speech was pressured and very rapid. Her ideas did not always make sense. Self-monitoring was impaired. She wanted to return to school and full-time work and could not understand why others did not think she was ready. Sensorimotor examination revealed a mild left hemiparesis and decreased coordination in her left hand. Neuropsychological evaluation indicated impaired attention and concentration, difficulty with registration and retrieval, and decreased verbal fluency.

MRI showed increased signal in the right subfrontal matter consistent with shearing axonal injury (Figure 10–5). When she was in the hospital, frequent mood swings were noted. She experienced a few brief episodes of impaired consciousness, during which she picked at her clothes. EEG showed mild sharp and spike transients over the right frontotemporal regions.

The patient and her family were educated about the neurobehavioral sequelae of head injury. She was assigned an outpatient case manager, and a highly structured cognitive rehabilitation program focusing on ADLs was begun. Psychotherapy was directed at setting small, realistic goals and suppressing negative behaviors. Partial complex seizures and mood lability were controlled with carbamazepine. This program worked well, and her level of independence and optimism climbed gradually over the next 12 months.

Comment: This case exemplifies the disorganized behavior pattern seen in patients with cognitive dysfunction that follows a major closed head injury. A variety of symptoms may develop. The patient had concrete and disorganized thinking, disinhibition, memory loss, mood lability, and seizures. Structural brain abnormalities on CT and MRI are quite variable in patients with significant postconcussive neurobe-

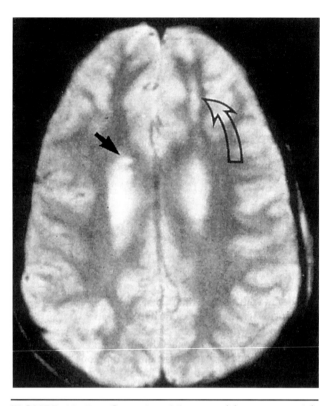

FIGURE 10–5. Case 6, a 25-year-old woman with cognitive disorganization, mood swings, and partial complex seizures following a closed head injury.
Proton density axial magnetic resonance imaging scan at the level of the centrum semiovale shows increased signal in the right subfrontal white matter consistent with diffuse axonal injury (open arrow) and a bright area representing a microhemorrhage in the left corpus callosum (dark arrow).

havioral syndromes. Her MRI showed subtle changes in the white matter related to axonal injury. Figure 10–6, in a patient with similar symptoms, shows prefrontal hemorrhagic contusions with subsequent dramatic encephalomalacia in the orbitofrontal regions following contracoup injury. Sometimes brain imaging has normal findings despite significant disturbance in behavior or cognition.

Prominent mood lability with a maniclike quality and pressured speech have been reported following right frontal injury.[16] Harrington and Salloway[17] recently reported a case of delayed onset of psychosis following a serious closed head injury. Patients with a personal or family history of affective disease are more vulnerable to developing a mood disturbance after a frontal lesion. Treatment requires a highly structured plan with close supervision. The program must include small steps, with a major emphasis on education for the patient and the family. Psychoactive medication, used judiciously, can be helpful.

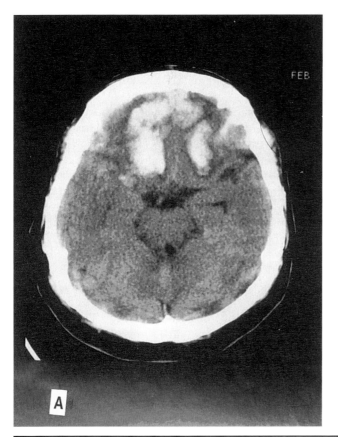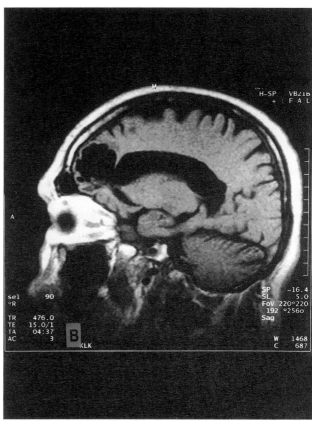

FIGURE 10–6. **A:** Noncontrast head computed tomography scan showing extensive orbitofrontal hemorrhagic contusions following contracoup injury. **B:** Noncontrast T$_1$-weighted magnetic resonance imaging scan showing a large black area of encephalomalacia in the right midline prefrontal cortex in the same patient 2 years after the head injury.

OTHER FRONTAL LOBE SYNDROMES

Late-Life Depression

Late-life-onset depression is a common problem seen in a geriatric psychiatry service. Patients with late-life-onset depression are more likely to have underlying neurological disease when compared with age-matched depressed patients with early-onset depression.[18,19] Late-life-onset depression may be a manifestation of frontal systems dysfunction.

Case 7: Late-Life Depression and Subcortical Vascular Disease

A 70-year-old right-handed man without any known history of psychiatric or neurological problems became depressed and anxious and had the urge to kill his family. He had a history of hypertension. Cognitive and neurological examination results were normal. MRI scan of the brain showed extensive periventricular and deep white matter

increased signal on T$_2$-weighted scans consistent with severe subcortical small vessel disease (Figure 10–7).

Treatment with nortriptyline, 10 mg/day, and haloperidol, 1 mg/day, brought relief of depressive symptoms and homicidal urges. Discontinuation of either medication caused return of depression and homicidal urges within 3 days. Resumption of medication caused swift resolution of symptoms. One enteric-coated aspirin per day was prescribed to help slow the progression of small vessel disease, although treatment of this disorder has not been carefully studied.

Comment: Binswanger and Alzheimer described subcortical encephalopathy caused by arteriosclerosis that leads to gliosis and demyelination in the subcortical white matter.[20] The clinical presentation is variable. Patients can develop dementia, depression, or focal sensorimotor signs. The main risk factors are age and hypertension. Frontal lobe symptoms predominate, with most signal abnormalities found in the subfrontal

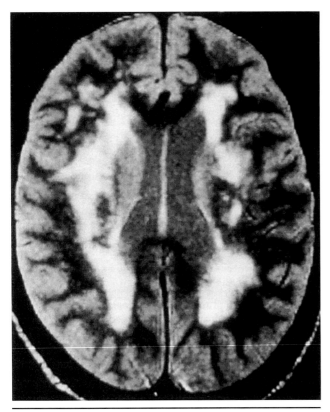

FIGURE 10–7.   Case 7, a 70-year-old man with the new onset of psychotic depression.

Axial proton density magnetic resonance imaging scan at the level of the lateral ventricles shows prominent areas of increased signal in periventricular and deep subcortical white and gray structures due to subcortical small vessel disease.

white matter.[21] Depression and cognitive impairment probably arise from disconnection of frontal subcortical circuits involving affect and cognitive timing.[22] Late-life depression caused by microvascular disease has been given the term *vascular depression*.[23,24]

Frontal Lobe Epilepsy

Another difficult clinical problem seen on a neuropsychiatry service and involving the frontal lobes is the evaluation of partial complex seizures arising from a prefrontal lobe focus. The behavioral episodes are often bizarre and irregular. Thrashing leg movements and even bicycle pedaling may be seen, and the patient may be semiconscious during the episode, giving the event the appearance of a psychogenic seizure. The EEG results may be normal if the epileptic focus is located deep in the frontal lobe. Prefrontal lobe seizures are frequently misdiagnosed as psychogenic events.[25,26]

Case 8: Frontal Partial Complex Seizures

A 28-year-old right-handed man was experiencing abnormal behavioral events during sleep. These events began during sleep and consisted of thrashing of his legs, occasional calling out, and confusion following the event. An event lasted about 1 minute, with several sometimes occurring in succession. His father could sometimes abort the events by focusing the patient's attention on specific objects in the room. The events occurred almost every night and sometimes many times per night. They never occurred during the day.

The events began about 6 months after he had a near-drowning accident at age 15 years. He had generalized tonic-clonic activity, with full loss of consciousness, on a few occasions in the first 2 years after the accident. He has had no witnessed generalized seizures in 10 years. Multiple anticonvulsants to control his sleep-related events had been tried as monotherapy and in combination, with only partial success.

He lived with his father and has never held sustained competitive employment. He had low normal intelligence. He had behavior problems in school and briefly received methylphenidate as a child for attention-deficit disorder. He had poor social judgment and often associated himself with peers who took advantage of him. He had no history of psychotic phenomena or aggressive behavior, although he did get very frustrated after a flurry of seizurelike events.

His EEG showed mild nonspecific slowing over the anterior regions bilaterally. MRI of the brain, based on an epilepsy protocol, had normal findings. A neurologist thought that these nocturnal events were psychogenic seizures, and his family sought a second opinion.

At the time of evaluation, he was taking carbamazepine, 1,800 mg/day, and primidone, 500 mg/day. His speech was somewhat thickened, and cognitive speed was slow. No focal cognitive deficits were noted. He appeared mildly sedated. His affect was flat, and he seemed discouraged. He had mild difficulty with rapid alternating movements with the left hand; otherwise, the sensorimotor examination results were normal.

On a 24-hour closed-circuit video-EEG, six episodes of seizurelike activity were seen occurring during sleep or immediately after waking. During the episodes, he had tonic and some clonic contractions of his trunk and arms as well as thrashing and jerking of the legs, followed by a period of confusion. Muscle artifact made EEG evaluation difficult. However, during Stage I sleep, numerous phase-reversing single spike-wave complexes were seen over midline frontal regions bilaterally. The patient and his father were told that these events were frontal partial complex seizures. The carbamazepine dose was raised to achieve a level at the top of the therapeutic range. Primidone was tapered gradually. When the dose of primidone was decreased to 125 mg/day, he had a secondarily generalized seizure. At 250 mg/day, no further generalized seizures were seen, and an overall increase in energy and motivation was noted. Self-care improved, and he began a regular exercise program at a local gym. Valproic acid was added to the carbamazepine but was not tolerated because of sedation. Felbamate caused visual hallucinations.

Comment: Frontal lobe seizures can be difficult to diagnose because of their bizarre appearance. The patient with partial complex seizures of frontal or limbic origin is rarely able to give a complete and accurate history. Information must be sought from people who have witnessed the events and who know their frequency, precipitating factors, and associated behavioral problems.

The thrashing leg movements were most likely caused by activation of leg fibers in the midline premotor areas. Partial complex seizures frequently occur during sleep or drowsiness, as in this case. This case illustrates the importance of simultaneous video and EEG monitoring in the evaluation. It is important to make the diagnosis so that proper treatment can be instituted and the family given accurate education and guidance. Learning and behavior problems are common in patients with refractory prefrontal lobe seizures because of dysfunction of frontal cognitive and regulatory systems. These patients frequently have difficulty in living independently and holding gainful employment. Treatment with barbiturates helped suppress the generalization of seizures in this case but made the patient feel lethargic and demoralized, which further decreased his level of productivity. He also was often demoralized because of his social isolation and lack of independence. Rehabilitation programs are needed that address the emotional and vocational needs of this patient population.

Case 9: Supplementary Motor Seizures

A 28-year-old right-handed woman experienced frequent seizurelike episodes that began with a premonition that something bad was going to happen. Her left arm became hyperextended, and her body was thrown toward the right. She began to scream and called for help; her emotions were heightened during the events, and her behavior appeared histrionic. Consciousness was not impaired, she had no postictal lethargy, and she had full recall for the events. She may have had a generalized seizure in the remote past. These events were quite stereotypic and occurred up to five

times per day. Treatment with carbamazepine partially decreased the frequency and intensity of these events.

A CT of the brain with and without contrast had normal findings. EEG showed some mild nonspecific slowing over the right anterior leads. At another facility, the patient was given the diagnosis of psychogenic seizures because of her histrionic behavior, preserved consciousness, and lack of automatisms and convulsive activity. Her seizurelike episodes persisted, and she sought further evaluation.

She was admitted for extended video-EEG monitoring. The carbamazepine was decreased. A number of more intense episodes were recorded, always with hyperextension of the left arm, screaming, and a histrionic manner; consciousness was preserved. Her body moved toward the right, and she would fall out of bed if the bed rail was down. EEG, at times, showed sharp waves phase reversing in the right frontal region. An MRI of the brain revealed a small, round homogeneous area of increased signal in the lateral region of the right supplementary motor area, most likely a low-grade glioma. She was given the diagnosis of right supplementary motor partial seizures caused by a small slow-growing neoplasm. She declined removal of the glioma, fearing surgical complications. The tumor did not change in size on MRI for 2 years. Her seizures have been better controlled on carbamazepine and sodium valproate.

Comment: Supplementary motor area seizures are often characterized by hyperextension of the contralateral arm and preservation of consciousness. Patients are often thrown toward one side of the bed. The patient's speech may be suppressed or activated during the event. The supplementary motor area and neighboring anterior cingulate gyrus play a role in the initiation of speech.[27] It can be difficult, however, to differentiate supplementary motor area seizures from psychogenic seizures. In this case, the striking emotionality during the events strongly influenced evaluators toward a diagnosis of psychogenic seizures, but the lateralized, stereotypic nature of the patient's events provided a helpful clue. Because of the patient's emotionality, this case raises the possibility that excess activation of the supplementary motor area and surrounding regions in the nondominant hemisphere can play a role in the genesis of histrionic behavior.

CONCLUSIONS

Frontal systems disorders provide an opportunity for understanding the pathophysiology of important human behaviors. Various disease processes can cause impairment in frontal lobe functions. The principal lesion that is producing executive dysfunction may actually be found outside the frontal lobe, as was seen in Cases 1, 2, and 7.

Three different types of frontal system dysfunction have been described—an apathetic type, a disinhibited type, and a disorganized type—based on the behavioral organization of specific regions of the frontal lobe and their subcortical and limbic connections. A mixture of symptoms from all three areas is often seen in patients with frontal system disease, but one type of symptom usually dominates.

Correct diagnosis makes possible appropriate treatment and accurate education for patients and their families. Review of the examination and treatment in the nine cases yields the following observations:

1. A careful history and examination were important in all nine of the cases presented. Eliciting the history from the patient alone is inadequate; information must be sought from family members and other informants as well.
2. Structural brain imaging, particularly MRI, is a key part of the diagnostic workup. MRI was considerably more informative than CT in six of the nine cases.
3. Neuropsychological testing was particularly helpful in four of the nine cases.
4. Routine EEG was diagnostic in the two cases with suspected mild partial complex seizures. Simultaneous videotaping and EEG was required to differentiate between frontal seizures and psychogenic seizures in two additional cases.
5. SPECT scanning was obtained in four of the nine cases but was not routinely ordered. SPECT showed marked frontal hypoperfusion in the case of frontal lobe dementia but was normal in the other three cases.
6. Educating the patient and the family about the illness and restructuring the patient's environment were helpful in all nine cases.
7. Psychotropic medication was prescribed for all patients in this sample and was helpful in treating depression, mood lability, epilepsy, and dyscontrol in five cases. Disinhibition in four patients with advanced and progressive neurodegenerative disorders was refractory to medication treatment.

In future research directed at treatment strategies and outcomes, controlled trials in which target symptoms can be reliably monitored are needed.

REFERENCES

1. Mega M, Cummings J: Frontal-subcortical circuits and neuropsychiatric disorders. J Neuropsychiatry Clin Neurosci 6:358–370, 1994
2. Campbell J, Duffy JD, Salloway S: Treatment strategies for patients with frontal systems dysfunction. J Neuropsychiatry Clin Neurosci 6:411–418, 1994
3. Guberman A, Stuss D: The syndrome of bilateral paramedian thalamic infarction. Neurology 33:540–546, 1983
4. Malamut BL, Graff-Radford N, Chawluk J, et al: Memory in a case of bilateral thalamic infarction. Neurology 42:163–169, 1992
5. Sandson TA, Daffner KR, Carvalho PA, et al: Frontal lobe dysfunction following infarction of the left-sided medial thalamus. Arch Neurol 48:1300–1303, 1991
6. Ross ED, Stewart RM: Akinetic mutism from hypothalamic damage: successful treatment with dopamine agonists. Neurology 31:1435–1439, 1981
7. Echiverri HC, Tattum WO, Merens TA: Akinetic mutism: pharmacologic probe of the dopaminergic mesencephalofrontal activating system. Pediatr Neurol 4:228–230, 1988
8. Fallon JH: Topographic organization of ascending dopaminergic projections. Ann N Y Acad Sci 537:1–9, 1988
9. Owen A, James M, Leigh PN, et al: Fronto-striatal cognitive deficits at different stages of Parkinson's disease. Brain 115:1727–1751, 1992
10. Albert ML, Feldman RG, Willis AL: The subcortical dementia of progressive supranuclear palsy. J Neurol Neurosurg Psychiatry 37:121–130, 1974
11. Lhermitte F, Pillon B, Serdaru M: Human autonomy and the frontal lobes, I: imitation and utilization behavior: a neuropsychological study of 75 patients. Ann Neurol 19:326–334, 1986
12. Lhermitte F: Human autonomy and the frontal lobes, II: patient behavior in complex and social situations. Ann Neurol 19:335–343, 1986
13. Pearson K, Kirschner K, Singh J, et al: Utilization behavior: environmental determinants and cognitive therapy (abstract). J Neuropsychiatry Clin Neurosci 6:297–298, 1994
13A. Teri L, Logsdon R, Peskind E, et al: Treatment of agitation in AD. Neurology 55:1271–1278, 2000
13B. Devanand DP, Marder K, Michaels KS, et al: A randomized placebo-controlled dose-comparison trial of haloperidol treatment for psychosis and disruptive behaviors in Alzheimer's disease. Am J Psychiatry 155:1512–1520, 1988

13C. Katz JR, Jeste DV, Mintzer JE, et al: Comparison of risperidone and placebo for psychosis and behavioral disturbances associated with dementia: a randomized, double-blind trial. J Clin Psychiatry 60:107–115, 1999

13D. Sultzer DL, Gray KF, Gunay I, et al: A double-blind comparison of trazadone and haloperidol for treatment of agitation in patients with dementia. Am J Geriatr Psychiatry 5:60–69, 1997

14. Neary D, Snowden J, Gustafson L, et al: Frontotemporal lobar degeneration. Neurology 51:1546–1554, 1998

15. Hutton M, Lendon CL, Rizzu P, et al: Association of missense and 5'-splice-site mutations in tau with the inherited dementia FTDP-17. Nature 393:702–705, 1998

16. Starkstein S, Pearlson G, Boston J, et al: Mania after brain injury. Arch Neurol 44:1069–1073, 1987

17. Harrington C, Salloway S: Dramatic neurobehavioral disorder in two cases following anteromedial frontal lobe injury. Neurocase 3:137–149, 1997

18. Coffey CE, Figiel GS, Djany WT, et al: Leukoencephalopathy in elderly depressed patients referred for ECT. Biol Psychiatry 24:143–161, 1988

19. Salloway S, Malloy P, Rogg J, et al: Clinical significance of subcortical encephalomalacia in early and late onset depression (abstract). Neurology 44 (suppl 2):A375, 1994

20. Schorer C: Alzheimer and Kraepelin describe Binswanger's disease. J Neuropsychiatry Clin Neurosci 4:55–58, 1992

21. Ischii N, Nishihara Y, Imamura T: Why do frontal lobe symptoms predominate in vascular dementia and lacunes? Neurology 36:340–345, 1986

22. Mayberg H: Frontal lobe dysfunction in secondary depression. J Neuropsychiatry Clin Neurosci 6:428–442, 1994

23. Salloway S, Malloy P, Rogg J, et al: MRI and neuropsychological differences in early and late-life onset geriatric depression. Neurology 46:1567–1574, 1996

24. Krishnan R, Hays J, Blazer D: MRI-defined vascular depression. Am J Psychiatry 154:497–501, 1997

25. Williamson P, Spencer DD, Spenser SS, et al: Complex seizures of frontal lobe origin. Ann Neurol 18:497–504, 1985

26. Saygi S, Katz A, Marks D, et al: Frontal lobe partial seizures and psychogenic seizures. Neurology 42:1274–1277, 1992

27. Jurgens U, Ploog D: Cerebral representation of vocalization in the squirrel monkey. Exp Brain Res 10:532–554, 1970

11

Treatment Strategies for Patients With Dysexecutive Syndromes

John J. Campbell III, M.D., James D. Duffy, M.B., Ch.B., Stephen P. Salloway, M.D., M.S.

Traumatic brain injury, neurodegenerative disorders, and other frontal systems disorders produce executive dysfunction and are a frequent cause of functional disability across the life span. Despite their frequency, the dysexecutive syndromes are often not recognized, and their significance is underappreciated. This is reflected in the virtual absence of substantive controlled research on appropriate treatment interventions for the dysexecutive syndromes.

This chapter offers a comprehensive approach to the treatment of the dysexecutive syndromes that makes use of pharmacological, environmental, cognitive, behavioral, and family strategies. The appropriate selection and integration of each of these treatment modalities are critical to developing an effective treatment plan. Although the dysexecutive syndromes are usually chronic and often progressive, their profoundly negative effect on the patient and his or her social constellation dictates an active treatment approach. The development of a comprehensive, multimodal treatment plan empowers the clinician and helps to mitigate the therapeutic nihilism that often surrounds these disorders. Indeed, as a result of using such an approach, one can expect meaningful and sustained improvements in the patient's functioning and the family's ability to cope. Patients with dysexecutive syndromes require a long-term treatment strategy that is consistent, durable, and predictable. A breakdown in the organization of the treatment team is likely to be translated into a decline in the patient's functioning.

The first and most important step in developing an effective treatment plan is the collection of adequate clinical data. In brief, information gathered should include the following:

1. Current cognitive and physical strengths and limitations
2. Evidence of past and present behavioral disturbances
3. Current social support characteristics and the effect of the patient's impairment on family functioning

Once this information is collected, the clinician must develop a comprehensive treatment plan that identifies both the patient's needs and potential resources. On the basis of this clinical distillation, the clinician must determine the potential usefulness and place in the treatment plan of each of the modalities discussed in the following sections.

PSYCHOPHARMACOLOGY

Our discussion of the psychopharmacological strategies in the dysexecutive syndromes requires a brief review of the neurochemistry of the prefrontal neural systems. This review can be limited to the neurotransmitters that are subject to manipulation by currently available psychotropic agents. No particular cognitive or behavioral function can be confidently ascribed to any one neurotransmitter, but through their influence on the facilitation, inhibition, and integration of different neural systems, neurotransmitters are particularly likely to influence the complex and plastic neural processes subserving the executive cognitive functions of the prefrontal cortex.

The rich noradrenergic (NA) projections to the cortical mantle arise from the pontine and medullary reticular formation and the locus coeruleus.[1] The NA fibers ascend by a direct hypothalamic route to the frontal poles of both hemispheres before fanning out posteriorly to innervate the entire cortex.[2] NA terminals are most dense in the anterior cortex and tend to localize predominantly in cortical layers IV and V.[3] Noradrenaline may have a role in regulating arousal and excitability.[4] Because ascending NA fibers are funneled through the frontal poles, lesions in this region are particularly likely to disrupt NA projections to the entire cortex.

The dopaminergic (DA) system consists of three primary clusters: the mesocortical, mesolimbic, and nigrostriatal.[5] The mesocortical system has targets in the prefrontal, piriform, and entorhinal cortices.[6] The mesocortical prefrontal system, originating in the ventral tegmentum and ascending through the ventral diencephalon, represents a distinct and separate system with DA projections to the prefrontal cortex that essentially overlap the projections of the mediodorsal nucleus of the thalamus.[7,8] DA mesocortical projections show the highest concentrations in the prefrontal cortex (including the premotor cortex). This distribution of projections suggests that dopamine plays an important role in the initiation, planning, temporal organization, and integration of motor behaviors.[4] In addition to the ascending DA systems described, a descending corticofugal tract arising in the prefrontal cortex is thought to maintain a regulatory control over subcortical DA fibers. The implications of this system for a theory of prefrontal dysfunction are reviewed by

Meyer-Lindenberg and Berman in Chapter 13 of this volume and elsewhere.[9]

Projections of the serotonergic system arise in the midline raphe nuclei of the pons and mesencephalon and ascend to multiple sites in the diencephalon, limbic system, and cortex. Serotonin (5-hydroxytryptamine; 5-HT) projections to the prefrontal regions are more diffuse than NA or DA projections and are most concentrated in the posterior somatosensory cortex.[10] This somatosensory innervation suggests that serotonin has a role in the processing of sensory information.[11] The significance of the high concentration of serotonin in the prefrontal cortex remains uncertain, but decreased serotonin levels in the prefrontal regions have been associated with completed suicide, aggression, and depression.[12–14]

Acetylcholine (ACh) projections are widely distributed throughout the peripheral and central nervous system.[15] In the context of this discussion, the system that arises in the basal forebrain nucleus basalis of Meynert and projects to the cortex is most pertinent.[16] The ACh system plays a major role in memory and, together with the NA system, modulates attention, thereby exerting a pervasive influence on almost all higher cognitive functioning.[4]

γ-Aminobutyric acid (GABA) is a ubiquitous neurotransmitter found in inhibitory interneurons throughout the central nervous system. Within the prefrontal cortex, GABA is thought to modulate excitatory neurotransmission.[17,18] The therapeutic implications of manipulating prefrontal GABAergic function are uncertain, although GABA modulates anxiety and seizures.[19]

Glutamate is the major excitatory neurotransmitter in the brain. There is a large glutaminergic output from the prefrontal cortex to the striatum. Glutamate plays a role in learning and memory and is implicated in psychosis.[20,21]

Virtually no well-controlled evidence supports the clinical utility of any particular psychotropic agent in the treatment of prefrontal dysfunction. Instruments for reliably measuring the signs and symptoms of prefrontal dysfunction are limited. It is hoped that a better understanding of the pharmacology of the frontal lobes and their subcorticolimbic connections will lead to a rational and effective approach to treatment. However, a review of the current literature does suggest that some psychotropic agents may provide symptomatic relief. We discuss the psychopharmacological treatment of each of the three subtypes of frontal systems dysfunction.

Dorsolateral Prefrontal Dysexecutive Syndrome

Patients showing the cognitive disorganization associated with dysfunction of the dorsolateral frontal convexity system are likely to become increasingly anxious and more disorganized when they are confronted with increased internal arousal and high levels of external sensory stimulation. Although environmental interventions are the most effective and benign method of reducing this subjective distress, psychopharmacological interventions may sometimes be helpful.

Neuroleptic medications diminish arousal and therefore will reduce the motor agitation shown by persons with the disorganized cognition of a dorsolateral convexity syndrome. Unfortunately, a high price is paid for this reduction in agitation. Neuroleptics are likely to exacerbate cognitive inertia and further impair executive cognitive functions.[22] In addition, patients with underlying neurological disease are at increased risk for developing tardive dyskinesia and akathisia.[23]

The use of neuroleptics should be limited whenever possible in favor of less intrusive and hazardous interventions. However, the atypical neuroleptic agents clozapine, olanzapine, risperidone, and quetiapine, through their combined serotonin-dopamine antagonism, may reduce agitation without untoward motor and cognitive effects.[24] Further investigation of these agents in the management of agitation associated with dysexecutive syndromes is warranted.

Benzodiazepines will reduce arousal and may be helpful in moderating agitation.[25] However, benzodiazepines also may produce disinhibition,[26] thereby aggravating impulsiveness and stimulus-driven behavior. Their use is warranted provided the patient is in a secure environment where any evidence of increased disinhibition can be rapidly identified and contained. Buspirone, a pure anxioselective agent of the azapirone chemical subgroup, has a very benign side-effect profile,[27] but its clinical efficacy in reducing the arousal of cognitively disorganized patients remains to be determined.

Antidepressants might theoretically exert a positive therapeutic effect by influencing the signal-to-noise ratio of sensory information processed by the cortex. The benefit of low-dose tricyclic antidepressants in attention-deficit disorder suggests that they may be useful in patients with the disorganized type of dysexecutive syndrome. The depression associated with lesions to the left anterior pole is responsive to nortriptyline and possibly other antidepressant agents.[28,29]

Psychostimulants have become the mainstay of treatment for attention-deficit disorder.[30] Given the overlap of symptoms between attention-deficit disorder and the disorganized type of dysexecutive syndrome, one might expect some benefit from these agents; however, no research or even any case reports are available to confirm the clinical utility of psychostimulants in patients with a frontal convexity syndrome. Because these agents may aggravate irritability and delusional thought content,[31] their use should be carefully monitored.

Dopamine agonists may improve executive cognition through their positive effect on motivation,[32] as discussed in the following section "Mesial Frontal (Apathetic) Dysexecutive Syndrome" in connection with apathy.[33]

Acetylcholinesterase inhibitors recently have been introduced as cognitive-enhancing agents in the treatment of mild to moderate Alzheimer's disease. Currently, tacrine and donepezil have been approved by the U.S. Food and Drug Administration, and other drugs are under review. These agents block the degradation of ACh, thus potentiating its effect on cerebral muscarinic receptors. The patterns of cognitive improvement observed in patients who respond to treatment suggest a primary effect on enhancing executive cognition.[34,35] These findings highlight a need for controlled trials to assess the efficacy of cholinergic enhancement for treating dorsolateral convexity syndromes of other etiologies, such as head injury or multiple sclerosis.

Alternative treatments for cognitive enhancement often include over-the-counter preparations such as Ginkgo biloba. This agent has not been adequately studied to date but appears to induce electroencephalogram (EEG) changes in some elderly individuals with cognitive impairment that suggests "cortical activation."[36] The cognitive implications of these EEG changes remain to be established. Potential roles for Ginkgo biloba in improving executive cognition must be elucidated in controlled trials before conclusions about its efficacy can be drawn.

Mesial Frontal (Apathetic) Dysexecutive Syndrome

Apathy arises from dysfunction of the mesial frontal neural network at the volitional-motor interface. Motivated behavior appears to be subserved by the functional balance between the anterior cingulum and the supplementary motor area.[37] Despite the neurochemical complexity of these networks, the treatment of acquired apathy syndromes rests heavily on DA augmentation.

The history of DA augmentation in the treatment of acquired apathy dates back to Ross and Stuart,[38] who treated a 36-year-old man with bromocriptine, an ergot derivative with affinity for the dopamine-2 receptor. Their case demonstrated the concept of DA deafferentation because levodopa/carbidopa, a presynaptic DA agent, did not diminish the apathy that resolved with bromocriptine. Since then, 40 cases have been reported in which apathetic-type dysexecutive syndromes have responded to bromocriptine, methylphenidate, lergotrile, ephedrine, amphetamine, bupropion, amantadine, selegiline, and lisuride.[39–51]

A review of these case reports reveals several points concerning the use of DA augmentation strategies:

1. Dopamine agonists are effective.
2. High doses are typically required.
3. Clinical improvement appears to proceed in a linear, dose-related pattern.
4. Some patients deteriorate rapidly when they miss a single dose, whereas others may be successfully weaned off their dopamine agonist.
5. Patients generally do not encounter significant side effects when the drugs are titrated slowly.
6. Only a single case of iatrogenic psychosis has been reported despite the use of high doses of dopamine agonists.
7. Children appear to benefit from lower doses of dopamine agonists.
8. Tachyphylaxis is rare.
9. High-dose therapies are expensive. The monthly cost of 40 mg of bromocriptine is more than $480.

Orbitofrontal (Disinhibited) Dysexecutive Syndrome

Patients with orbitofrontal lesions are characterized by poor impulse control and stimulus-bound behavior.[52] The jocularity and emotional lability shown by these patients are often misinterpreted as mania. The most disturbing behavior in such individuals is impulsive and short-lived aggression. Although an extensive literature addresses the pharmacological treatment of aggression in general, little attempt has been made to characterize the particular treatment response of different types of aggression. With this caveat in mind, the explosive aggression often shown by patients after a significant traumatic brain injury has

been reported to respond to high-dose β-adrenergic receptor blockade.[53] Other agents with apparent efficacy for this type of aggression include valproic acid,[54] carbamazepine,[55] serotonin reuptake inhibitors,[56] and lithium.[57]

Although these psychopharmacological treatments offer some symptomatic relief, they should be only one part of a comprehensive treatment plan. Any treatment plan that does not include some of the following psychosocial interventions is unlikely to succeed.

ENVIRONMENTAL TREATMENT STRATEGIES

Environmental manipulation is the most effective strategy for improving the function of the patient with a dysexecutive syndrome. Although this approach has a benign side-effect profile, it requires considerable time on the clinician's part and coordination among key people actively involved in the patient's care. The levels of commitment and consistency required of the patient's caregivers are likely to wear down even the most determined of social supports. Few families are able to shoulder this responsibility alone, and it is important that a wide range of social support services be identified for the patient, including rehabilitation programs, workshops, day programs, personal aides, and respite care. Under the guidance of a clinical team leader, these social resource providers must be involved in a dialogue about environmental strategies that will offer the patient the highest possible level of function.

It is helpful to bear in mind the nature of executive cognition, which includes initiation, planning, temporal organization, and self-monitoring, when deciding what environmental interventions are necessary to maintain and improve the function of patients with dysexecutive syndromes.

Environmental Modification

The patient's environment should be characterized by consistency and low sensory stimulation. Patients with dysexecutive syndromes are likely to become anxious and overwhelmed by novel or ambiguous situations. They will benefit from a predictable routine. Patients having difficulty with multistep tasks may benefit from cue cards that break tasks down and list their basic components. For example, chores can be listed separately and scheduled on a daily planner. The patient's caregivers play the central role in ensuring consistency in the environment. They should therefore be empowered to take the lead in the design and execution of an environmental modification plan.

Patients with dysexecutive syndromes have difficulty driving and frequently present a risk to themselves or others. They may have to curtail driving because of impulsivity or poor judgment. Many states authorize physicians to report such persons to the Department of Motor Vehicles. It is important to be aware of these laws, which differ from state to state.

Advocacy and Resources

Many practical aspects of the patient's care require attention. A source of adequate income for the patient must be identified. Disability from Social Security or other sources must be sought. A custodian or durable power of attorney for person and property may need to be arranged to protect the patient's interests.

Specific Skills Training

Highly focused training protocols have been reviewed by Sohlberg et al.[58] and Mateer[59] as part of a comprehensive rehabilitation program for patients with dysexecutive syndromes. These protocols are based on behavioral approaches and include task-specific routines for activities of daily living, external compensatory systems such as cue cards,[60] social skills training,[61] and metacognitive skills training to increase awareness and self-monitoring.[62,63] The authors report that these interventions are still in the experimental phase. Given the severe impairments brought on by executive dysfunction, however, therapeutic trials of these modalities may be of significant benefit to affected patients.

Hospitalization

The life of an individual with a dysexecutive syndrome is often characterized by series of crises. Whenever possible, attempts should be made to resolve these crises in the patient's social milieu rather than resorting to multiple hospitalizations. Unfortunately, all too often these patients are trapped in a revolving door, constantly moving into and out of the inpatient psychiatric unit, where they frequently receive incorrect diagnoses of a personality disorder. When a chaotic social environment cannot be simplified, hospitalization is frequently inevitable.

It is important to note that the person with a dysexecutive syndrome is likely to improve rapidly on admission to a structured, consistent, supportive inpatient milieu. Such prompt improvement can mislead the treatment team into underestimating the patient's impairment. This quiescent period is a useful time to identify and address the factors that led to the patient's decompensation. Facilitating occasional periods of respite for caregivers often makes good therapeutic sense.

PSYCHOTHERAPY

The presence of a dysexecutive syndrome does not mitigate the experience of emotional pain and discomfort. Indeed, the emotional lability and impulsiveness that characterize the syndrome are likely to heighten the individual's distress. Executive dysfunction seriously impairs one's flexibility in dealing with emotional and interpersonal challenges. Yet, the patient with a dysexecutive syndrome frequently encounters the grief, confusion, and, occasionally, hostility of a family and social circle who are themselves attempting to understand the profound changes that have occurred in the patient.

Therapeutic interventions are most beneficial when focused on supportive psychotherapy. Psychotherapy has to address the decreased self-esteem that stems from the patient's vanquished dreams and loss of productivity. The caring, understanding atmosphere that this mode of therapy offers is a powerful source of support for the patient. Therapy is most effective when it is brief, directive, reality based, and focused on immediate concerns.

FAMILY THERAPY

Family therapy is an important and often neglected treatment modality in managing dysexecutive syndromes. The significant personality changes induced by frontal lobe impairment clearly destabilize the family system. When this is not recognized, optimal treatment cannot be achieved. A destabilized family system represents an ambiguous, emotionally charged, toxic environment, which affects the treatment plan in a decidedly negative way.

Family therapy begins with education. Families must understand the patient's changed behavior. As described earlier, signs of executive dysfunction appear to the family as willful behavior. Apathetic patients are frequently accused of being lazy or uncaring. Disinhibited patients are provocative and volatile. Disorganized patients generate frustration given the appearance of normal cognition. This adds considerable burden to family members who are struggling to cope with loss of the premorbid family system.

The McMaster model of problem-centered systems family therapy provides an ideal assessment and treatment tool for the families of patients with dysexecutive syndromes.[64] This model relies on a clear and concise conceptual framework that facilitates participation of the patient in the treatment.

The McMaster model requires a careful assessment of six essential areas of family functioning: roles, problem solving, behavior control, communication, affective involvement, and affective responsiveness.[65] All areas are affected by executive dysfunction (Table 11–1). The model provides the basis for a structured treatment approach that focuses on the specific problems identified by the assessment. Active collaboration of the family is required, with the therapist acting as facilitator. The major objectives of therapy include family openness, clarity of communication, and the development of active problem-solving skills. Families find the therapy to be clear and logical and to foster responsibility and efficacy.

Patients are typically unable to fulfill their prior roles within the family. The allocation of role responsibilities in families is an implicit or explicit process that, in a healthy system, optimizes use of a family member's skills. The need to reallocate roles can be quite destabilizing for families lacking flexibility or resources. The turmoil may be diminished by finding new, adaptive roles for the patient. A significant new role for the family will be that of caregiver. This responsibility is usually taken on with some mixed feelings, which may interfere with family functioning. Families have particular ambivalence around role reallocation for apathetic patients, who appear lazy and unconcerned. Therapy sessions provide a forum for families to deal with their frustrations constructively.

Executive impairment has a negative effect on problem-solving skills. The stepwise assessment of problem solving offered by the McMaster model clarifies this process for families. Steps include identifying the problem, communicating the problem to the appropriate person, developing solutions, choosing a solution, and implementing, monitoring, and reviewing the outcome. Disorganized patients respond well to the breakdown of problems into steps. They are able to

participate in the process, increasing their sense of efficacy and self-worth.

Behavior control involves physically dangerous situations, situations that involve meeting and expressing needs and drives, and social comportment. Patients with disinhibited-type dysexecutive syndromes have significant dysfunction in all three spheres and continually violate family standards of acceptable behavior.

Communication is focused on verbal exchange along two axes: clear versus masked and direct versus indirect. Communication is divided into affective and instrumental areas. The optimal communicative style is clear and direct. Patients with executive impairment have great difficulty with styles that are masked and indirect. The ambiguity created by suboptimal communication styles generates confusion and dysphoria in impaired patients. Agitation and catastrophic reactions then occur.

Patients with dysexecutive syndromes most easily follow concrete language. Yet families are frequently uncomfortable speaking concretely with the impaired member because they consider it demeaning to the person. The therapist can demonstrate effective communicative styles through modeling and may then teach the family these approaches. Furthermore, many families have difficulty with effective communication of affect. Given the emotional instability associated with executive dysfunction, optimal affective communication is therapeutically desirable. Patients are then able to express their feelings to their support network, and family members can clarify their feelings to the patient, who is at a disadvantage in interpreting and reacting appropriately to affect.

Affective involvement is equated with family members' emotional investment in one another. Apathetic patients appear underinvolved with others. Families often misinterpret this as emotional abandonment. Therapy sessions provide an opportunity for family members to express their feelings as they tend to personalize this situation. Acceptance of the apathetic state as a sign of brain dysfunction, and not as willful behavior, is an important goal.

Affective responsiveness concerns the emotional behavior of family members. As a rule, patients with dysexecutive syndromes have impaired affective responsiveness. This takes the form of lability, or excessively high or low emotional output. The emotional atmosphere of the home has been shown to have a significant effect on the course of psychiatric illness, particularly schizophrenia.[66–68] Families must be

TABLE 11–1. Cardinal features of family dysfunction associated with frontal lobe syndromes

	Apathetic type	Disinhibited type	Disorganized type
Roles	Ability to generate income and participate in chores is inherently limited by apathy. The need to reallocate roles is commonly an unpleasant experience for families.	Patients' behavior is usually too inappropriate to maintain gainful employment. They may participate in chores, but performance is variable, particularly when the patient "doesn't feel like it."	Patients' cognitive impairments are frequently minimized through compensatory strategies such that they can occasionally hold a job and participate in family chores to varying degrees.
Behavior control	Behavioral repertoire is universally limited. Families often erroneously interpret this as a deliberate behavior.	Lack of self-monitoring and low frustration tolerance lead to verbal and physical acting out. Family efforts to modify the behavior are usually rebuffed.	Behavior is more appropriate. Problematic behaviors are usually limited to situations of high stress and emotion that contribute to impulsive acts.
Communication	Communications are sparse and dysprosodic. This communicative style is inherently unsatisfying to family members, who gradually diminish their involvement.	Communications are typically direct and unmasked to the point of being inappropriately frank and vulgar. Patients' ability to listen and not interrupt others is quite impaired.	Ability to comprehend implied meanings is diminished. Patients do best with a direct and unmasked style of communication that borders on concrete.
Affective responsiveness	Affective responsiveness declines profoundly. Family members often mistakenly interpret patient's apathy as deliberate and respond to the patient with frustration and sadness.	Patients have a wide range of affects typically in excess of what the situation deems as appropriate. Anger and frustration are disproportionately expressed at the expense of the more tender affects.	Patients' affects fall into a more appropriate range, with the exception of times of stress, when the patient can become impulsive and irrational. Efforts to lower expressed emotion can be helpful.
Affective involvement	Family members commonly interpret the apathetic patient's emotional blunting as a lack of caring and withdraw from him or her.	The patient's irritability and tendency to be verbally abusive and hostile push family members away. Marital and family discord are common.	Emotional ties to family members are generally intact. Families more easily become invested in supporting the patient through his or her struggles.
Problem solving	Symptoms of inertia and lack of motivation diminish the patient's ability to participate in problem solving. Families are forced to compensate by taking on a greater share of this task.	Patients are frequently left out of family efforts at problem solving for reasons detailed above. Their participation is additionally impaired by the common occurrence of comorbid dysexecutive symptoms.	The dysexecutive syndrome impairs independent problem solving. Family members can act as "auxiliary executive systems" to help the patient remain organized enough to contribute to solving problems.

made aware of the toxic effects of high expressed emotion on the vulnerable patient with executive impairment. The use of time-out periods is one method to help restabilize the environment. If issues cannot be approached with appropriate affect, then the discussion should take place away from the patient. Family work on communication skills also contributes to a more stable emotional milieu.

The treatment of executive dysfunction is a long-term investment making full use of the biopsychosocial model. No single model of disease is sufficient in approaching these patients. Reductionism distances the physician from the patient and stifles the creativity needed to truly understand and provide help. The neuropsychiatrist is able to comprehend illness from multiple perspectives and to intervene at multiple levels. In this sense, neuropsychiatry is not an esoteric subspecialty devoted to the study of unusual brain disorders. It is perhaps better understood as a celebration of what it is to be human.

Case Report

Mr. A is a 43-year-old man with an 8-year history of relapsing-remitting multiple sclerosis. As his illness progressed, he found himself more fatigued and less able to sustain concentration over the workday such that he was not able to continue full-time work and was placed on disability. He presented to the neuropsychiatry service in the context of a recent temper outburst that resulted in him damaging furniture in the house and threatening family members. He had significant remorse and noted that he had become progressively more irritable, listless, and depressed, feeling that his situation was hopeless.

His cognitive examination revealed difficulties with a two-step Luria motor sequence and problems with sustained concentration and cognitive efficiency. Peripheral neurological examination showed mild bilateral internuclear opthalmoplegia, right gaze diplopia, and hyperreflexia in both legs with mild proximal right leg weakness. A magnetic resonance image of the brain identified numerous plaques in the frontal white matter, periventricular areas, and brain stem.

Parenteral steroids were begun, with improvement noted in the diplopia and leg weakness. A trial of bupropion was begun to treat his depression. Within 2 weeks, his mood improved, and his lack of energy diminished considerably. Supportive psychotherapy was initiated and focused on the loss of his health and current struggles within the family.

A family assessment was done. He had been married for 18 years to his current wife, who was

employed part time as a restaurant hostess. They had five children: one girl, age 5 years, and four boys, ages 4, 7, 14, and 17 years. They lived in a four-bedroom home, which they owned. The oldest son slept in a room he built in the basement.

The family had to shuffle their roles following Mr. A's inability to work. His wife began working full time at the restaurant in the evening. The patient assumed the parental roles at home. He struggled greatly with being organized. He had to do laundry, clean the home, cook meals, do food shopping, tend to the yard, and send the children off to school. His wife was a perfectionist and always maintained a well-organized, neat home. The patient was considerably less successful because of fatigue and disorganization despite the obvious benefits of the bupropion. He again found himself irritable and feeling like a failure.

The area of behavior control was notable for the patient's explosive outbursts and also for the oldest son, whose grades at school were declining. He was defiant with his parents and would frequently provoke his father into shouting matches, adding to Mr. A's dysphoria and proneness to outbursts. The patient found it difficult to approach his son with patience and consistency.

The family's communication skills were generally excellent. Mr. and Mrs. A spoke comfortably about instrumental and affective concerns. The style was direct and unmasked. The exception to this was the oldest son, who preferred to remain quiet at home and keep his concerns to himself. The other children were quite verbal but avoided subjects that might provoke irritation in their father.

Problematic areas in affective responsiveness were Mr. A's explosive outbursts and the oldest son's anger. The wife had a pervasive sense of guilt that she could not control the home situation more effectively, even though she was working more than 50 hours per week. There was a sense of sadness among all of the family members over the loss of the former stable, effective system. The younger children feared their father's losses of control.

The family members were genuinely interested in one another and showed their affective involvement with words and actions. They were comfortable showing affection and empathy and valued the experience of nurturing. The oldest son and his father had enjoyed a particularly close relationship, and both were painfully aware that they were no longer "buddies."

The family was generally effective at problem solving. The patient became easily flustered in reporting problems at home because he felt that he should be able to handle them. The wife tended to "take over" the process in an effort to solve the problem by herself. Otherwise, solutions were discussed, implemented, and monitored for effectiveness in a flexible manner.

The family situation was plainly contributing to and perpetuating the identified problem of Mr. A's explosive behaviors. The family therapy component of Mr. A's treatment plan elicited and addressed the issues described above. His housework was clarified by creating a weekly schedule for him on a dry-erase board on the refrigerator, which allowed a reasonable time frame to accomplish tasks such as laundry and housecleaning throughout the week. His struggles with finding a sense of value as a homemaker were discussed and were appreciated by the family, who could then be more supportive. During treatment, the oldest son refused to participate in individual counseling, ran away several times, and eventually moved in with his girlfriend. No suitable solution was found, and the family continues to struggle with this problem as they resolve others. The parents and family as a whole scheduled regular times when they would be together to talk. The family sessions helped put the issues "on the table" and made it easier for the children to share their concerns with their parents.

This case illustrates the value that a comprehensive, biopsychosocial approach to frontal lobe syndromes offers to affected individuals and their families. The family has endured several flare-ups of Mr. A's multiple sclerosis, which required hospitalization. His need for brief inpatient psychiatric stays caused by behavioral outbursts has diminished. The family appreciates that their struggles will continue, but they have grown closer as a response to this.

CONCLUSIONS

Frontal lobe dysfunction presents as a challenging group of cognitive and behavioral disorders. A therapeutic plan that addresses the biological, psychological, and social aspects of the patient's presentation can offer significant improvement. New pharmacological, psychotherapeutic, and rehabilitative treatments for patients with dysexecutive syndromes clearly need to be developed. Evaluating the efficacy of these treatments will be simplified by the development of reliable rating instruments to measure various aspects of executive impairment.

REFERENCES

1. Ungerstedt U: Stereotaxic mapping of the monoamine pathways in the rat brain. Acta Physiol Scand 367 (suppl):1–22, 1971

2. Morrison JH, Molliver ME, Grzanna R: Noradrenergic innervation of the cerebral cortex: widespread effect of cortical lesions. Science 205:313–316, 1979

3. Morrison JH, Magistretti PJ: Monoamines and peptides in cerebral cortex: contrasting principles of cerebral organization. Trends Neurosci 6:146–151, 1983

4. Fuster JM: The Prefrontal Cortex. New York, Raven, 1989

5. Glowinski J: The mesocortico-prefrontal dopaminergic neurons. Trends Neurosci 7:415–418, 1984

6. Bannon MJ, Roth RH: Pharmacology of mesocortical dopamine neurons. Pharmacol Rev 35:53–68, 1983

7. Beckstead RM: Convergent thalamic and mesencephalic projections to the anterior medial cortex in the rat. J Comp Neurol 166:403–416, 1976

8. Bjorklund A, Divac I, Lindvall O: Regional distribution of catecholamines in the cerebral cortex, evidence for a dopaminergic innervation of the primate prefrontal cortex. Neurosci Lett 7:115–119, 1978

9. Weinberger DR, Berman KF, Zec RF: Physiological dysfunction of the dorsolateral prefrontal cortex in schizophrenia. Arch Gen Psychiatry 43:114–124, 1986

10. Brown RM, Crane AM, Goldman PS: Regional distribution of monoamines in the cerebral cortex and subcortical structures of the rhesus monkey: concentrations and in vivo synthesis rates. Brain Res 168:133–150, 1979

11. Lewis DA, Campbell MJ, Foote SL, et al: The monoaminergic innervation of the primate neocortex. Human Neurobiology 5:181–188, 1986

12. Owens F, Chambers D, Cooper S: Serotonergic mechanisms in the brains of suicide victims. Brain Res 362:185–188, 1986

13. Ferrier I, McKeith I, Cross A: Postmortem neurochemical studies in depression. Ann N Y Acad Sci 487:128–142, 1986

14. Palmer AM, Stratman GC, Procter AW, et al: Possible neurotransmitter basis of behavioral change in Alzheimer's disease. Ann Neurol 23:616–620, 1988

15. MacKay AVP, Davies P, Dewar AJ, et al: Regional distribution of enzymes associated with neurotransmission by monoamines, acetylcholine, and GABA in the human brain. J Neurochem 30:827–839, 1978

16. Mesulam M-M, Mufson EJ, Levey AI, et al: Cholinergic innervation of the cortex by the basal forebrain. J Comp Neurol 214:170–197, 1983

17. Hendry SHC, Jones EG, Emson PC: Morphology, distribution, and synaptic relations of somatostatin- and neuropeptide gamma-immunoreactive neurons in rat and monkey neocortex. J Neurosci 4:2497–2517, 1984

18. Dykes RW, Landry P, Metherate R: Functional role of GABA in cat primary somatosensory cortex: shaping receptive fields of cortical neurons. J Neurophysiol 52:1006–1093, 1984

19. Paul SM, Crawley JN, Sklonic P: The neurobiology of anxiety, in American Handbook of Psychiatry. Edited by Berger PR, Brodie KH. New York, Basic Books, 1980, pp 591–596

20. Hyman S, Nestler E: Molecular Foundations of Psychiatry. Washington, DC, American Psychiatric Press, 1994

21. Lipton SA, Rosenberg PA: Excitatory amino acids as a final common pathway for neurological disorders. N Engl J Med 330:613–622, 1994

22. Medalia A, Gold J, Merriam A: The effects of neuroleptics on neuropsychological test results of schizophrenics. Arch Clin Neuropsychol 3:249–271, 1988

23. Rifkin A, Quitkin F, Klein D: Akinesia: a poorly recognized drug-induced extrapyramidal behavioral disorder. Arch Gen Psychiatry 32:672–674, 1975

24. Meltzer HY, McGurk SR: The effects of clozapine, risperidone, and olanzapine on cognitive function in schizophrenia. Schizophr Bull 25:233–255, 1999

25. Fogel BS, Eslinger PJ: Diagnosis and management of patients with frontal lobe syndrome, in Medical Psychiatric Practice. Edited by Stoudmire A, Fogel BS. Washington, DC, American Psychiatric Press, 1991, pp 450–452

26. Klein D, Gittleman R, Quitken F, et al: Diagnosis and Treatment of Psychiatric Disorders: Adults and Children, 2nd Edition. Baltimore, MD, Williams & Wilkins, 1980

27. Ratey JJ, Sovner R, Mikkelsen E: Buspirone therapy for maladaptive behavior and anxiety in developmentally disabled persons. J Clin Psychiatry 50:382–384, 1989

28. Robinson RG, Kubos KL, Starr LB: Mood disorders in stroke patients: importance of location of lesion. Brain 107:81–93, 1984

29. Reding MJ, Orto LA, Winter SW: Antidepressant therapy after stroke: a double blind trial. Arch Neurol 43:763–765, 1986

30. Donnelly M: Attention-deficit hyperactivity disorder and conduct disorder, in Treatment of Psychiatric Disorders, Vol 1. Edited by the American Psychiatric Task Force on Treatments of Psychiatric Disorders. Washington, DC, American Psychiatric Press, 1989, pp 365–398

31. Bowers M: The role of drugs in the production of schizophreniform psychoses and related disorders, in Psychopharmacology: The Third Generation of Progress. Edited by Meltzer HJ. New York, Raven, 1987, pp 819–824

32. Tariot P, Sunderland T, Weingartner H, et al: Cognitive effects of L-deprenyl on Alzheimer's disease. Psychopharmacology 91:489–495, 1987

33. Campbell JJ, Duffy JD. Treatment strategies in amotivated patients. Psychiatric Annals 27:44–49, 1997

34. Friedman JI, Temporini H, Davis KL. Pharmacologic strategies for augmenting cognitive strategies in schizophrenia. Biol Psychiatry 45:1–16, 1999

35. Cummings JL: Cholinesterase inhibitors: a new class of psychotropic compounds. Am J Psychiatry 157:4–15, 2000

36. Itil TM, Eralp E, Ahmed I, et al: The pharmacological effects of ginkgo biloba, a plant extract, on the brain of dementia patients in comparison with tacrine. Psychopharmacol Bull 34:391–397, 1998

37. Duffy JD, Campbell JJ: The regional prefrontal syndromes: a clinical and theoretical overview. J Neuropsychiatry Clin Neurosci 6:379–387, 1994

38. Ross ED, Stuart RM: Akinetic mutism from hypothalamic damage: successful treatment with a dopamine agonist. Neurology 31:1435–1439, 1981

39. Echiverri HC, Tatum WO, Merens TA, et al: Akinetic mutism: pharmacologic probe of the dopaminergic mesencephalofrontal activating system. Pediatr Neurol 4:228–230, 1988

40. Campagnolo DI, Katz RT: Successful treatment of akinetic mutism with a post synaptic dopamine agonist (case report). Arch Phys Med Rehabil 73:975, 1992

41. Parks RW, Crockett DJ, Manji HK, et al: Assessment of bromocriptine intervention for the treatment of frontal lobe syndrome: a case study. J Neuropsychiatry Clin Neurosci 4:109–111, 1992

42. Catsman-Berrevoets CE, van Harskamp F: Compulsive presleep behavior and apathy due to bilateral thalamic stroke: response to bromocriptine. Neurology 38:647–649, 1988

43. Anderson B: Relief of akinetic mutism from obstructive hydrocephalus using bromocriptine and ephedrine: case report. J Neurosurg 76:152–155, 1992

44. Stewart JT, Leadon M, Gonzalez-Rothi LJ: Treatment of a case of akinetic mutism with bromocriptine. J Neuropsychiatry Clin Neurosci 2:462–463, 1990

45. Barret K: Treating organic abulia with bromocriptine and lisuride: four case studies. J Neurol Neurosurg Psychiatry 54:718–721, 1991

46. Fleet WS, Valenstein E, Watson RT, et al: Dopamine agonist therapy for neglect in humans. Neurology 37:1765–1770, 1987

47. Crimson ML, Childs A, Wilcox RE, et al: The effect of bromocriptine on speech dysfunction in patients with diffuse brain injury (akinetic mutism). Clin Neuropharmacol 11:462–466, 1988

48. Marin RS: Apathy: a neuropsychiatric syndrome. J Neuropsychiatry Clin Neurosci 3:243–254, 1991

49. Muller U, von Cramon DY: The therapeutic potential of bromocriptine in neuropsychological rehabilitation of patients with brain damage. Prog Neuropsychopharmacol Biol Psychiatry 53:1103–1120, 1994

50. Watanabe MD, Martin EM, DeLeon OA: Successful methylphenidate treatment of apathy after subcortical infarcts. J Neuropsychiatry Clin Neurosci 7:502–504, 1995

51. Dombovy ML, Wong A, Schneider W, et al: Clinical use of amantadine in brain injury rehabilitation. Arch Phys Med Rehabil 73:975–976, 1992

52. Mesulam M-M: Frontal cortex and behavior. Ann Neurol 19:320–324, 1986

53. Fava M: Psychopharmacologic treatment of pathologic aggression. Psychiatr Clin North Am 20:427–451, 1997

54. Giakas W, Siebly J, Mazure C: Valproate in the treatment of temper outbursts. J Clin Psychiatry 51:525–556, 1990

55. McAllister TW: Carbamazepine in mixed frontal lobe and psychiatric disorders. J Clin Psychiatry 46:393–394, 1985

56. Fava M, Rosenbaum JF, Pava JA: Anger attacks in unipolar depression, I: clinical correlates and response to fluoxetine treatment. Am J Psychiatry 150:1158–1163, 1993

57. Glenn MB, Wroblewski B, Parziale J: Lithium carbonate for aggressive behavior or affective instability in ten brain injured patients. Am J Phys Med Rehabil 68:221–226, 1989

58. Sohlberg KM, Mateer CA, Stuss DT: Contemporary approaches to the management of executive control dysfunction. J Head Trauma Rehabil 8:45–58, 1993

59. Mateer CA: Executive function disorders: rehabilitation challenges and strategies. Seminars in Clinical Neuropsychiatry 4:50–59, 1999

60. Craine SF: The retraining of frontal lobe dysfunction, in Cognitive Rehabilitation: Conceptualization and Intervention. Edited by Trexler LE. New York, Plenum, 1982, pp 240–255

61. Sohlberg KM, Mateer CA: Training use of compensatory memory books: a three stage behavioral approach. J Clin Exp Neuropsychol 11:871–891, 1989

62. Wood RL: Brain Injury Rehabilitation: A Neurobehavioral Approach. Rockville, MD, Aspen, 1987

63. Cicerone KD, Giacino JT: Remediation of executive function deficits after traumatic brain injury. Neuropsychological Rehabilitation 2:12–22, 1992

64. Epstein NB, Bishop DS: Problem-centered systems therapy of the family, in Handbook of Family Therapy. Edited by Gurman A, Kniskern D. New York, Brunner/Mazel, 1981, pp 444–482

65. Epstein NB, Bishop DS, Levin S: The McMaster model of family functioning. Journal of Marriage and Family Counseling 4:19–31, 1978

66. Leff JP: Schizophrenia and sensitivity to the family environment. Schizophr Bull 2:566–574, 1976

67. Leff JP, Vaughn CE: The role of maintenance therapy and relatives' expressed emotion in relapse of schizophrenia: a two year followup. Br J Psychiatry 138:40–45, 1981

68. Vaughn CE, Synder KS, Jones S, et al: Family factors in schizophrenic relapse: replication in California of British expressed emotion. Arch Gen Psychiatry 41:1169–1177, 1984

PART 4

Frontal Lobe Dysfunction in Neuropsychiatric Disorders

12

Frontal Lobe Dysfunction in Secondary Depression

Helen S. Mayberg, M.D., F.R.C.P.C.

Many neurological disorders are accompanied by depression. Because the clinical presentations of mood symptoms in neurological patients are similar to those seen in primary affective illness, it has been argued that neurological depressions are appropriate and useful models in the study of the pathophysiology of mood disorders in general. A group of hypotheses based on evidence from descriptive, experimental, and theoretical studies have in fact been proposed suggesting involvement of specific neural pathways and a variety of neurotransmitters in depression associated with particular neurological syndromes.[1–13] Although a single unifying mechanism for these depressions has not yet been established, the presence of affective symptoms in specific neurological diseases provides a framework for examining the basic neural systems regulating mood and emotions.

CLINICAL OBSERVATIONS

Clinical studies of depression in neurological patients have focused on three categories of disorders: 1) diseases with generalized or randomly distributed pathologies, such as Alzheimer's disease, multiple sclerosis, and systemic illness with central nervous system involvement[14–25]; 2) conditions in which neurochemical or neurodegenerative changes are reasonably well defined, as in Parkinson's disease, Huntington's disease, progressive supranuclear palsy, Fahr's disease,

I thank my collaborators at the Johns Hopkins Medical Institutions, Sergio Starkstein, M.D., Ph.D., Robert Robinson, M.D., Robert Dannals, Ph.D., and Henry Wagner, M.D., and at the University of Texas Health Science Center at San Antonio, Stephen Brannan, M.D., Roderick Mahurin, Ph.D., Mario Liotti, M.D., Ph.D., and Peter Fox, M.D., who made significant contributions to the collective body of research discussed in this chapter. This work was supported by National Institute of Mental Health Grants MH00163 and MH49553; National Institute of Health Grants NS15080 and NS15178; Young Investigator and Independent Investigator Awards from the National Alliance for Research in Schizophrenia and Depression (NARSAD), a Clinical Hypothesis Award from the Charles A. Dana Foundation, and a grant from Eli Lilly and Company.

Wilson's disease, and carbon monoxide poisoning[7,26–38]; and 3) discrete brain lesions, as seen with trauma, ablative surgery, stroke, tumors, or focal epilepsy.[39–57]

A prominent role for the frontal and temporal lobes and the striatum in the expression and modulation of mood and affect has emerged from these various studies. Classic lesion-deficit correlations, found by using quantitative X-ray computed tomography (CT) or magnetic resonance imaging (MRI), consistently support an association between lesions disrupting frontostriatal or basal-limbic pathways and depressed mood. No consensus exists, however, as to whether the left or the right hemisphere is dominant in these behaviors. Reports of patients with traumatic frontal lobe injury indicate a high correlation between affective disturbances and right hemisphere pathology.[40] Studies in stroke, however, suggest that left-sided lesions of both frontal cortex and the basal ganglia are more likely to result in depressive symptoms than are right-sided lesions,[47,48,50] after which displays of euphoria or indifference predominate.[44,46,49] This view, however, is not shared by all investigators.[45,58] Further evidence supporting the lateralization of emotional behaviors is provided in studies of pathological laughing and crying. Crying is more common with left hemisphere lesions, whereas laughter is seen in patients with right hemisphere lesions,[59] consistent with subsequent reports of poststroke mood changes. Lateralization of mood symptoms also has been examined in patients with temporal lobe epilepsy, although here again there is no consensus. Affective disorders have been described with left,[53,54,57] right,[52] and nonlateralized temporal lobe foci.[56] More precise identification of the sites within the temporal lobes most critical for the development of mood symptoms in these patients awaits further study. Studies of plaque loci in multiple sclerosis also have suggested an association of depression with lesions in the temporal lobe,[22] but these reports have not shown lateralized effects.

Despite the many clear similarities, much variability remains in the location of lesions associated with depression in different neurological conditions. This variability is in part due to the methodological and theoretical limitations of anatomical imaging techniques, which, by definition, restrict lesion identification to those brain areas that are structurally damaged. Functional imaging offers a complementary perspective from which the consequences of anatomical or chemical lesions on global and regional brain function also can be examined. One can use these methods to probe how similar mood symptoms occur with ana-tomically or neurochemically distinct disease states, as well as evaluate the paradox that seemingly comparable lesions do not always result in comparable behavioral phenomena.

FUNCTIONAL BRAIN IMAGING STUDIES

Positron-emission tomography (PET) is widely used to measure a variety of physiological variables in vivo, including regional brain blood flow,[60,61] oxygen metabolism,[60,62] glucose utilization,[63–65] blood–brain barrier permeability,[66] tissue pH, and amino acid transport.[67] Methods are also available to map and quantify presynaptic and postsynaptic neuroreceptor densities and affinities for many neurotransmitters and neuropeptides, notably benzodiazepines, dopamine, serotonin, acetylcholine, and opiates.[68–70]

An important application of PET and single photon emission computed tomography (SPECT) scanning since their introduction has been to study patterns of abnormal function in patients with well-characterized and, generally, pathologically confirmed diseases.[71,72] The results have had a tremendous effect on both diagnosis and management of epilepsy, brain tumors, and dementia,[73–75] as well as a growing role in the evaluation of stroke, movement disorders, and head trauma.[76–78] Scan abnormalities also have been identified in groups of patients with certain well-defined psychiatric diagnoses, including depression; schizophrenia; panic, attention-deficit, anxiety, and obsessive-compulsive disorders; alcoholism; and substance abuse.[79–88] Although the sensitivity and specificity of these patterns have not been fully established, these types of studies provide unrivaled tools for identifying previously unrecognized brain abnormalities and potential disease mechanisms in a variety of neuropsychiatric illnesses, including depression.

Functional abnormalities in primary affective disorder patients have been described in several published reports. Studies to date, measuring regional glucose metabolism and blood flow, have examined both young and old patients, drug-naive and medication-refractory disease, state and trait abnormalities, and a variety of patient subgroups.[79,89–96] Despite the obvious clinical heterogeneity of the patient populations examined and differences in data analysis strategies among investigators, abnormalities involving the frontal cortex and, less commonly, temporal cortex have been consistently reported, although the regional localizations within the lobe differ somewhat (Figure 12–1). All of these studies

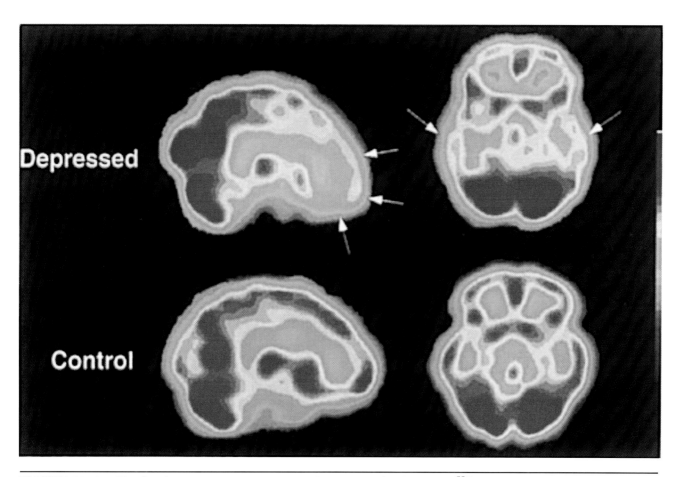

FIGURE 12–1. Single photon emission computed tomography (SPECT) ^{99m}Tc-hexamethylpropyleneamine oxime (HMPAO) images.

Sagittal (*left* images) and axial (*right* images) views are shown normalized to each subject's cerebellar perfusion for visual comparisons. Symmetric frontal and temporal hypoperfusion is present in the depressed subject (arrows, axial view). Note that frontal perfusion is most abnormal inferiorly (arrows, sagittal view). Patient: 30-year-old woman. Control subject: 28-year-old woman.

support a role for specific frontal cortical-striatal-thalamic loops[97–100] or paralimbic pathways[3,101–103] in the pathophysiology of depression, although no abnormality is yet considered pathognomonic.

A parallel tactic is to examine the regional localization of depression by using PET in selected neurological patients—specifically, in those with diseases in which the predominant gross pathology spares the frontal and temporal cortices, the areas repeatedly implicated in the lesion-deficit literature. Changes in both mood and cognitive performance are extremely common in diseases affecting the basal ganglia, most notably in Parkinson's disease, in Huntington's disease, and following ischemic lesions of the striatum.[8,28,30,48] Bradyphrenia with impaired psychomotor and cognitive performance is often present in basal ganglia disease patients, and it may actually obscure the recognition of a coexisting depressive disorder in some patients.[12,38,104–107] Deficits in attention and motivation, as well as more profound impairments on tasks classically localized to the frontal lobes, are also prominent in these patient groups and appear more pronounced in depressed subjects.

Depressions in patients who are not neurologically impaired share many of the clinical features characteristic of basal ganglia disease, including apathy, bradyphrenia, psychomotor slowing, and disturbed frontal lobe function. These clinical similarities may indicate the involvement of common neuroanatomical and neurochemical systems in the genesis of idiopathic depression and depression associated with basal ganglia disease.

The combination of motor, mood, and cognitive symptoms in these patients and their postulated regional localization provide the basis for focused hypothesis testing with PET. One can specifically examine whether depressed and nondepressed patients are discriminated by their respective brain glucose metabolic patterns. One can also test the hypothesis that depression is associated with selective dysfunction of frontal subcortical and paralimbic systems, consistent with the anatomical observations made in other neurological patient populations.

Mayberg and colleagues[6,10,108–110] studied three basal ganglia disorders to address these hypotheses of selective dysfunction: Parkinson's disease, Huntington's disease, and unilateral ischemic lesions of the striatum. In each disease group, patients with and without depression were matched for age, disease stage, symptom severity, cognitive performance, and medications. CT scans were screened to exclude patients with gross cortical atrophy or coexisting conditions. Our goal was to match, as closely as possible, two sets of patients with a given neurological disease who differed only by the presence or absence of mood symptoms. Patients for all experiments were studied in the awake, resting state in a quiet room, with eyes closed and covered. Scans were acquired by using a preselected imaging plane, parallel to the anterior commissure–posterior commissure (AC-PC) line, determined with X-ray CT.[111] Absolute metabolic rates for glucose were calculated for average whole brain and individual cortical and subcortical regions with standard methods.[63] All intersubject comparisons were made by using regional metabolic rates normalized to the whole brain average. Individual regions of interest were grouped into functional cortical subdivisions derived from human and primate anatomical and physiological studies.[3,97,98] Frontal lobe groupings were specifically selected to differentiate primary motor and premotor areas from dorsolateral prefrontal and inferior prefrontal/paralimbic cortex regions (Figure 12–2).

We used this strategy to first examine each clinical disorder separately to identify disease-specific regional abnormalities for depression. A second analysis compared the pattern of regional abnormalities in depressed patients independent of the underlying disease etiology, testing the hypothesis that mood symptoms correlate with abnormalities in specific brain regions regardless of the underlying pathological condition. We then postulated potential mechanisms for these depressions in relation to the identified functional imaging abnormalities, based on the known pathophysiology of each illness.

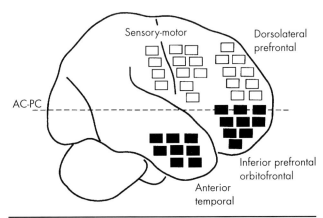

FIGURE 12–2.   Positron-emission tomography (PET) region of interest template, frontal lobe subdivisions. Frontal lobe regions used for PET data analysis were defined by using standardized landmarks and classification schemes. Shaded regions of interest delineate paralimbic cortex. AC-PC = anterior commissure–posterior commissure line.

Parkinson's Disease

Depression is the most common behavioral disturbance seen in patients with Parkinson's disease, affecting an estimated 50% of patients.[30,112] The cause of depression in Parkinson's disease is unknown. The loss of mesocortical and mesolimbic dopamine connections to the frontal lobe and the disruption of monoaminergic afferents from the mesencephalon have been implicated in the pathogenesis of depression in Parkinson's disease on the basis of the reduced brain serotonin, nigral and ventral tegmental area (VTA) dopamine, and locus coeruleus norepinephrine in patients who die with Parkinson's disease.[113–116] Loss of these brain stem monoaminergic neurons, with degeneration of their respective cortical and subcortical projections, is a plausible mechanism for depression in these patients.[2,4,5,7,30,116]

Clinically, depression in Parkinson's disease has been reported most commonly in patients with right hemiparkinsonism (left-brain dysfunction); this is consistent with the widely supported view that associates depression with left-sided lesions.[29,117–119] Despite these observations, no anatomical differences have been identified that distinguish depressed from nondepressed patients with Parkinson's disease.

Although structural imaging studies have been relatively unhelpful, there is a large PET literature in patients with the disease.[120–124] The findings of increased cerebral blood flow and glucose metabolism in the posterolateral basal ganglia seem proportional to the severity of motor symptoms and are thought to reflect disinhibition of striatal neurons associated with loss of dopamine cell bodies in the substantia nigra. Global cortical decreases also have been observed, as have selective changes in dopamine-innervated regions of frontal cortex. Temporal-parietal hypometabolism, a pattern similar to that seen in Alzheimer's disease, also has been identified in patients with dementia and Parkinson's disease[125]; the specificity of regional changes for specific cognitive features, however, are not yet fully delineated.[126]

Using the strategies and methods outlined above, Mayberg and colleagues[6] examined the relation between mood and regional glucose metabolism in Parkinson's disease. We found bilateral caudate and orbital–inferior frontal hypometabolism in the depressed Parkinson's disease patients compared with both nondepressed patients and control subjects (Figure 12–3). The magnitude of the metabolic change in the inferior prefrontal–orbital frontal region is inversely correlated with depression severity, as rated by the Hamilton Rating Scale for Depression, but not with measures of cognitive performance. The regional localization is consistent, although not identical, with lesion locations in patients with poststroke depressions and with patterns of hypometabolism described in primary affective disorders. This finding supports a selective frontostriatal or paralimbic defect in the depression of these patients. Because of the strong interaction of depression and cognition,[107,127,128] further studies are needed to separate the relative contributions of specific cognitive deficits to the frontostriatal and basolimbic localization of mood symptoms. In our study, patients were matched for performance on a group of frontal lobe tests as well as overall cognitive functioning, so there were no obvious confounds of these behaviors. Studies to test these issues explicitly with PET are under way.

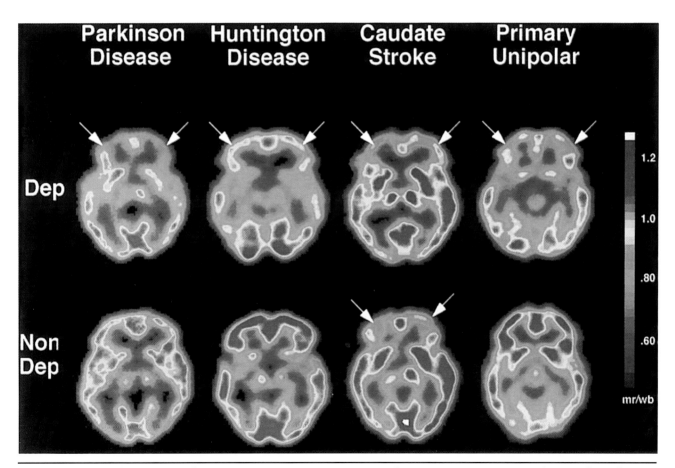

FIGURE 12–3. Fluorodeoxyglucose positron-emission tomography images in primary and secondary depression, basal ganglia level.

All depressed patients have bilateral frontal lobe hypometabolism, independent of disease etiology (arrows, *top row*). Frontal cortex metabolism is normal in nondepressed patients, except those with strokes (arrows, *bottom row*). Scale: relative metabolic rate (regional absolute metabolic rate/whole brain metabolic rate).

Findings with respect to biochemical mechanisms for depression in Parkinson's disease have focused on three systems—dopamine, serotonin, and norepinephrine—thus paralleling studies in primary affective disorder.[129–131] Selective involvement of mesocortical or mesolimbic dopamine pathways is an appealing hypothesis for the mechanism of depression in Parkinson's disease, given the prominence of the dopamine deficiency in the illness and the critical role of the ventral tegmental–nucleus accumbens dopaminergic circuit in modulating motivation and reward in general.[132,133] In support of this theory, depressed Parkinson's disease patients, in contrast to nondepressed Parkinson's disease patients and unipolar depressed patients, do not show the expected euphoric response to the central stimulant methylphenidate,[7] a pharmacological effect dependent on the functional integrity of mesocorticolimbic dopamine neurons.[132–136] Morphological and biochemical studies in Parkinson's disease have identified abnormalities in these brain regions, but results have varied.[113,137–139] Disproportionate degeneration of dopamine neurons in the VTA has, however, been found in Parkinson's disease patients with predominant mood and cognitive symptoms.[116] Cortical projections from this region selectively distribute to the orbitofrontal and prefrontal cortex,[99,140] the areas of hypometabolism observed in the PET studies just described.[6] Despite these compelling lines of evidence, cerebrospinal fluid (CSF) homovanillic acid levels do not correlate with mood,[141] and dopamine agonists have little effect on depressive or cognitive symptoms.[142] These inconsistencies may be explained, however, by the poor correlation between CSF dopamine metabolites and regional brain dopamine metabolism.[143] In addition, levodopa replacement may selectively improve nigrostriatal function at the expense of the mesolimbic system—a phenomenon observed experimentally in rats.[144]

Serotonergic and noradrenergic mechanisms are also strongly implicated, and depression in Parkinson's disease responds, like primary depression, to standard antidepressant therapies.[145,146] Electroconvulsive therapy also improves mood (as well as some of the other motor features of Parkinson's disease), although the neurochemical mechanisms are likely multidimensional.[147–149] Converging data, however, strongly favor a more selective serotonergic etiology for depression in Parkinson's disease. CSF levels of the serotonin metabolite 5-hydroxyindoleacetic acid (5-HIAA) have been reduced in depressed but not in non-depressed Parkinson's disease patients withdrawn from dopaminergic agonist therapy,[5,128,150] a finding consistent with studies in depressed patients without Parkinson's disease.[151] Treatment with 5-hydroxytryptophan and L-tryptophan also improves mood symptoms in Parkinson's disease; as in primary affective disorder, this improvement correlates with increases in CSF 5-HIAA levels.[141,152–154] Selective serotonin reuptake blockers such as fluoxetine and fluvoxamine are also effective in treating depression.[155,156] In total, these observations support a more critical role for serotonin than for norepinephrine in modulating mood symptoms in Parkinson's disease. These findings also suggest strategies for future studies.

The question remains of whether a common mechanism can account for both 1) the selective orbital and inferior prefrontal hypometabolism and 2) the evidence of dopaminergic and serotonergic dysfunction documented in depressed patients with Parkinson's disease. The regional localization of the metabolic abnormalities is consistent with both the orbital frontal–basal ganglia–thalamic pathways[98] and the basotemporal limbic circuit[102,103,157] (Figure 12–3). These particular brain areas have several relevant neurochemical properties. Available evidence in primates, rodents, and humans suggests that ascending monoaminergic projections from the dorsal raphe and VTA terminate in the cortex but in different regions. Dopaminergic efferents from the VTA show regional specificity for the orbitofrontal and prefrontal cortex,[140] whereas serotonergic projections are more widely distributed.[158] Furthermore, the major cortical outflow to the dorsal raphe originates in the orbitofrontal cortex.[101] It might be postulated, then, that primary degeneration of mesocorticolimbic dopamine neurons in patients with Parkinson's disease may lead to dysfunction of the orbitofrontal cortex, which secondarily affects serotonergic cell bodies in the dorsal raphe. Theoretically, disruption of connections at any point along these pathways might result in the metabolic and biochemical defects previously observed, focusing attention on both dopamine and serotonin and their interactions in the depression of Parkinson's disease[159,160] (Figure 12–4).

Huntington's Disease

George Huntington, in his 1872 description of hereditary chorea, was the first to observe that "the tendency to insanity and sometimes to that form of insanity which leads to suicide is marked" (p. 320)[161] Depres-

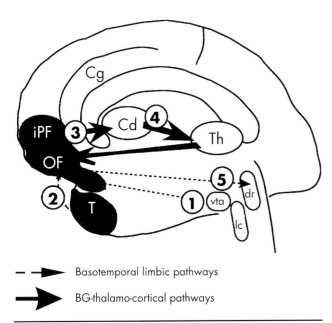

— ▶ Basotemporal limbic pathways

━▶ BG-thalamo-cortical pathways

FIGURE 12–4. Secondary depression model.
Possible mechanisms for common paralimbic cortex hypometabolism in primary and secondary depressions include **(1)** degeneration of mesencephalic monoamine neurons (vta, dr, lc) and their cortical projections; **(2)** remote changes in basotemporal limbic regions, with or without involvement of the amygdala; **(3)** and **(4)** anterograde or retrograde disruption of cortico–basal ganglia (BG) circuits from striatal degeneration or injury; **(5)** secondary involvement of serotonergic neurons via disruption of orbitofrontal outflow to the dorsal raphe. Cd=caudate; Cg=anterior cingulate; dr=dorsal raphe; iPF=inferior prefrontal cortex; lc=locus coeruleus; OF=orbitofrontal cortex; T=temporal cortex; Th=thalamus; vta=ventral tegmental area.

sion occurs in up to 40% of patients with Huntington's disease[32,33] and often precedes the more familiar motor and cognitive features that characterize the illness. The consistent association of involuntary movements, dementia, and mood change with striatal degeneration has given rise to hypotheses in which dysfunction of specific motor and nonmotor basal ganglia–thalamic–cortical pathways is implicated in the pathogenesis of these symptoms.[8,162] Motor pathways have been studied in the most detail; in these studies, loss of spiny neurons in the caudate and putamen as well as neurochemical changes in the pallidum and substantia nigra are described.[163–165] Although the mechanisms underlying the cognitive and mood disorders are less well understood, selective involvement of limbic and prefrontal striatal pathways has been proposed.

No detailed anatomical studies of regional atrophy and mood disturbance in Huntington's disease have

been done, although CT studies have shown correlations between cognitive performance and subcortical atrophy, as measured with the bicaudate ratio.[166] As in Parkinson's disease, there are many published PET studies in patients with Huntington's disease, and decreases in striatal, frontal, and cingulate cortex glucose metabolism have been reported.[167–172]

The relation between the mood disorder and regional metabolic abnormalities also has been tested by Mayberg et al.,[10] who used methods identical to those in the study of patients with Parkinson's disease described earlier.[6] Depressed and nondepressed patients with Huntington's disease, matched for age, years of duration of involuntary movements, functional disability, and measures of apathy, irritability, and global and frontal cognitive function, were studied with [18]fluorodeoxyglucose PET. Caudate, putamen, and cingulate metabolism was significantly lower in the patients with Huntington's disease compared with the control subjects, independent of mood state; these results were comparable with previously published studies. Orbital–inferior prefrontal cortex and thalamic hypometabolism, on the other hand, differentiated depressed patients from both the nondepressed patients with Huntington's disease and the healthy control subjects, in a pattern similar to that seen in the depressed parkinsonian patients (Figure 12–4). These findings again suggested that disruption of pathways linking paralimbic frontal cortex and the basal ganglia is integral to the development of depression in Huntington's disease but that the disruption occurs via different mechanisms than those proposed for Parkinson's disease.

The predominant chemical and anatomical changes in Huntington's disease occur in the striatum. Pathological changes in cortex have not been appreciated in early stages of the disease, although both cortical atrophy[173] and cell loss in the frontal cortex[174] have been documented in more advanced cases. Atrophy alone, however, did not explain the findings in the described PET study; depressed and nondepressed patients had comparable quantitative measures of atrophy by MRI.

The established connections between specific striatal subnuclei and exclusive regions of cortex, via the pallidum and thalamus, provide a cogent physiological mechanism by which specific cortical areas are selectively affected in the depressed group of patients with Huntington's disease (Figure 12–3). Primary dysfunction or degeneration of neurons in the frontal cortex is one explanation for the hypometabolism seen in this region in depressed patients with Huntington's disease. Although specific neuroreceptor changes in frontal cortex, seen at autopsy, have been shown to correlate with the atrophy that occurs late in the course of the disease,[173,175] differences between depressed and nondepressed patients have not been studied. Alternatively, disproportionate involvement of the dorsomedial caudate, which undergoes early degeneration in Huntington's disease,[173] may be present in some, but not all, patients, accounting for the affective disorder seen in a significant subset of Huntington's disease patients. Preferential involvement of the dorsomedial caudate can also be directly addressed by postmortem pathological studies in psychiatrically well-characterized Huntington's disease patients who die early in the course of illness. Anterograde or retrograde degeneration of pathways linking dorsomedial caudate, dorsomedial thalamus, and orbitofrontal–inferior prefrontal cortex might similarly result in remote hypometabolism in appropriate regions of thalamus and cortex.[174] Changes in basotemporal limbic pathways linking the orbitofrontal cortex with the amygdala, temporal pole, and dorsomedial thalamus[157,176] also would explain the observed pattern of focal hypometabolism. Although amygdala metabolism was not reliably sampled in our PET study, atrophy of the amygdala has been reported in Huntington's disease.[177] Correlations with depression have yet to be explored.

Neurochemical mechanisms are more obscure. Degeneration of VTA neurons or their projections has not been reported in Huntington's disease, although dopaminergic projections from the VTA have regional specificity for the orbitofrontal and prefrontal cortex. Striatal monoaminergic, peptidergic, and glutamatergic changes, however, are well documented,[164,165] but no systematic studies of these pathways have been done in depressed patients with Huntington's disease. Future in vitro and in vivo neurochemical studies targeting these specific brain regions may help to delineate further the pathophysiological mechanisms specific to depression in Huntington's disease.

Stroke Studies

Clinicians have long recognized that depression is a frequent consequence of stroke.[51] Systematic studies examining the relation between changes in mood, alterations in specific neurotransmitters, and discrete lesion locations have evolved more recently. Results suggest that the development of clinically significant

depression after stroke depends on two variables: the location of the brain injury and the time elapsed since the stroke.[46] Although severe depressions have been described with lesion sites in both hemispheres, left frontal and left basal ganglia lesions appear more likely to be associated with mood changes than any other lesion location.[47–49]

The prevailing hypotheses concerning mechanisms for depressions following stroke involve direct injury to midbrain catecholamine neurons or disruption of their cortical projections. Experimental stroke lesions in rodents and primates have resulted in decreased norepinephrine, dopamine, and serotonin concentrations early after brain injury. Changes in central monoamines and their metabolites in the spinal fluid of stroke patients also have been measured.[178,179] Levels of 3-methoxy-4-hydroxyphenylglycol (MHPG) were lower in patients with left compared with right hemisphere strokes and correlated with clinical measures of depression severity. These neurochemical changes support the theory that mood disorders result from changes in functionally available biogenic amines.[129]

It is also postulated that mood changes do not result solely from the stroke lesion but are due to the interruption of well-established subcortical-cortical connections—"remote diaschisis."[180] This thesis readily explains the high association of both basal ganglia and frontal lesions with depression. Functional imaging can be used to test this disconnection theory directly and offers a complementary approach to lesion-mapping studies in the evaluation of brain areas critical for the maintenance of normal mood after brain injury. These methods enable us to ask what pattern of cortical or subcortical dysfunction is common among patients with similar phenomena and different brain lesions or what is different about patients with seemingly similar lesions but different mood symptoms.

The examination of regional changes in metabolism or blood flow in patients with specific clinical deficits is a well-described strategy. The pattern of cortical hypometabolism has been shown to correlate with persistent disturbances of language, memory, and attention.[180–182] Applying this strategy to subcortical lesions has definite advantages over studies of patients with cortical infarctions; with subcortical lesions, there are no confounding effects of direct tissue damage or atrophy in brain areas where metabolic measurements are of the greatest interest. The high association of behavioral sequelae, including mood disorders, with lesions of the striatum makes these patients highly suitable for these types of studies. Finally, the known pathways linking the basal ganglia and specific areas of frontal cortex, which have been studied in primates,[97,98,101] provide a logical analysis strategy. The hypothesis that disruption of specific motor and nonmotor loops linking the basal ganglia, thalamus, and cortex accounts for specific clinical deficits can be tested by examining the patterns of regional glucose metabolism in relation to specific lesions.[108,109,183]

To this end, Mayberg et al.[109] divided patients with chronic unilateral subcortical strokes into two groups: 1) those with lesions of motor nuclei (putamen with or without posterior internal capsule) and 2) those with lesions of nonmotor nuclei (head of the caudate alone or caudate plus anterior limb of internal capsule). Patients with putamen lesions had widespread ipsilateral cortical and thalamic hypometabolism and were clinically identified by motor deficits (Figure 12–5). In contrast, patients with caudate lesions had ipsilateral hypometabolism involving more restricted areas of frontal, temporal, or cingulate cortex (Figure 12–5). Clinically, these patients as a group had selective disturbances of cortical function without motor impairment. Although the pattern of remote cortical hypometabolism was not identical among individual patients with nonmotor clinical deficits, all subjects had focal rather than hemispheric changes in metabolism ipsilateral to their stroke lesions. The clinical and metabolic phenomenology seen in this small group of patients[109] is consistent with segregated motor and nonmotor behavioral circuits described in primates.[98,100] The data suggest that precise localization of structural lesions with MRI, combined with mapping of remote metabolic phenomena with PET, may be useful in differentiating functionally separate pathways connecting the basal ganglia and cortex and may contribute to understanding the mechanisms underlying lesion-induced disturbances of motor control, mood, and cognition.

A similar strategy was then used to examine patients with comparable basal ganglia lesions but variable mood symptoms.[108,183] Patients with single lesions of the basal ganglia restricted to the head of the caudate, with or without extension into the anterior limb of the internal capsule, were identified from an ongoing clinical study of patients with poststroke mood disorders. Patients were subdivided by DSM-III mood disorder diagnosis into three groups: euthymic, depressed, and manic. Patients in the euthymic and depressed groups all had left-sided lesions, whereas manic patients all had right-sided lesions.

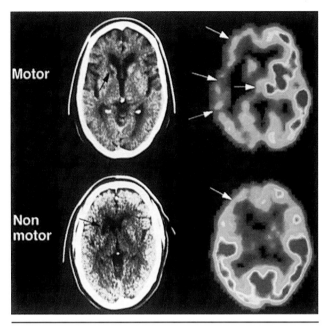

FIGURE 12–5. X-ray computed tomography and fluorodeoxyglucose positron-emission tomography scans in two patients with unilateral basal ganglia strokes.

The motor stroke (black arrow, *top left* image) is associated with diffuse hypometabolism involving the entire ipsilateral hemisphere (white arrows, *top right* image). Note change in the ipsilateral thalamus. The nonmotor stroke (black arrow, *bottom left* image) is associated with a more restricted abnormality of cortical metabolism—in this case, ipsilateral prefrontal cortex (arrow, *lower right* image).

Patients with mood changes (depressed and manic patients together) were compared with euthymic patients, and bilateral hypometabolism was seen in all the limbic regions of interest: orbital–inferior frontal cortex, anterior temporal cortex, and cingulate cortex. The most pronounced changes occurred in the temporal lobes, and metabolism in this region differentiated patients by mood diagnosis (Figure 12–6). Manic patients showed temporal hypometabolism ipsilateral to the lesion only. Depressed patients had bilateral temporal as well as cingulate hypometabolism. Euthymic patients had normal temporal and cingulate metabolism. Interestingly, lesion location did not predict mood change, although the precision of lesion localization was limited by the structural imaging techniques used. Furthermore, the role of lesion side was not fully addressed because patients with right-sided lesions and depression were not available for this study. Notably, bilateral inferior frontal hypometabolism was seen in all subjects and was not useful in differentiating depressed from nondepressed stroke

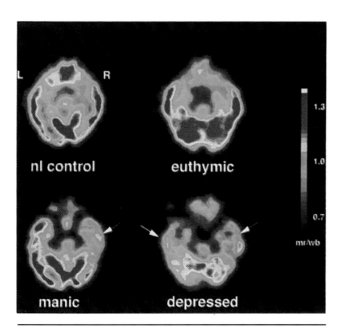

FIGURE 12–6. Fluorodeoxyglucose positron-emission tomography scans in patients with single caudate lesions and varying mood states.

Single scans at the level of the temporal lobe are shown in four subjects. Euthymic stroke patients, like healthy control subjects, have normal, symmetric temporal lobe metabolism. In contrast, manic patients show unilateral (right-sided) temporal hypometabolism, and depressed patients show bilateral temporal hypometabolism. Scale: relative metabolic rate (regional absolute metabolic rate/whole brain metabolic rate).

patients, as was clearly demonstrated in the studies of Parkinson's disease[6] and Huntington's disease[10] (Figure 12–4).

The mechanisms underlying these cortical changes remain uncharacterized. It nonetheless can be postulated that the remote metabolic effects that occurred in the orbital–inferior frontal cortex may be lesion-specific because they disrupted orbitofrontal–striatal–thalamic circuits in all patient subgroups. These bilateral changes were unexpected and have no obvious explanation. Temporal lobe abnormalities, however, appear to be mood state–specific, implicating selective disruption of basotemporal limbic pathways in the patients with mood changes. Undercutting of the medial forebrain bundle as it passes ventral to the caudate, with disruption of selective ascending monoaminergic cortical projections, also might result in secondary changes in regional limbic metabolism. Further studies, including selective lesion studies in animals, are necessary to test these hypotheses.

COMPARISON OF PRIMARY AND SECONDARY DEPRESSIONS

From this series of studies of depression in Parkinson's disease, Huntington's disease, and isolated basal ganglia lesions, it became apparent that basolimbic regions (anterior temporal cortex, orbitofrontal–inferior prefrontal cortex) had consistent abnormalities in the depressed, but not the nondepressed, patients in each disease group.

A subsequent study by Mayberg et al.[184] tested the hypothesis that primary and secondary depressions, regardless of disease etiology, have comparable patterns of abnormal metabolism involving brain areas with limbic connections. In this study, groups of patients with the three neurological diseases were compared with a group of patients with primary affective disorder. Depressed patients, independent of disease group, had significantly decreased metabolism bilaterally in both paralimbic frontal and temporal cortex (Figures 12–4 and 12–7). Further analyses showed no statistical differences between patients with primary and secondary depression—although the magnitude of the abnormalities was greatest in patients with basal ganglia disease. Unlike the original studies performed in each disease independently, these studies showed the frontal and temporal changes in all three depressed patient groups. The temporal lobe abnormalities were not appreciated when each disease was analyzed separately, probably because of inadequate statistical power.

As hypothesized, depressed mood correlated with changes in stereotypic brain regions and was state-specific rather than disease-specific. The potential confound of associated cognitive impairments in these patients was not directly addressed. However, depressed and nondepressed patients were matched for their cognitive performance in all experiments. Although no published studies have explicitly tested these mood–cognitive function interactions, primate experiments have examined the effects of precise cortical lesions on tasks such as delayed response and delayed alternation (behavioral deficits also described in depressed and basal ganglia disease patients), and these primate studies identified selective involvement of dorsolateral prefrontal and orbitofrontal cortex in these behaviors.[185,186] Preliminary studies in primary affective disorder patients have shown that global cognitive impairment is highly correlated with medial prefrontal hypoperfusion, whereas psychomotor

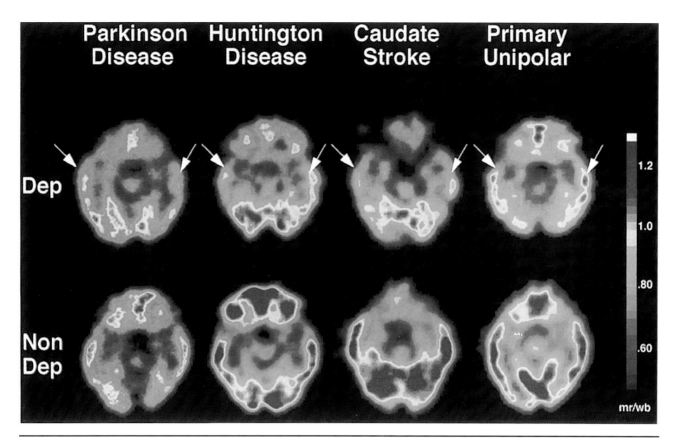

FIGURE 12–7. Fluorodeoxyglucose positron-emission tomography images in primary and secondary depression, temporal lobe level.

The depressed patients have symmetric bitemporal hypometabolism, independent of disease diagnosis (arrows, *top row*). Temporal metabolism is normal in all nondepressed patients. Scale: relative metabolic rate (regional absolute metabolic rate/ whole brain metabolic rate).

slowing correlates most strongly with blood flow decreases in the dorsolateral prefrontal cortex.[187,188] Prospective examination of specific cognitive deficits awaits future studies in both unipolar depression and depression in neurological patients.

A UNIFYING VIEW OF SECONDARY DEPRESSION

The repeated observation from these independent studies of patients with Parkinson's disease, Huntington's disease, and caudate strokes is the common involvement of paralimbic regions (orbital–inferior prefrontal and temporal cortex) in patients with mood disorders, independent of disease diagnosis.[110] These findings have been replicated in Parkinson's disease and subcortical stroke, as well as in patients with temporal lobe epilepsy and Alzheimer's disease.[189–193] These findings make it possible to propose a functional

lesion-deficit map of brain areas involved in depression. The regional localization of the metabolic abnormalities matches two known pathways: the orbito-frontal–basal ganglia–thalamic circuit[97,98] and the basotemporal limbic circuit that links the orbitofrontal cortex and anterior temporal cortex via the uncinate fasciculus.[99–103] Unfortunately, the precise mechanisms responsible for these metabolic changes cannot be delineated by these experiments.

Hypotheses based on the known neurochemical and degenerative defects present in these three disorders can, however, be offered to account for the selective disruption of these corticostriatal and basotemporal limbic pathways (Figure 12–4):

1. Primary degeneration of the VTA, seen in Parkinson's disease, with disruption of dopamine projections to the mesolimbic frontal cortex
2. Primary degeneration of the basal amygdaloid nucleus, also reported in Huntington's disease, which

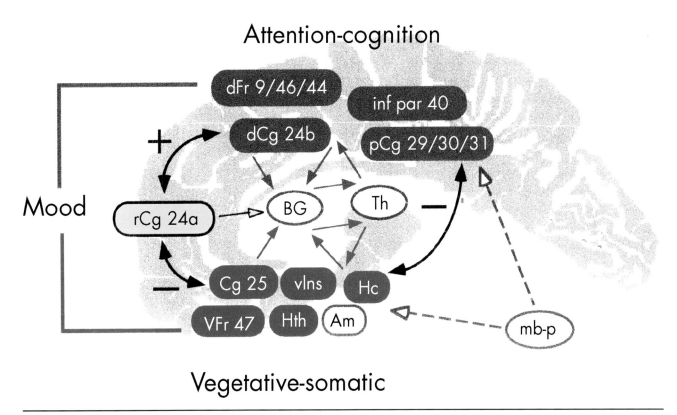

FIGURE 12–8.   Comprehensive depression model.

Brain regions consistently identified in positron-emission tomography (PET) studies of depression are represented in this schematic model. Regions with known anatomical interconnections that also show synchronized changes (using PET) in three behavioral states—normal transient sadness (control subjects), baseline depressed (patients), and post–fluoxetine treatment (patients)—are grouped into three main compartments: dorsal (red), ventral (blue), and rostral (yellow). The dorsal-ventral segregation also identifies those brain regions where an inverse relationship is seen across the different PET paradigms. Sadness and depressive illness are both associated with decreases in dorsal limbic and neocortical regions (red areas) and relative increases in ventral paralimbic areas (blue areas); with successful treatment, these findings reverse.

   White regions delineate brain regions potentially critical to the evolution of the model but in which changes have not been consistently identified across PET studies. Black arrows indicate reciprocal connections through the anterior and posterior cingulate linking the dorsal and ventral compartments. Colored arrows identify segregated ventral and dorsal compartment afferents and efferents to and from the striatum (caudate, putamen, nucleus accumbens) and thalamus (predominantly mediodorsal and anterior thalamus), although individual cortico-striatal-thalamic pathways are not delineated. Dotted lines indicate serotonergic projections to limbic, paralimbic, subcortical, and cortical regions in both compartments. *Red:* dFr=dorsolateral prefrontal; inf par=inferior parietal; dCg=dorsal anterior cingulate; pCg=posterior cingulate. *Blue:* Cg 25=subgenual (infralimbic) cingulate; vIns=ventral anterior insula; Hc=hippocampus; vFr=ventral frontal; Hth=hypothalamus. *Yellow:* rCg=rostral anterior cingulate. *White:* mb-p=midbrain-pons; BG=basal ganglia; Th=thalamus; Am=amygdala. Numbers are Brodmann's designations.[194][188]

has direct connections with both the orbitofrontal and the basotemporal areas via limbic pathways

3. Cell dropout in frontal cortex, which has been reported in Huntington's disease

4. Anterograde or retrograde degeneration along basal ganglia–thalamic–cortical pathways secondary to caudate degeneration in either Huntington's disease or stroke lesions

5. Secondary changes in brain stem monoamines from dysfunction of the orbitofrontal cortex, the major cortical outflow to the mesencephalon

Disease-specific interruptions of individual connections could explain the characteristic paralimbic frontal and temporal metabolic defects that have been identified and could reconcile the presence of similar clinical symptomatology in the settings of different disease etiologies.

   In summary, patients with depression and neurological disease are useful models in the study of the functional neuroanatomy of mood. Imaging techniques provide a focused and novel approach for exploring the biological similarities and differences between primary and secondary depression. Future studies designed to identify specific in vivo neurochemical markers in patients with depression of different etiologies may advance our understanding of the pathogenesis of these disorders and contribute to the full characterization of neural systems regulating normal mood and emotions.

NEW RESEARCH AND PROGRESS TOWARD A COMPREHENSIVE THEORY OF DEPRESSION

A recent series of studies has been completed, which has resulted in an expanded and more comprehensive theory and working model of depression.[194] This new model (Figure 12–8), developed from the earlier prototype illustrated in Figure 12–4, includes data from experiments examining blood flow changes with induced sadness in healthy subjects, resting state patterns of regional metabolism in patients with both primary and secondary depression, and changes in metabolism with antidepressant treatment.[194–201] The convergence of findings from these experiments with other clinical, anatomical, neurochemical, and functional imaging studies[79,89–103,202–232] is the basis for this model, which implicates failure of the coordinated interactions of a distributed network of limbic-cortical pathways in the pathogenesis of depression. The model (Figure 12–8) proposes that dorsal neocortical decreases and ventral paralimbic increases characterize both healthy sadness and depressive illness. It is further postulated that concurrent inhibition of overactive paralimbic regions and normalization of hypofunctioning dorsal cortical sites are necessary for disease remission, whether facilitated by psychotherapy, medication, electroconvulsive therapy, or surgery. Integrity of the rostral anterior cingulate, with its direct connections to both dorsal and ventral areas, is also required for the observed reciprocal compensatory changes because pretreatment metabolism in this region uniquely predicts antidepressant treatment response.[195]

Although all clinical and biological features of the depression syndrome cannot be fully accounted for by this or any model at our present stage of knowledge, this formulation[194] has been offered as an evolving and adaptable framework to facilitate the continued integration of clinical functional imaging findings with complementary basic human and animal research in the study of the pathogenesis of primary major depression and other affective disorders.[233–238]

REFERENCES

1. Bear DM: Hemispheric specialization and the neurology of emotion. Arch Neurol 40:195–202, 1983
2. Fibiger HC: The neurobiological substrates of depression in Parkinson's disease: a hypothesis. Can J Neurol Sci 11:105–107, 1984
3. Mesulam M-M: Patterns in behavioral neuroanatomy: association areas, the limbic system, and hemispheric specialization, in Principles of Behavioral Neurology. Edited by Mesulam M-M. Philadelphia, PA, FA Davis, 1985, pp 1–70
4. Holcomb HH: Parkinsonism and depression: dopaminergic mediation of neuro-pathologic processes in human beings, in The Catecholamines in Psychiatric and Neurologic Disorders. Edited by Lake CR, Ziegler MG. Boston, MA, Butterworth, 1985, pp 269–282
5. Mayeux R, Stern Y, Sano M, et al: The relationship of serotonin to depression in Parkinson's disease. Mov Disord 3:237–244, 1988
6. Mayberg HS, Starkstein SE, Sadzot B, et al: Selective hypometabolism in the inferior frontal lobe in depressed patients with Parkinson's disease. Ann Neurol 28:57–64, 1990
7. Cantello R, Aguaggia M, Gilli M, et al: Major depression in Parkinson's disease and the mood response to intravenous methylphenidate: possible role of the "hedonic" dopamine synapse. J Neurol Neurosurg Psychiatry 52:724–731, 1989
8. McHugh PR: The basal ganglia: the region, the integration of its systems and implications for psychiatry and neurology, in Function and Dysfunction of the Basal Ganglia. Edited by Franks AJ, Ironside JW, Mindham RHS, et al. Manchester, UK, Manchester University Press, 1990, pp 259–269
9. Zubenko GS, Moossy J, Kopp U: Neurochemical correlates of major depression in primary dementia. Arch Neurol 47:209–214, 1990
10. Mayberg HS, Starkstein SE, Peyser CE, et al: Paralimbic frontal lobe hypometabolism in depression associated with Huntington's disease. Neurology 42:1791–1797, 1992
11. Cummings JL: Neuroanatomy of depression. J Clin Psychiatry 54 (suppl):14–20, 1993
12. Rogers D, Lees AJ, Smith E, et al: Bradyphrenia in Parkinson's disease and psychomotor retardation in depressive illness: an experimental study. Brain 110:761–776, 1987
13. Taylor AE, Saint-Cyr JA, Lang AE: Frontal lobe dysfunction in Parkinson's disease: the cortical focus of the neostriatal outflow. Brain 109:845–883, 1986
14. Knesevich JW, Martin RL, Berg L, et al: Preliminary report on affective symptoms in the early stages of senile dementia of the Alzheimer type. Am J Psychiatry 140:233–235, 1983

15. Lazarus LW, Newton N, Cohler B, et al: Frequency and presentation of depressive symptoms in patients with primary degenerative dementia. Am J Psychiatry 144:41–45, 1987

16. Cummings JL, Victoroff JI: Noncognitive neuropsychiatric syndromes in Alzheimer's disease. Neuropsychiatry Neuropsychol Behav Neurol 2:140–158, 1990

17. Zubenko GS, Moossy J: Major depression in primary dementia. Arch Neurol 45:1182–1186, 1988

18. Jagust WJ, Reed BR, Seab JP, et al: Clinical-physiological correlates of Alzheimer's disease and frontal lobe dementia. Am J Physiol Imaging 4:89–96, 1989

19. Zubenko GS, Sullivan P, Nelson JP, et al: Brain imaging abnormalities in mental disorders of late life. Arch Neurol 47:1107–1111, 1990

20. Goodstein RK, Ferrel RB: Multiple sclerosis presenting as depressive illness. Diseases of the Nervous System 38:127–131, 1977

21. Mathews WB: Multiple sclerosis presenting with acute remitting psychiatric symptoms. J Neurol Neurosurg Psychiatry 42:859–863, 1979

22. Honer WG, Hurwitz T, Li DKB, et al: Temporal lobe involvement in multiple sclerosis patients with psychiatric disorders. Arch Neurol 44:187–190, 1987

23. Hietaharju A, Yli-Kerttula U, Hakkinen V, et al: Nervous system manifestations in Sjögren's syndrome. Acta Neurol Scand 81:144–152, 1990

24. Nemeroff CB: Clinical significance of psychoneuroendocrinology in psychiatry: focus on the thyroid and adrenal. J Clin Psychiatry 50 (suppl):13–22, 1989

25. Omdal R, Mellgren SI, Husby G: Clinical neuropsychiatric and neuromuscular manifestations in systemic lupus erythematosus. Scand J Rheumatol 17:113–117, 1988

26. Mindham RHS: Psychiatric symptoms in parkinsonism. J Neurol Neurosurg Psychiatry 33:188–191, 1970

27. Mayeux R, Stern Y, Rosen J, et al: Depression, intellectual impairment, and Parkinson's disease. Neurology 31:645–650, 1981

28. Mayeux R: Emotional changes associated with basal ganglia disorders, in Neuropsychology of Human Emotion. Edited by Heilman KM, Satz P. New York, Guilford, 1983, pp 141–164

29. Starkstein SE, Preziosi TH, Bolduc PL, et al: Depression in Parkinson's disease. J Nerv Ment Dis 178:27–31, 1990

30. Mayberg HS, Solomon DH: Depression in Parkinson's disease: a biochemical and organic viewpoint, in Behavioral Neurology of Movement Disorders (Advances in Neurology Series, Vol 65). Edited by Weiner WJ, Lang AE. New York, Raven, 1995, pp 49–60

31. Caine E, Shoulson I: Psychiatric syndromes in Huntington's disease. Am J Psychiatry 140:728–733, 1983

32. Folstein SE, Abbott MH, Chase GA, et al: The association of affective disorder with Huntington's disease in a case series and in families. Psychol Med 13:537–542, 1983

33. Shoulson I: Huntington's disease: cognitive and psychiatric features. Neuropsychiatry Neuropsychol Behav Neurol 3:15–22, 1990

34. Peyser CE, Folstein SE: Huntington's disease as a model for mood disorders: clues from neuropathology and neurochemistry. Mol Chem Neuropathol 12:99–119, 1990

35. Albert ML, Feldman RG, Willis AL: The subcortical dementia of progressive supranuclear palsy. J Neurol Neurosurg Psychiatry 37:121–130, 1974

36. Seidler GH: Psychiatrisch-psychologische Aspekte des Fahr-Syndroms. Psychiatr Prax 12:203–205, 1985

37. Dening TR, Berrios GE: Wilson's disease: psychiatric symptoms in 195 patients. Arch Gen Psychiatry 46:1126–1134, 1989

38. Laplane D, Levasseur M, Pillon B, et al: Obsessive-compulsive and other behavioural changes with bilateral basal ganglia lesions: a neuropsychological, magnetic resonance imaging and positron tomography study. Brain 12:699–725, 1989

39. Damasio AR, Van Hoesen GW: Emotional disturbances associated with focal lesions of the limbic frontal lobe, in Neuropsychology of Human Emotion. Edited by Heilman KM, Satz P. New York, Guilford, 1983, pp 85–110

40. Grafman J, Vance SC, Weingartner H, et al: The effects of lateralized frontal lesions on mood regulation. Brain 109:1127–1148, 1986

41. Lishman WA: Brain damage in relation to psychiatric disability after head injury. Br J Psychiatry 114:373–375, 1966

42. Blumer D, Benson DF: Personality changes with frontal and temporal lobe lesions, in Psychiatric Aspects of Neurological Disease. Edited by Benson DF, Blumer D. New York, Grune & Stratton, 1975, pp 151–170

43. Eslinger PJ, Damasio AR: Severe bilateral disturbance of higher cognition after bilateral frontal lobe ablation: patient EVR. Neurology 35:1731–1741, 1985

44. Gainotti G: Emotional behavior and hemispheric side of the lesion. Cortex 8:41–55, 1972

45. Ross ED, Rush AJ: Diagnosis and neuroanatomical correlates of depression in brain-damaged patients. Arch Gen Psychiatry 39:1344–1354, 1981

46. Robinson RG, Kubos KL, Starr LB, et al: Mood disorders in stroke patients: importance of location of lesion. Brain 107:81–93, 1984

47. Parikh RM, Lipsey JR, Robinson RG, et al: Two-year longitudinal study of post-stroke mood disorders: dynamic changes in correlates of depression at one and two years. Stroke 18:579–584, 1987

48. Mendez MF, Adams NL, Lewandowski KS: Neurobehavioral changes associated with caudate lesions. Neurology 39:349–354, 1989

49. Starkstein SE, Robinson RG, Price TR: Comparison of cortical and subcortical lesions in the production of post-stroke mood disorders. Brain 110:1045–1059, 1987

50. Starkstein SE, Robinson RG, Berthier ML, et al: Differential mood changes following basal ganglia versus thalamic lesions. Arch Neurol 45:725–730, 1988

51. Robinson RG: The Clinical Neuropsychiatry of Stroke. Cambridge, UK, Cambridge University Press, 1998

52. Flor-Henry P: Psychosis and temporal lobe epilepsy. Epilepsia 10:363–395, 1969

53. Bear D, Fedio P: Quantitative analysis of interictal behavior in temporal lobe epilepsy. Arch Neurol 34:454–467, 1977

54. Perini G, Mendius R: Depression and anxiety in complex partial seizures. J Nerv Ment Dis 172:287–290, 1984

55. Mendez MF, Cummings UL, Benson DF: Depression in epilepsy. Arch Neurol 43:766–770, 1986

56. Robertson MM, Trimble MR, Townsend HRA: Phenomenology of depression in epilepsy. Epilepsia 28:364–368, 1987

57. Altshuler LL, Devinsky O, Post RM, et al: Depression, anxiety, and temporal lobe epilepsy: laterality of focus and symptoms. Arch Neurol 47:284–288, 1990

58. Sinyor D, Jacques P, Kaloupek DG, et al: Post stroke depression and lesion location: an attempted replication. Brain 109:537–546, 1986

59. Sackeim H, Greenberg MS, Weiman AL, et al: Hemispheric asymmetry in the expression of positive and negative emotions. Arch Neurol 39:210–218, 1982

60. Frackowiak RSJ, Lenzi GL, Jones T, et al: Quantitative measurements of regional cerebral blood flow and oxygen metabolism in man using ^{15}O and positron emission tomography: theory, procedure and normal values. J Comput Assist Tomogr 4:727–736, 1980

61. Raichle ME, Martin MRW, Herscovitch P, et al: Brain blood flow measures with intravenous H$_2$^{15}O: implementation and validation. J Nucl Med 24:790–798, 1983

62. Baron JC, Bouser MG, Comar D, et al: Noninvasive tomographic study of cerebral blood flow and oxygen metabolism in vivo. Eur Neurol 20:273–284, 1981

63. Phelps ME, Huang SC, Hoffman EH, et al: Tomographic measurement of local cerebral glucose metabolic rate in humans with (F-18)2-fluoro-2-deoxy-D-glucose: validation of method. Ann Neurol 6:371–388, 1979

64. Reivich M, Kuhl D, Wolf A, et al: The ^{18}F-fluorodeoxyglucose method for the measurement of local cerebral glucose utilisation in man. Circ Res 44:127–137, 1979

65. Sokoloff L: Localization of functional activity in the central nervous system by measurement of glucose utilization with radioactive deoxyglucose. J Cereb Blood Flow Metab 1:7–36, 1981

66. Yen CK, Budinger TF: Evaluation of blood-brain barrier permeability changes in rhesus monkeys and humans using 82Rb and positron emission tomography. J Comput Assist Tomogr 5:792–799, 1981

67. Comar D, Cartron JC, Maziere M, et al: Labelling and metabolism of methionine-methyl-^{11}C. Eur J Nucl Med 1:11–14, 1976

68. Sedvall G, Farde L, Persson A, et al: Imaging of neurotransmitter receptors in the living brain. Arch Gen Psychiatry 43:995–1005, 1986

69. Luciagnani G, Moresco RM, Fazio F: PET-based neuropharmacology: state of the art. Cerebrovascular and Brain Metabolism Reviews 1:271–287, 1989

70. Dannals RF, Ravert HT, Wilson AA: Radiochemistry of tracers for neurotransmitter receptor studies, in Quantitative Imaging: Neuroreceptors, Neurotransmitters and Enzymes. Edited by Frost JJ, Wagner HN. New York, Raven, 1990, pp 19–35

71. Therapeutics and Technology Assessment Subcommittee of the American Academy of Neurology: Assessment: positron emission tomography. Neurology 41:163–167, 1991

72. Holman BL, Devous MD: Functional Brain SPECT: the emergence of a powerful clinical method. J Nucl Med 33:1888–1904, 1992

73. Fisher RS, Frost JJ: Epilepsy. J Nucl Med 32:651–659, 1991

74. Coleman RE, Hoffman JM, Hanson MW: Clinical Application of PET for the evaluation of brain tumors. J Nucl Med 32:616–622, 1991

75. Duara R (ed): Positron Emission Tomography in Dementia (Frontiers of Clinical Neuroscience, Vol 10). New York, Wiley, 1990

76. Baron JC: Positron tomography in cerebral ischemia. Neuroradiology 27:509–516, 1985

77. Brooks DJ: Functional imaging of movement disorders, in Movement Disorders, Vol 3. Edited by Marsden CD, Fahn S. Boston, MA, Butterworth, 1993, pp 65–87

78. Ichise M, Chung DG, Wang P, et al: Technetium-99m-HMPAO SPECT, CT and MRI in the evaluation of patients with chronic traumatic brain injury: a correlation with neuropsychological performance. J Nucl Med 35: 217–226, 1994

79. Baxter LR, Schwartz JM, Phelps ME, et al: Reduction of prefrontal cortex glucose metabolism common to three types of depression. Arch Gen Psychiatry 46:243–250, 1989

80. Reiman EM, Raichle ME, Butler FK, et al: A focal brain abnormality in panic disorder, a severe form of anxiety. Nature 310:683–685, 1984

81. Gur RE, Resnick SM, Gur RC: Laterality and frontality of cerebral blood flow and metabolism in schizophrenia: relationship to symptom specificity. Psychiatry Res 27:325–334, 1989

82. Buchsbaum MS: The frontal lobes, basal ganglia and temporal lobes as sites for schizophrenia. Schizophr Bull 16:379–391, 1990

83. Zametkin AJ, Nordahl TE, Gross M, et al: Cerebral glucose metabolism in adults with hyperactivity of childhood onset. N Engl J Med 323:1361–1366, 1990

84. Baxter LR Jr, Schwartz JM, Mazziotta JC, et al: Cerebral glucose metabolic rates in nondepressed patients with obsessive-compulsive disorder. Am J Psychiatry 145: 1560–1563, 1988

85. Rauch SL, Jenike MA, Alpert NM, et al: Regional cerebral blood flow measured during symptom provocation in obsessive-compulsive disorder using oxygen 15-labeled carbon dioxide and positron emission tomography. Arch Gen Psychiatry 51:62–70, 1994

86. Volkow ND, Hitzemann R, Wang GJ, et al: Decreased brain metabolism in neurologically intact healthy alcoholics. Am J Psychiatry 149:1016–1022, 1992

87. Volkow ND, Fowler JS, Wolf AP, et al: Changes in brain glucose metabolism in cocaine dependence and withdrawal. Am J Psychiatry 148:621–626, 1991

88. Holman BL, Garada B, Johnson KA, et al: Comparison of brain perfusion SPECT in cocaine abuse and AIDS dementia complex. J Nucl Med 33:1312–1315, 1992

89. Post RM, DeLisi LE, Holcomb HH, et al: Glucose utilization in the temporal cortex of affectively ill patients: positron emission tomography. Biol Psychiatry 22:545–553, 1987

90. Buchsbaum MS, Wu J, DeLisi LE, et al: Frontal cortex and basal ganglia metabolic rates assessed by positron emission tomography with 18F-2-deoxyglucose in affective illness. J Affect Disord 10:137–152, 1986

91. Delvenne V, Delecluse F, Hubaine PP, et al: Regional cerebral blood flow in patients with affective disorders. Br J Psychiatry 157:359–365, 1990

92. Sackeim HA, Prohovnik I, Moeller JR, et al: Regional cerebral blood flow in mood disorders. Arch Gen Psychiatry 47:60–70, 1990

93. Martinot JL, Hardy P, Feline A, et al: Left prefrontal glucose hypometabolism in the depressed state: a confirmation. Am J Psychiatry 147:1313–1317, 1990

94. Bench CJ, Friston KJ, Brown RG, et al: The anatomy of melancholia-focal abnormalities of cerebral blood flow in major depression. Psychol Med 22:607–615, 1992

95. Drevets WC, Videen TO, Price JL, et al: A functional anatomical study of unipolar depression. J Neurosci 12:3628–3641, 1992

96. Mayberg HS, Lewis PJ, Regenold W, et al: Paralimbic hypoperfusion in unipolar depression. J Nucl Med 35:929–934, 1994

97. Alexander GE, DeLong MR, Strick PL: Parallel organization of functionally segregated circuits linking basal ganglia and cortex. Annu Rev Neurosci 9:357–381, 1986

98. Alexander GE, Crutcher MD, De Long MR: Basal ganglia-thalamocortical circuits: parallel substrates for motor, oculomotor, "prefrontal" and "limbic" functions. Prog Brain Res 85:119–146, 1990

99. Nauta WJA, Domesick VB: Afferent and efferent relationships of the basal ganglia, in Functions of the Basal Ganglia. Edited by Evered D, O'Connor M. London, Pitman, 1984, pp 3–29

100. Goldman-Rakic PS, Selemon LD: Topography of corticostriatal projections in nonhuman primates and implications for functional parcellation of the neostriatum, in Cerebral Cortex. Edited by Jones EG, Peters A. New York, Plenum, 1984, pp 447–466

101. Nauta WJH: The problem of the frontal lobe: a reinterpretation. J Psychiatr Res 8:167–187, 1971

102. Maclean PD: The Triune Brain in Evolution: Role in Paleocerebral Function. New York, Plenum, 1990

103. Papez JW: A proposed mechanism of emotion. Archives of Neurology and Psychiatry 38:725–743, 1937

104. Gotham AM, Brown RG, Marsden CD: Depression in Parkinson's disease: a quantitative and qualitative analysis. J Neurol Neurosurg Psychiatry 49:381–389, 1986

105. Levin BE, Llabre MM, Weiner WJ: Parkinson's disease and depression: psychometric properties of the Beck Depression Inventory. J Neurol Neurosurg Psychiatry 51:1401–1404, 1988

106. Starkstein SE, Preziosi TJ, Forrester AW, et al: Specificity of affective and autonomic symptoms of depression in Parkinson's disease. J Neurol Neurosurg Psychiatry 53:869–873, 1990

107. Taylor AE, Saint-Cyr JA, Lang AE: Idiopathic Parkinson's disease: revised concepts of cognitive and affective status. Can J Neurol Sci 15:106–113, 1988

108. Mayberg HS, Starkstein SE, Morris PL, et al: Remote cortical hypometabolism following focal basal ganglia injury: relationship to secondary changes in mood (abstract). Neurology 41 (suppl):266, 1991

109. Mayberg HS, Starkstein SE, Sadzot B, et al: Patterns of remote hypometabolism (FDG-PET) in subcortical strokes differentiates grey and white matter lesions (abstract). J Cereb Blood Flow Metab 9 (suppl):621, 1989

110. Mayberg HS: Neuro-imaging studies of depression in neurological disease, in Depression in Neurologic Diseases. Edited by Starkstein SE, Robinson RG. Baltimore, MD, Johns Hopkins University Press, 1993, pp 186–216

111. Talairach J, Tournoux P: Co-planar Stereotaxic Atlas of the Brain. New York, Thieme Medical, 1988

112. Cummings JL: Depression and Parkinson's disease: a review. Am J Psychiatry 149:443–454, 1992

113. Agid Y, Cervera P, Hirsch E, et al: Biochemistry of Parkinson's disease 28 years later: a critical review. Mov Disord 4 (1, suppl):S126–S144, 1989

114. Jellinger K: Overview of morphological changes in Parkinson's disease. Adv Neurol 45:1–18, 1986

115. Scatton B, Javoy-Agid F, Rouquier L, et al: Reduction of cortical dopamine, noradrenaline, serotonin and their metabolites in Parkinson's disease. Brain Res 275:321–328, 1983

116. Torack RM, Morris JC: The association of ventral tegmental area histopathology with adult dementia. Arch Neurol 45:211–218, 1988

117. Barber J, Tomer R, Sroka H, et al: Does unilateral dopamine deficit contribute to depression? Psychiatry Res 15:17–24, 1985

118. Spicer KB, Roberts RJ, Le Witt PA: Neuropsychological performance in lateralized parkinsonism. Arch Neurol 45:429–432, 1988

119. Huber SJ, Freidenberg DL, Shuttleworth EC, et al: Neuropsychological similarities in lateralized parkinsonism. Cortex 25:461–470, 1989

120. Kuhl DE, Metter EJ, Riege WH: Patterns of local cerebral glucose utilization determined in Parkinson's disease by the [¹⁸F]fluorodeoxyglucose method. Ann Neurol 15:419–424, 1984

121. Martin WRW, Beckman JH, Calne DB, et al: Cerebral glucose metabolism in Parkinson's disease. Can J Neurol Sci 11:169–173, 1984

122. Metter EJ, Riege WH, Kuhl DE, et al: Cerebral metabolic relationships for selected brain regions in Alzheimer's, Huntington's, and Parkinson's diseases. J Cereb Blood Flow Metab 4:500–506, 1984

123. Perlmutter JS, Raichle ME: Regional blood flow in hemiparkinsonism. Neurology 35:1127–1134, 1985

124. Wolfson LI, Leenders KL, Brown LL, et al: Alterations of regional cerebral blood flow and oxygen metabolism in Parkinson's disease. Neurology 35:1399–1405, 1985

125. Kuhl DE, Metter EJ, Benson DF, et al: Similarities of cerebral glucose metabolism in Alzheimer's and parkinsonian dementia (abstract). J Cereb Blood Flow Metab 5 (suppl 1):169, 1985

126. Jagust WJ, Reed BR, Martin EM, et al: Cognitive function and regional cerebral blood flow in Parkinson's disease. Brain 115:521–537, 1992

127. Starkstein SE, Preziosi TJ, Berthier ML, et al: Depression and cognitive impairments in Parkinson's disease. Brain 112:1141–1153, 1989

128. Sano M, Stern Y, Williams J, et al: Coexisting dementia and depression in Parkinson's disease. Arch Neurol 46:1284–1286, 1989

129. Schildkraut JJ: The catecholamine hypothesis of affective disorders: a review of supporting evidence. Am J Psychiatry 122:509–522, 1965

130. Van Praag HM, Korf J, Lakke JPWF, et al: Dopamine metabolism in depressions, psychoses, and Parkinson's disease: the problem of the specificity of biological variables in behaviour disorders. Psychol Med 5:138–146, 1975

131. Siever LJ, Davis KL: Overview: toward a dysregulation hypothesis of depression. Am J Psychiatry 142:1017–1031, 1985

132. Wise RA: Catecholamine theories of reward: a critical review. Brain Res 152:215–247, 1978

133. Wise RA: The dopamine synapse and the notion of "pleasure centers" in the brain. Trends Neurosci 4:91–95, 1980

134. Phillips AG, Fibiger HC: The role of dopamine in maintaining intracranial self-stimulation in the ventral tegmentum, nucleus accumbens, and prefrontal cortex. Can J Psychol 32:58–66, 1978

135. Martin WR, Sloan JW, Sapira JD, et al: Physiologic subjective, and behavioural effects of amphetamine, methamphetamine, ephedrine, phenmetrazine, and methylphenidate in man. Clin Pharmacol Ther 32:632–637, 1975

136. Lyness WH, Friedle NM, Moore KE: Destruction of dopaminergic terminals in nucleus accumbens: effect on d-amphetamine self-administration. Pharmacol Biochem Behav 11:553–556, 1979

137. Javoy-Agid F, Agid Y: Is the mesocortical dopaminergic system involved in Parkinson's disease? Neurology 30:1326–1330, 1980

138. Hornykiewicz O: Biochemical abnormalities in some extrastriatal neuronal systems in Parkinson's disease, in Parkinson's Disease: Current Progress, Problems, and Management. Edited by Rinne UK, Klinger M, Stamm G. New York, Elsevier North-Holland, 1980

139. Uhl GR, Hedreen JC, Price DL: Parkinson's disease: loss of neurons from the ventral tegmental area contralateral to therapeutic surgical lesions. Neurology 35:1215–1218, 1985

140. Simon H, LeMoal M, Calas A: Efferents and afferents of the ventral tegmental-A₁₀ region studied after local injection of [³H]-leucine and horseradish peroxidase. Brain Res 178:17–40, 1979

141. Mayeux R, Stern Y, Williams JBW, et al: Clinical and biochemical features of depression in Parkinson's disease. Am J Psychiatry 143:756–759, 1986

142. Marsh GG, Markham CH: Does levodopa alter depression and psychopathology in parkinsonism patients? J Neurol Neurosurg Psychiatry 36:925–935, 1973

143. Hildebrand J, Bourgeois F, Buyse M, et al: Reproducibility of monoamine metabolite measurements in human cerebrospinal fluid. Acta Neurol Scand 81:427–430, 1990

144. Kelly PH, Seviour PW, Iversen SD: Amphetamine and apomorphine responses in the rat following 6-OHDA lesions of the nucleus accumbens septi and corpus striatum. Brain Res 94:507–522, 1975

145. Andersen J, Aabro E, Gulmann N, et al: Anti-depressive treatment in Parkinson's disease: a controlled trial of the effect of nortriptyline in patients with PD treated with L-dopa. Acta Neurol Scand 62:210–219, 1980

146. Stark P, Hardison CD: A review of multicenter controlled studies of fluoxetine versus imipramine and placebo in outpatients with major depressive disorder. J Clin Psychiatry 46:53–58, 1985

147. Yudofsky SC: Parkinson's disease, depression, and electroconvulsive therapy: a clinical and neurobiologic synthesis. Compr Psychiatry 20:579–581, 1979

148. Young RC, Alexopoulos GS, Shamoian CA: Dissociation of motor response from mood and cognition in a parkinsonian patient treated with ECT. Biol Psychiatry 20:566–569, 1985

149. Burke WJ, Peterson J, Rubin EH: Electroconculsive therapy in the treatment of combined depression and Parkinson's disease. Psychosomatics 29:341–346, 1988

150. Kostic VS, Dijuric BM, Covickovic-Sternic N, et al: Depression and Parkinson's disease: possible role of serotonergic mechanisms. J Neurol 234:94–96, 1987

151. Van Praag HM: Depression. Lancet 2:1259–1264, 1982

152. Coppen A, Metcalve M, Carroll JD, et al: Levodopa and L-tryptophan therapy in parkinsonism. Lancet 1:654–657, 1972

153. Sano I, Taniguchi K: L-5-Hydroxytryptophan treatment of Parkinson's disease. Munchener Medizinische Wochenschrift 114:1717–1719, 1972

154. Van Praag HM: Serotonin precursors in the treatment of depression. Adv Biochem Psychopharmacol 34:259–286, 1982

155. Delgado PL, Charney DS, Price LH, et al: Serotonin function and the mechanism of antidepressant action: reversal of antidepressant-induced remission by rapid depletion of plasma tryptophan. Arch Gen Psychiatry 47:411–418, 1990

156. McCance-Katz EF, Marek KL, Price LH: Serotonergic dysfunction in depression associated with Parkinson's disease. Neurology 42:1813–1814, 1992

157. Porrino LJ, Crane AM, Goldman-Rakic PS: Direct and indirect pathways from the amygdala to the frontal lobe in rhesus monkeys. J Comp Neurol 198:121–136, 1981

158. Azmitia EC, Gannon PJ: Primate serotonergic system: a review of human and animal studies and a report on Macaca fascicularis, in Myoclonus (Advances in Neurology Series, Vol 43). Edited by Fahn S. New York, Raven, 1986, pp 407–468

159. Ng LKY, Chase TN, Colburn RW, et al: Release of 3H-dopamine by L-5-hydroxytryptophan. Brain Res 45:499–505, 1972

160. Dray A: Serotonin in the basal ganglia: functions and interactions with other neuronal pathways. J Physiol Paris 77:393–403, 1981

161. Huntington G: On chorea. Medical and Surgical Report 26:317–321, 1872

162. Albin RL, Young AB, Penney JB: The functional anatomy of basal ganglia disorders. Trends Neurosci 12:366–375, 1989

163. Albin RL, Young AB, Penney JB, et al: Abnormalities of striatal projection neurons and N-methyl-D-aspartate receptors in presymptomatic Huntington's disease. N Engl J Med 322:1293–1298, 1990

164. Beal MF, Martin JB: Neuropeptides in neurological disease. Ann Neurol 20:547–565, 1986

165. Young AB, Greenamyre JT, Hollingsworth Z, et al: NMDA receptor losses in putamen from patients with Huntington's disease. Science 241:981–983, 1988

166. Starkstein SE, Folstein SE, Brandt J, et al: Brain atrophy in Huntington's disease. Neuroradiology 31:156–159, 1989

167. Berent S, Giordani B, Lehtinen S, et al: Positron emission tomography scan investigation of Huntington's disease: cerebral metabolic correlations of cognitive function. Ann Neurol 23:541–546, 1988

168. Hayden MR, Martin WR, Stoessl AJ, et al: PET in early diagnosis of Huntington's disease. Neurology 36:888–894, 1986

169. Kuhl DE, Phelps ME, Markham CH, et al: Cerebral metabolism and atrophy in Huntington's disease determined by [18]FDG and computed tomographic scans. Ann Neurol 12:425–434, 1982

170. Kuwert T, Lange HW, Langen K-J, et al: Cerebral glucose consumption measured by PET in patients with and without psychiatric symptoms of Huntington's disease. Psychiatry Res 29:361–362, 1989

171. Leenders KL, Frackowiak RSJ, Quinn N, et al: Brain energy metabolism and dopaminergic function in Huntington's disease measured in vivo using positron emission tomography. Mov Disord 1:69–75, 1986

172. Young AB, Penney JB, Starosta-Rubinstein S, et al: PET scan investigations of Huntington's disease: cerebral metabolic correlates of neurological features and functional decline. Ann Neurol 20:296–303, 1986

173. Vonsattel JP, Meyers RH, Stevend TJ, et al: Neuropathological classification of Huntington's disease. J Neuropathol Exp Neurol 44:559–577, 1985

174. Sotrel A, Myers RH: Morphometric analysis of prefrontal cortex in Huntington's disease. Neurology 41:1117–1123, 1991

175. London ED, Yamamura HI, Bird ED, et al: Decreased receptor-binding sites for kainic acid in brains of patients with Huntington's disease. Biol Psychiatry 16:155–162, 1981

176. Cassell MD, Wright DJ: Topography of projections from the medial prefrontal cortex to the amygdala in the rat. Brain Res Bull 17:321–333, 1986

177. Zech M, Roberts GW, Bogerts B, et al: Neuropeptides in the amygdala of controls, schizophrenics and patients suffering from Huntington's chorea: an immunohistochemical study. Acta Neuropathol (Berl) 71:259–266, 1986

178. Meyer JS, Welch KMA, Okamoto S, et al: Disordered neurotransmitter function: demonstration by measurement of norepinephrine and 5-hydroxydopamine in CSF of patients with recent cerebral infarction. Brain 97:655–664, 1984

179. Robinson RG, Parikh, Rodriguez RA, et al: CSF monoamine metabolite measures in post-stroke depression (abstract). Society for Neuroscience Abstracts 301:S7, 1988

180. Baron JC: Depression of energy metabolism in distant brain structures: studies with positron emission tomography in stroke patients. Semin Neurol 9:281–285, 1989

181. Metter EJ, Riege WH, Hanson WR, et al: Subcortical structures in aphasia: an analysis based on FDG, PET and CT. Arch Neurol 45:1229–1234, 1988

182. Pappata S, Tran DS, Baron JC, et al: Remote metabolic effects of cerebrovascular lesions: magnetic resonance and positron tomography imaging. Neuroradiology 29:1–26, 1987

183. Starkstein SE, Mayberg HS, Berthier ML, et al: Mania after brain injury: neuroradiological and metabolic findings. Ann Neurol 27:652–659, 1990

184. Mayberg HS, Starkstein SE, Jeffery PJ, et al: Limbic cortex hypometabolism in depression: similarities among patients with primary and secondary mood disorders (abstract). Neurology 42 (suppl 3):181, 1992

185. Goldman PS, Rosvold HE, Vest B, et al: Analysis of the delayed-alternation deficit produced by dorsolateral prefrontal lesions in the rhesus monkey. Journal of Comparative Physiology and Psychology 77:212–220, 1971

186. Divac I, Rosvole E, Szwarcbart MK: Behavioral effects of selective ablation of the caudate nucleus. Journal of Comparative Physiology and Psychology 63:184–190, 1967

187. Dolan RJ, Bench CJ, Brown RG, et al: Regional cerebral blood flow abnormalities in depressed patients with cognitive impairment. J Neurol Neurosurg Psychiatry 55:768–773, 1992

188. Bench CJ, Friston KJ, Brown RG, et al: Regional cerebral blood flow in depression measured by positron emission tomography: the relationship with clinical dimensions. Psychol Med 23:579–590, 1993

189. Jagust WJ, Reed BR, Martin EM, et al: Cognitive function and regional cerebral blood flow in Parkinson's disease. Brain 115:521–537, 1992

190. Ring HA, Bench CJ, Trimble MR, et al: Depression in Parkinson's disease: a positron emission study. Br J Psychiatry 165:333–339, 1994

191. Grasso MG, Pantano P, Ricci M, et al: Mesial temporal cortex hypoperfusion is associated with depression in subcortical stroke. Stroke 25:980–985, 1994

192. Bromfield EB, Altschuler L, Leiderman DB, et al: Cerebral metabolism and depression in patients with complex partial seizures. Arch Neurol 49:617–623, 1992

193. Hirono N, Mori E, Ishii K, et al: Frontal lobe hypometabolism and depression in Alzheimer's disease. Neurology 50:380–383, 1998

194. Mayberg HS: Limbic-cortical dysregulation: a proposed model of depression. J Neuropsychiatry Clin Neurosci 9:471–481, 1997

195. Mayberg HS, Brannan SK, Mahurin RK, et al: Cingulate function in depression: a potential predictor of treatment response. Neuroreport 8:1057–1061, 1997

196. Mayberg HS, Liotti M, Jerabek PA, et al: Induced sadness: a PET model of depression. Hum Brain Mapp 1 (suppl):396, 1995

197. Mayberg HS, Mahurin RK, Brannan SK, et al: Parkinson's depression: discrimination of mood-sensitive and mood-insensitive cognitive deficits using fluoxetine and FDG PET (abstract). Neurology 45 (suppl):Al66, 1995

198. Mayberg HS, Liotti M, Brannan SK, et al: Reciprocal limbic-cortical function and negative mood: converging PET findings in depression and normal sadness. Am J Psychiatry 156:675–682, 1999

199. Mayberg HS, Brannan SK, Liotti M, et al: The role of the cingulate in mood homeostasis (abstract). Society for Neuroscience Abstracts 22:267, 1996

200. Mayberg HS, Liotti M, Brannan SK, et al: Disease and state-specific effects of mood challenge on rCBF (abstract). Neuroimage 7:S901, 1998

201. Mayberg HS, Brannan SK, Tekell JL, et al: Regional metabolic effects of fluoxetine in major depression: serial changes and relationship to clinical response. Biol Psychiatry 48:830–843, 2000

202. Bench CJ, Frackowlak RSJ, Dolan RJ: Changes in regional cerebral blood flow on recovery from depression. Psychol Med 25:247–251, 1995

203. Goodwin GM, Austin NM, Dougall N, et al: State changes in brain activity shown by the uptake of 99mTc-exametazime with single photon emission tomography in major depression before and after treatment. J Affect Disord 29:243–253, 1993

204. Bremner JD, Innis RB, Salomon RM, et al: Positron emission tomography measurement of cerebral metabolic correlates of tryptophan depletion-induced depressive relapse. Arch Gen Psychiatry 54: 364–374, 1997

205. Bonne O, Krausz Y: Pathophysiological significance of cerebral perfusion abnormalities in major depression: trait or state marker? Eur Neuropsychopharmacol 7: 225–233, 1997

206. Buchsbaum MS, Wu J, Siegel BV, et al: Effect of sertraline on regional metabolic rate in patients with affective disorder. Biol Psychiatry 41:15–22, 1997

207. Passero S, Nardini M, Battistini N: Regional cerebral blood flow changes following chronic administration of antidepressant drugs. Prog Neuropsychopharmacol Biol Psychiatry 19:627–636, 1995

208. Drevets WC, Price JL, Simpson JR Jr, et al: Subgenual prefrontal cortex abnormalities in mood disorders. Nature 386:824–827, 1997

209. Sheline YI, Wang PW, Gado MH, et al: Hippocampal atrophy in recurrent major depression. Proc Natl Acad Sci U S A 93:3908–3913, 1996

210. Wu JC, Gilin JC, Buchsbaum MS, et al: Effect of sleep deprivation on brain metabolism of depressed patients. Am J Psychiatry 149:538–543, 1992

211. Wu J, Buchsbaum MS, Gillin JC, et al: Prediction of antidepressant effects of sleep deprivation by metabolic rates in the ventral anterior cingulate and medial prefrontal cortex. Am J Psychiatry 156:1149–1158, 1999

212. Malizia A: Frontal lobes and neurosurgery for psychiatric disorders. J Psychopharmacol 11:179–187, 1997

213. Pardo JV, Pardo PJ, Raichel NM: Neural correlates of self-induced dysphoria. Am J Psychiatry 150:713-719, 1993

214. George MS, Ketter TA, Parekh PI, et al: Brain activity during transient sadness and happiness in healthy women. Am J Psychiatry 152:341–351, 1995

215. Schneider F, Gur RE, Mozley LH, et al: Mood effects on limbic blood flow correlate with emotional self-rating: a PET study with oxygen-15 labeled water. Psychiatry Res 61:265–283, 1995

216. Gemar MC, Kapur S, Segal Z, et al: Effects of self-generated sad mood on regional cerebral activity: a PET study in normal subjects. Depression 4:81–88, 1996

217. Reiman EM, Lane RD, Ahern GL, et al: Neuroanatomical correlates of externally and internally generated human emotion. Am J Psychiatry 154:918–925, 1997

218. Lane RD, Reiman EM, Ahern GL, et al: Neuranatomical correlates of happiness, sadness and disgust. Am J Psychiatry 154:926–933, 1997

219. Cosgrove GR, Rausch SL: Psychosurgery. Neurosurg Clin N Am 6:167–176, 1995

220. Nauta WJH: Circuitous connections linking cerebral cortex, limbic system, and corpus striatum, in The Limbic System: Functional Organization and Clinical Disorders. Edited by Doane BK, Livingston KE. New York, Raven, 1986, pp 43–54

221. Carmichael ST, Price JL: Architectonic subdivision of the orbital and medial prefrontal cortex in the macaque monkey. J Comp Neurol 346:366–402, 1994

222. Carmichael ST, Price JL: Limbic connections of the orbital and medial prefrontal cortex in macaque monkeys. J Comp Neurol 363:615–641, 1995

223. Carmichael ST, Price JL: Connectional networks within the orbital and medial prefrontal cortex of macaque monkeys. J Comp Neurol 371:179–207, 1996

224. Morecraft RJ, Geula C, Mesulam M-M: Cytoarchitecture and neural afferents of orbitofrontal cortex in the brain of the monkey. J Comp Neurol 323:341–358, 1992

225. Mesulam M-M, Mufson EJ: Insula of the Old World monkey I, II, III. J Comp Neurol 212:1–52, 1992

226. Kunishio K, Haber SN: Primate cingulostriatal projection: limbic striatal versus sensorimotor striatal input. J Comp Neurol 350:337–356, 1994

227. Baleydier C, Mauguiere F: The duality of the cingulate gyrus in the rhesus monkey: neuroanatomical study and functional hypotheses. Brain 103:525–554, 1980

228. Vogt BA, Pandya DN: Cingulate cortex of the rhesus monkey, II: cortical afferents. J Comp Neurol 262:271–289, 1987

229. Vogt BA, Nimchinsky EA, Vogt LJ, et al: Human cingulate cortex: surface features, flat maps, and cytoarchitecture. J Comp Neurol 359:490–506, 1995

230. Morecraft RJ, Geula C, Mesulam MM: Architecture of connectivity within a cingul-fronto-parietal neurocognitive network for directed attention. Arch Neurol 50:279–284, 1993

231. Pandya DN, Yeterian EH: Comparison of prefrontal architecture and connections. Philos Trans R Soc Lond B Biol Sci 351:1423–1432, 1996

232. Rolls ET: Connections, functions and dysfunctions of limbic structures, the prefrontal cortex and hypothalamus, in The Scientific Basis of Clinical Neurology. Edited by Swash M, Kennard C. London, Churchill Livingstone, 1985, pp 201–213

233. Dias R, Robbins TW, Roberts AC: Dissociation in prefrontal cortex of affective and attentional shifts. Nature 380:69–72, 1996

234. Rolls ET: The orbitofrontal cortex. Philos Trans R Soc Lond B Biol Sci 351:1433–1444, 1996

235. Overstreet DH. The Flinders sensitive line rats: a genetic animal model of depression. Neurosci Biobehav Rev 17:51–68, 1993

236. Nibuya M, Nestler EJ, Duman RS: Chronic antidepressant administration increases the expression of CAMP response element binding protein (CREB) in rat hippocampus. J Neurosci 16:2365–2372, 1996

237. Duncan GE, Knapp DJ, Johnson KB, et al: Functional classification of antidepressants based on antagonism of swim stress-induced fos-like immunoreactivity. J Pharmacol Exp Ther 277:1076–1089, 1996

238. Hyman SE, Nestler EJ: Initiation and adaptation: a paradigm for understanding psychotropic drug action. Am J Psychiatry 153:151–162, 1996

13

The Frontal Lobes and Schizophrenia

A. Meyer-Lindenberg, M.D., Ph.D., Karen F. Berman, M.D.

FRONTAL LOBE INVOLVEMENT IN SCHIZOPHRENIA: HISTORICAL PERSPECTIVE

Schizophrenia has been called the "graveyard of neuropathology." If that is so, it is one quite frequently visited: a MEDLINE search for the key words "schizophrenia" and "frontal lobes" listed more than 750 papers written on this subject in the last 10 years. Given this impressive amount of information and interest, we restrict this chapter to citing current overviews of subtopics in the field; individual papers are referenced only if they are of historical importance or too recent (1997–1999) to have been covered by previous summaries.

From the time of Kraeplin's[1] and Bleuler's[2] initial conceptualizations, schizophrenia has been regarded as a disease of the brain. Given the often devastating and pervasive nature of the disorder and the huge toll it exerts on both the individual and the society, it was surprising and frustrating that no gross brain abnormality could be identified either on the structural level (giving rise to the quip cited above) or with simple measures of brain function, such as the electroencephalogram (EEG)[3] or global blood flow.[4] In this situation, inferences about possible brain structures involved in the disease were primarily made by clinical analogy, and it was natural to compare the known symptomatology of frontal lobe lesions, including behavioral disorganization, apathy, and failure to plan ahead, with similar phenomena in schizophrenic patients. In addition, other subtle neurological features ("soft signs") of patients with schizophrenia[5] have been linked to a dysfunction of prefrontal cortex. These include motor and practic difficulties, reflex abnormalities, a very well-characterized difficulty[6] with smooth pursuit eye movements, and failure to inhibit saccades. Out of this clinical impression emerged an impressive database indicating that tests initially developed to assess frontal lobe disorders (such as the Wisconsin Card Sorting Test [WCST]) had markedly abnormal results in schizophrenic patients but not in many other severe mental illnesses. Landmark studies by Milner[7] linked this impairment more specifically to the dorsolateral prefrontal cortex, making this the frontal lobe region most implicated and studied in the pathophysiology of schizophrenia.

Enormous advances in the available scientific armamentarium have brought the subtle functional and structural alterations of the prefrontal cortex in schizophrenia increasingly into focus. A first major advance was made by Ingvar and Franzen,[8] who observed that nonschizophrenic subjects in the resting state tended to show relatively greater regional cerebral blood flow prefrontally than did patients with schizophrenia. They coined the term *hypofrontality* to describe this phenomenon. Importantly, they also linked this to the phenomenology of the illness by showing that the more withdrawn, mute, socially isolative, and severely afflicted patients were, the more hypofrontal they were. The importance of this finding was extended by the introduction of activation study paradigms,[9] in which the inherently ill-defined and variable resting state was replaced by an activation task performed by the subject while being scanned, preferably in comparison to a control task differing in a specific psychological subcomponent of interest that could thereby be studied. This method showed that schizophrenic patients activated dorsolateral prefrontal cortex significantly less than nonschizophrenic control subjects did. This functional hypofrontality has become one of the best-confirmed findings in schizophrenia research and a point of departure for several of the structural-functional and pathogenetic models advanced since and reviewed below.

FRONTAL LOBE STRUCTURE IN SCHIZOPHRENIA

Postmortem Studies

Several reviews of postmortem studies of schizophrenia discussing alterations of the frontal lobes are available.[10–13] With regard to gross anatomy, the findings seem to be more impressive in the temporal than in the frontal lobe structures, confirming the in vivo neuroimaging findings of enlarged ventricles, decreased size of ventromedial temporal lobe structures, and decreased parahippocampal cortical thickness, whereas alterations of prefrontal cortex are less reliably found. In contrast, morphometric microscopy studies have been more successful in uncovering alterations in neuronal density, possibly reflecting a loss of neuropil[14] and decreased neuron size in frontal, limbic, and temporal regions (the latter would include reports of histological disarray in the entorhinal cortex, consistent with a developmental abnormality).[15] Investigations of connectivity are at an early stage but describe abnormal dendritic spine densities in the cortex as well as various changes in synaptic vesicle protein expression in limbic, temporal, and frontal cortices. A review of new morphometric methods is given by Rajkow-

ska.[16] Investigations of aberrant neurodevelopment in schizophrenia[17] describe abnormalities in cortical cytoarchitecture and several developmentally regulated proteins in the hippocampal region suggesting abnormal neuronal migration, differentiation, and/or cell pruning. Important recent findings include a report by Selemon et al.,[18] who found increased neuronal density, interpreted as decrease in neuropil, in the prefrontal area in schizophrenic patients. Garey et al.[19] reported a reduction in the numerical density of spines in schizophrenia (13 brains) in temporal and frontal cortex. As a negative result regarding a possible pathogenic mechanism for these microstructural alterations, Webster et al.[20] could not find differences in cell adhesion molecule expression in the prefrontal cortex of schizophrenic patients compared with control subjects.

A well-replicated finding of considerable theoretical importance is the general lack of neurodegenerative disease lesions or ongoing astrocytosis-gliosis, which is consistent with the notion that neural injury in schizophrenia would be prematurational and is not progressive. Recent studies confirming the absence of indicators for neurodegeneration include those by Arnold and Trojanowski[21] and Falkai et al.[22]

Structural Neuroimaging

Recent reviews of structural brain imaging findings in schizophrenia include Buckley,[23] Okazaki,[24] and Lawrie and Abukmeil.[25] As in the case of neuropathology, ventricular enlargement (greatest in the body and temporo-occipital horns) is the most replicated finding, followed by temporal lobe volume loss, whereas no unequivocal support for frontal lobe changes is found in meta-analysis. However, the most recent studies, which used an increasingly sophisticated methodology, did tend to find volume alterations that were primarily the result of gray matter reduction, in accordance with the neuropathological results reported above. Recent studies indicating this include those by Buchanan et al.,[26] who found relatively selective reductions in inferior prefrontal cortex gray matter volumes, Sullivan et al.,[27] and Wright et al.[28] A correlation between psychomotor poverty and prefrontal gray matter volume deficit was reported by Chua et al.[29] A question of considerable importance is whether the structural changes are progressive over time. Such a progression in the frontal lobes in patients was found in a recent follow-up study by Gur et al.[30] In contrast, ventricular volumes, including the anterior portion, were found to be stable over time by Vita et al.[31] After reviewing the literature, Woods[32] and DeLisi[33] (who in her own data found temporal lobe atrophy) argued in favor of progressive structural changes in schizophrenia. At present, the literature is inconsistent, and the issue must be regarded as in need of further study, especially because alterations seen on structural neuroimaging with magnetic resonance techniques are sensitive to confounding variables such as blood volume and hydration status, which may obscure or falsely suggest a structural alteration. It is probably safe to say that any progressive changes are certainly very subtle and that several important confounds, including medication effects, in these studies have not been addressed.

Advances continue to be made in moving from global measures, such as volume, to more qualitatively sensitive indices of alterations of anatomical structures, such as the gyrification index.[34] Toward the goal of a better definition of the schizophrenia phenotype(s), studies including unaffected siblings are also of importance. One large recent study[35] of this type found reductions of frontal gray matter volumes in patients and their siblings.

FUNCTIONAL ALTERATION OF THE FRONTAL LOBES IN SCHIZOPHRENIA

Neuroimaging Studies

Functional neuroimaging studies depend on the fact that neuronal activation results in regionally increased blood flow that can be measured either directly by radiotracer methods (positron-emission tomography [PET], single photon emission computed tomography [SPECT]) or indirectly by a regional effect on the ratio of deoxy- to oxyhemoglobin that can be imaged by magnetic resonance techniques (BOLD effect). Metabolic correlates of neural activity are studied with [18F]fluorodeoxyglucose-PET.

Resting Condition Studies

Studies of brain blood flow and metabolism in the resting state do not show a clear-cut abnormality in the frontal (or any other) brain region; both hypo- and hyperactivation of various frontal areas have been reported.[36,37] The main reason for this, in our opinion, is that the resting state is physiologically and psychologically too variable to permit reliable group comparison studies.

Positron-Emission Tomography

Cognitive activation paradigms have been reliable in showing prefrontal hypofunction in patients. Starting with work by Weinberger et al.[38] and Berman et al.,[9] tasks involving working memory or other cognitive operations related to the frontal lobe have been widely used and have consistently elicited hypoactivation in frontal lobe structures in patients compared with control subjects. Working memory, the system used to hold information in temporary storage to complete a task,[39] has been closely linked to prefrontal structures,[40] especially a subcomponent dubbed the *central executive* that is assumed to play a crucial role in monitoring, allocating, and scheduling cortical processing resources.[41] Working memory impairment may lie at the core of schizophrenic cognitive dysfunction[42] and also has been hypothesized to play an important role in schizophrenic symptomatology, in that negative symptoms and behavioral disorganization in the disorder can be understood as a failure in the working memory functions of the prefrontal cortex by which information is updated on a moment-to-moment basis or retrieved from long-term stores, held in mind, and used to guide behavior by ideas, concepts, and stored knowledge. Recent studies have begun to investigate the question of the relation of prefrontal cortex activation to the workload imposed by the task,[40,42] a relation that may be altered in schizophrenia.[43]

Studies that used radioactive tracer methods to evaluate brain-activation-related blood flow changes were recently reviewed by Velakoulis and Pantelis[37] and Weinberger and Berman.[44] Hypoactivation is also found when performance deficits in the patient group are controlled for or not present.[45] In a study of monozygotic twins discordant for schizophrenia, all affected twins showed hypoactivation of the frontal lobes during a working memory task relative to their unaffected sibling.[46] Recent studies confirming hypoactivation of the frontal cortex in schizophrenic patients under cognitive activation include those by Crespo-Facorro et al.[47] (PET, word list recall), Parellada et al.[48] (SPECT, WCST), Ragland et al.[49] (PET, WCST), Scottish Schizophrenia Research Group[50] (SPECT, verbal fluency), Gracia Marco et al.[51] (SPECT, WCST), and Fletcher et al.[45] (PET, word list recall). McGuire et al.[52] found, with PET, an inverse correlation between verbal disorganization (thought disorder) and the inferior frontal cortex. A negative result was reported by Mellers et al.,[53] who could not find a difference in frontal lobe activation on SPECT between

11 patients and 16 control subjects with temporal lobe epilepsy during a verbal fluency paradigm.

Functional Magnetic Resonance Imaging

The comparatively new imaging modality of functional magnetic resonance imaging, offering increased temporal and spatial resolution, the ability to scan subjects repeatedly, and an increasingly wide availability to researchers, has added substantially to our knowledge about functional brain alterations in schizophrenia. Recent reviews of psychiatric applications of the technique include those by Kindermann et al.[54] and Weinberger et al.[55] The great majority of studies that used cognitive activation paradigms confirmed the results found in PET/SPECT measurements, the most recent additions being studies by Stevens et al.[56] (auditory working memory for tones and words), Callicott et al.[57] ("*n*-back" working memory task), Curtis et al.[58] (verbal fluency), Volz et al.[59] (WCST), and Yurgelun-Todd et al.[60] (verbal fluency). In the *n*-back task, subjects are presented with a sequence of numbers from 1 to 4. In the control condition, "0-back," they respond by pressing one of four response buttons that corresponds to the number presented on the screen. In the "1-back" condition, subjects must respond with the number seen in the previous presentation, necessitating holding one number at a time in working memory storage. In the "2-back" condition, the correct response is the numbers seen in the two previous presentations, and so forth. In this technique, the working memory load can be varied across a dynamic range while the stimulus presentation and responses remain the same.

Verbal fluency paradigms, another example of experimental conditions that reliably activate the dorsolateral prefrontal cortex, present the subject with a cue (e.g., a letter or a category, such as "A" or "body parts") usually displayed verbally on a screen. The subject then responds with as many words that begin with this letter or that belong to the displayed category as possible.

In contrast to these cognitive activation studies, Mattay et al.[61] used a simple motor paradigm and reported a less lateralized and localized lateral premotor area activation in patients, indicating that hypoactivation may be specific to cognitive activation paradigms and/or dorsal prefrontal structures in schizophrenia.

Other Modalities

The ability of proton magnetic resonance spectroscopy to assay in vivo the neuronal integrity marker *N*-acetyl-

aspartate, combined with improvements in the resolution and coverage area of the technique, have added considerably to our knowledge about frontal lobe alterations in schizophrenia. Bertolino et al.[62] found that patients had significant reductions of *N*-acetylaspartate bilaterally in the hippocampal region and in the dorsolateral prefrontal cortex but in no other cortical area. The same pattern has subsequently been identified in childhood-onset schizophrenia[63–65] and in drug-naive patients.[62,66] Because *N*-acetylaspartate is a neuronal integrity marker, this finding would indicate diminished neuronal integrity in these areas. The functional significance of this finding is underscored by the fact that a tight correlation was found between dorsolateral prefrontal cortex (DLPFC) activation on the WCST and the *N*-acetylaspartate level in this region in patients.[66A] Because most intracortical excitatory neurons are glutamatergic and these are the primary population represented in the *N*-acetylaspartate measure, this might reflect a decrease in intracortical excitatory neurotransmission (see also next section, "Neurochemical Alterations in Schizophrenia Involving the Frontal Lobe").

The EEG literature in schizophrenia is markedly inconsistent, reflecting both the sensitivity and the lack of specificity of this method in its commonly applied form. Recent reviews are not available; Gerez and Tello[67] provide a starting point for further reading. An interesting recent EEG study[68] found decreased coherence in the frontal lobe region in schizophrenic patients, consistent with a loss of regional intracortical connectivity.

NEUROCHEMICAL ALTERATIONS IN SCHIZOPHRENIA INVOLVING THE FRONTAL LOBES

Neurochemical alterations in schizophrenia recently have been reviewed by Weickert and Kleinman.[69] After decades in which the monoamines, primarily dopamine, were the focus of interest in schizophrenia research, recent interests have shifted toward complex dysregulation of neurotransmitters and G proteins.[70] Recent theories also have emphasized cortical amino acid neurotransmitter systems such as glutamate and γ-aminobutyric acid (GABA).

Dopamine

The frontal lobe receives a prominent dopaminergic innervation by the ventral tegmental area,[71] and dopamine release is regulated, in turn, by the frontal area.[72,73] This feedback loop is complex, and the dopamine hypothesis in its original form, which assumed a hyperdopaminergic state as the cause of schizophrenia, has been difficult to prove; the assumption that schizophrenia combines a hyperdopaminergic state in the striatum with a diminished dopaminergic innervation in the frontal lobe has been promoted.[74,75] In this structure, evidence from a variety of studies is accumulating[39] to indicate that dopamine has a major role in regulating the excitability of the cortical neurons on which the working memory function of the prefrontal cortex depends.

The neuroimaging evidence for alterations in the dopamine system in schizophrenia has been reviewed by Laruelle[76] and Volkow et al.[77] Some 15 studies over the last 10 years led to the conclusion that compared with healthy control subjects, patients with schizophrenia have a significant but mild elevation of D_2 dopamine receptor density parameters in the striatum and a significant larger variability of these indices. Laruelle et al.[78] and Breier et al.[79] found elevated amphetamine-induced synaptic dopamine concentrations in the basal ganglia in schizophrenia. Studies of presynaptic activity reported an increase in dopamine transmission response to amphetamine challenge and an increase in dopa-decarboxylase activity. Together, these data are compatible with both pre- and postsynaptic alterations of dopamine transmission in schizophrenia. Recent studies mostly reaffirm a diminished dopaminergic innervation of the frontal cortex. Stefanis et al.[80] reported a threefold higher level of D_4 mRNA in the frontal cortex of schizophrenic patients compared with control subjects. Some degree of specificity of this effect on the receptor level was suggested by a negative finding of Dean et al.,[81] who found no alterations in D_1 receptors and the dopamine transporter in the frontal lobe. In a study suggesting a link between structural pathology and dopaminergic alterations, Bertolino et al.[82] found correlations, in patients, between striatal dopamine SPECT measures and dorsolateral prefrontal cortex neuronal integrity as measured by *N*-acetylaspartate.

Serotonin

Interest in serotonergic mechanisms in schizophrenia has been furthered to a large degree by the finding that many so-called atypical antipsychotic drugs have a large serotonin type 2 (5-HT$_2$) receptor binding component.[83] Regulatory interactions between the dopa-

minergic and the serotonergic systems at the level of the prefrontal cortex (but also in the brain stem) have been proposed (reviewed in Lieberman et al.[84]). The serotonin system appears to inhibit dopaminergic function at the terminal dopaminergic fields in the forebrain. Serotonergic antagonists release the dopamine system from this inhibition. Several postmortem studies (reviewed in Gerez and Tello[67]) described a reduction of 5-HT$_2$ receptor density in the prefrontal cortex of patients with schizophrenia. A recent report by Dean et al.[81] also found decreased 5-HT$_2$-related binding in the DLPFC of schizophrenic patients. No in vivo evidence for this, however, was found in a well-done recent neuroimaging study.[85] On the gene expression level, Kouzmenko et al.[86] did not find an association of a 5-HT$_{2A}$ receptor gene polymorphism A(-1438)G and the density of this receptor in patients or control subjects.

Glutamate and GABA

The role of the glutamatergic and GABAergic systems in schizophrenia has been reviewed by Tamminga[87] and Weinberger.[88] In keeping with the increasing focus on cortical, as opposed to subcortical, abnormalities in the disorders, these transmitters acquire a special interest because they are the primary cortical excitatory and inhibitory signaling systems. Several observations implicate brain glutamatergic abnormalities in the pathophysiology of this illness. This evidence includes both human neurochemical and clinical pharmacological data.[89] Furthermore, the psychotomimetic action of phencyclidine and ketamine, *N*-methyl-D-aspartate (NMDA)–sensitive glutamate receptor antagonists, suggests an association between human psychosis and the NMDA receptor. One glutamatergic hypothesis of schizophrenia postulates a diminished glutamatergic transmission in the hippocampal glutamate-mediated efferent pathways and cerebral dysfunction in the hippocampus and its target areas, which would include the frontal lobe. Recently, Dean et al.[81] and Benes et al.[90] reported increased GABA$_A$ receptors in the DLPFC of schizophrenic patients, whereas the density of NMDA receptors and nitric oxide synthase activity were not altered. Sokolov[91] found decreased levels of NMDAR1, GluR1, GluR7, and KA1 mRNAs, encoding glutamate receptor subunits, in the frontal cortex of 21 patients with schizophrenia. Simpson et al.[92] reported slight increases in glutamate and GABA uptake sites in prefrontal, but not temporal, areas in schizophrenia, consistent with a locally overabundant glutamate system in prefrontal cortex in schizophrenia. Magnetic resonance spectroscopic imaging studies of glutamate and GABA have been inconclusive.[93] Interactions between dopaminergic and glutamatergic neurotransmission were reported by Breier et al.,[94] who used PET to identify increased striatal dopamine release after administration of ketamine.

Second Messenger Systems

The study of second messenger systems and intracellular metabolites in schizophrenia has been furthered recently by the availability of noninvasive in vivo imaging modalities, such as magnetic resonance spectroscopic imaging.[91] This method has consistently identified decreased phosphomonoesters and increased phosphodiesters in frontal lobes, although one group[95] could not confirm this finding in drug-naive patients. In agreement with the in vivo studies, increases in phosphoinositide signaling activity and G protein levels in postmortem brain from eight subjects with schizophrenia were recently reported by Jope et al.[96] The second messenger inositol phosphate was reduced in the brains of 10 schizophrenic patients in a postmortem study by Shimon et al.[97] (although this was not specific to the frontal lobes).

TOWARD A NETWORK APPROACH TO SCHIZOPHRENIC NEUROBIOLOGY

The frontal lobe functions as part of a network, as is evident from the large body of functional neuroimaging research cited above, as well as by its extensive connectivity with other cortical and thalamic relay areas and the plethora of neuropsychological functions in which it is implicated. The specifics of this network obviously vary by task, but a consistent finding in studies of working memory is a coactivation of prefrontal, anterior cingulate, parietal, and cerebellar structures that is associated with a task-related decrease in superior temporal areas. It is therefore both a natural and an important step in the development of thinking about the involvement of this structure in schizophrenia that increased attention is being paid to possible functional-structural networks that include the frontal lobes and that may be involved in this disease.

(Temporal) Hippocampal–Prefrontal Interactions

The evidence that schizophrenia may be understood as a neurodevelopmental disorder has gained wide-

spread support. The evidence was reviewed by Raedler et al.[98] Numerous recent studies implicate frontohippocampal dysfunction within the framework of a neurodevelopmental abnormality, with the evidence pointing toward primary disturbance in the hippocampus. Besides the dorsolateral prefrontal cortex, the hippocampus and the adjacent medial temporal lobe structures are the most commonly implicated areas with regard to structural or functional pathology. Saunders et al.[99] reported that in the monkey, early injury to the primate medial temporal lobe disrupts the normal regulation of striatal dopamine activity by the dorsolateral prefrontal cortex during adulthood. Bertolino et al.[100] showed with proton magnetic resonance spectroscopic imaging that early mesial temporolimbic lesions in the monkey led to specific alterations of prefrontal cortex neuronal N-acetylaspartate. Heritability of hippocampal reductions in N-acetylasparate in relatives of schizophrenic patients was reported by Callicott et al.[101] Poland et al.[102] reported a reduction of frontal N-acetylaspartate by perinatal stress in a rat model. Disconnection between the hippocampus and the prefrontal lobe may be mediated by glutamatergic mechanisms.[103] Of interest in this context is an elegant study of structural magnetic resonance imaging data by Bullmore et al.,[104] who found significantly reduced dependencies between frontal and hippocampal volumes in schizophrenic patients.

Frontotemporal Disconnection

Given the interest in a network approach, neuroimaging methods that directly address the question of interregional connectivity are of interest.[105] Few of these have been published so far. Mallet et al.[106] calculated correlations between various regions of glucose metabolic rate in PET and found decreased intrafrontal, as well as frontal posterior, connectivity. Although correlation between left and right frontal lobes was absent in a depressed and obsessive-compulsive patient population, schizophrenic patients were characterized by having more extensive and more widespread correlation decrease. A frontotemporal uncoupling also was the result of an earlier study by Friston and Frith,[107] who used PET data from a verbal fluency experiment. They used a method that allowed them to assess patterns of activation most different between control subjects and patients and found that the prefrontal and temporal activations were uncoupled (did not appear in the same pattern) in the patients but did appear in the same pattern in the control subjects. Jennings et al.[108] used path analysis and reported significantly different neural interactions among frontal regions and between the frontal and temporal cortices in schizophrenic patients during a semantic processing task. Norman et al.[109] found that frontotemporal connectivity was disrupted with an EEG coherence measure. Friston[110] reviewed the frontotemporal disconnection hypothesis.

Interactions of the Prefrontal Lobe With Subcortical Structures: Striatum, Thalamus, Cerebellum

Andreasen et al.[111] advanced a hypothesis that implicates compromised connectivity among nodes located in prefrontal regions, several thalamic nuclei, and the cerebellum as the cause of a fundamental cognitive deficit in schizophrenia and called the disruption in this circuitry *cognitive dysmetria*, signifying "poor mental coordination" that manifests itself in difficulty in prioritizing, processing, coordinating, and responding to information. This hypothesis is based on several studies from Andreasen's group (the latest published being Crespo-Facorro et al.[47] and Wiser et al.[112]) in which the structures enumerated above differed in activation between schizophrenic patients and control subjects on several unrelated tasks and in different cohorts and on the fact that the circuit described is anatomically connected. A review of cerebellar involvement in schizophrenia is given by Martin and Albers[113] and by Katsetos et al.[114] Thalamic pathology was reviewed by Jones[115] and Andreasen.[116]

CONCLUSIONS

An enormous body of work on schizophrenia and the frontal lobes in the last decade has confirmed the importance of this structure in the disease but has not yielded a coherent picture. However, certain trends have emerged that—by emphasizing interactions of frontal and other brain structures, developmental alterations leading to subtle structural abnormalities, and complex neurotransmitter regulatory interdependencies—come closer to the clinically multifaceted and etiologically complex entity that is schizophrenia. The following hypotheses are attractive.

Frontal structural and functional abnormalities are present in schizophrenia. They may develop as a consequence of a prenatal hippocampal dysfunction (which itself may arise from an interaction of environmental and genetic factors). They manifest themselves

clinically in cognitive and psychotic symptoms that relate to the involvement of the prefrontal cortex in central executive functions.

In this view, neurochemical alterations would primarily arise for two reasons: as secondary (to the structural alterations) and in part as compensatory, arising either from altered prefrontal regulation of (monoaminergic) subcortical release sites or in the context of a disturbed excitatory-inhibitory balance in structurally abnormal cortical areas insofar as the glutamate/GABA system is concerned.

REFERENCES

1. Kraepelin E: Dementia Praecox and Paraphenia (1919). Melbourne, FL, RE Krieger, 1971
2. Bleuler E: Dementia Praecox or the Group of Schizophrenias (German original 1911, English translation 1950). New York, International Universities Press, 1950
3. Berger H: On the electroencephalogram of man: fourteenth report. Electroencephalogr Clin Neurophysiol 28 (suppl):299, 1969
4. Kety SS, Woodford RB, Harmel MH, et al: Cerebral blood flow and metabolism in schizophrenia: the effects of barbiturate semi-narcosis, insulin coma and electroshock. Am J Psychiatry 151 (6 suppl):203–209, 1994
5. Ismail BT, Cantor-Graae E, Cardenal S, et al: Neurological abnormalities in schizophrenia: clinical, etiological and demographic correlates. Schizophr Res 30:229–238, 1998
6. Sweeney JA, Luna B, Srinivasagam NM, et al: Eye tracking abnormalities in schizophrenia: evidence for dysfunction in the frontal eye fields. Biol Psychiatry 44:698–708, 1998
7. Milner B: Aspects of human frontal lobe function. Adv Neurol 66:67–81, 81–84 (discussion), 1995
8. Ingvar DH, Franzen G: Abnormalities of cerebral blood flow distribution in patients with chronic schizophrenia. Acta Psychiatr Scand 50:425–462, 1974
9. Berman KF, Zec RF, Weinberger DR: Physiologic dysfunction of dorsolateral prefrontal cortex in schizophrenia, II: role of neuroleptic treatment, attention, and mental effort. Arch Gen Psychiatry 43:126–135, 1986
10. Heckers S: Neuropathology of schizophrenia: cortex, thalamus, basal ganglia, and neurotransmitter-specific projection systems. Schizophr Bull 23:403–421, 1997
11. Arnold SE, Trojanowski JQ, Gur RE, et al: Absence of neurodegeneration and neural injury in the cerebral cortex in a sample of elderly patients with schizophrenia. Arch Gen Psychiatry 55:225–232, 1998
12. Bachus SE, Kleinman JE: The neuropathology of schizophrenia. J Clin Psychiatry 57 (suppl 11):72–83, 1996

13. Bogerts B: Recent advances in the neuropathology of schizophrenia. Schizophr Bull 19:431–445, 1993

14. Selemon LD, Goldman-Rakic PS: The reduced neuropil hypothesis: a circuit based model of schizophrenia. Biol Psychiatry 45:17–25, 1999

15. Arnold SE, Hyman BT, Van Hoesen GW, et al: Some cytoarchitectural abnormalities of the entorhinal cortex in schizophrenia. Arch Gen Psychiatry 48:625–632, 1991

16. Rajkowska G: Morphometric methods for studying the prefrontal cortex in suicide victims and psychiatric patients. Ann N Y Acad Sci 836:253–268, 1997

17. Lewis DA: Development of the prefrontal cortex during adolescence: insights into vulnerable neural circuits in schizophrenia. Neuropsychopharmacology 16:385–398, 1997

18. Selemon LD, Rajkowska G, Goldman-Rakic PS: Elevated neuronal density in prefrontal area 46 in brains from schizophrenic patients: application of a three-dimensional, stereologic counting method. J Comp Neurol 392:402–412, 1998

19. Garey LJ, Ong WY, Patel TS, et al: Reduced dendritic spine density on cerebral cortical pyramidal neurons in schizophrenia [see comments]. J Neurol Neurosurg Psychiatry 65:446–453, 1998

20. Webster MJ, Vawter MP, Freed WJ: Immunohistochemical localization of the cell adhesion molecules Thy-1 and L1 in the human prefrontal cortex of patients with schizophrenia, bipolar disorder, and depression. Mol Psychiatry 4:46–52, 1999

21. Arnold SE, Trojanowski JQ: Recent advances in defining the neuropathology of schizophrenia. Acta Neuropathol (Berl) 92:217–231, 1996

22. Falkai P, Honer WG, David S, et al: No evidence for astrogliosis in brains of schizophrenic patients: a post-mortem study. Neuropathol Appl Neurobiol 25:48–53, 1999

23. Buckley PF: Structural brain imaging in schizophrenia. Psychiatr Clin North Am 21:77–92, 1998

24. Okazaki Y: Morphological brain imaging studies on major psychoses. Psychiatry Clin Neurosci 52 (suppl): S215–S218, 1998

25. Lawrie SM, Abukmeil SS: Brain abnormality in schizophrenia: a systematic and quantitative review of volumetric magnetic resonance imaging studies. Br J Psychiatry 172:110–120, 1998

26. Buchanan RW, Vladar K, Barta PE, et al: Structural evaluation of the prefrontal cortex in schizophrenia. Am J Psychiatry 155:1049–1055, 1998

27. Sullivan EV, Mathalon DH, Lim KO, et al: Patterns of regional cortical dysmorphology distinguishing schizophrenia and chronic alcoholism. Biol Psychiatry 43:118–131, 1998

28. Wright IC, Ellison ZR, Sharma T, et al: Mapping of grey matter changes in schizophrenia. Schizophr Res 35:1–14, 1999

29. Chua SE, Wright IC, Poline JB, et al: Grey matter correlates of syndromes in schizophrenia: a semi-automated analysis of structural magnetic resonance images. Br J Psychiatry 170:406–410, 1997

30. Gur RE, Cowell P, Turetsky BI, et al: A follow-up magnetic resonance imaging study of schizophrenia: relationship of neuroanatomical changes to clinical and neurobehavioral measures. Arch Gen Psychiatry 55:145–152, 1998

31. Vita A, Dieci M, Giobbio GM, et al: Time course of cerebral ventricular enlargement in schizophrenia supports the hypothesis of its neurodevelopmental nature. Schizophr Res 23:25–30, 1997

32. Woods BT: Is schizophrenia a progressive neurodevelopmental disorder? Toward a unitary pathogenetic mechanism. Am J Psychiatry 155:1661–1670, 1998

33. DeLisi LE: Is schizophrenia a lifetime disorder of brain plasticity, growth and aging? Schizophr Res 23:119–129, 1997

34. Kulynych JJ, Luevano LF, Jones DW, et al: Cortical abnormality in schizophrenia: an in vivo application of the gyrification index. Biol Psychiatry 41:995–999, 1997

35. Cannon TD, van Erp TG, Huttunen M, et al: Regional gray matter, white matter, and cerebrospinal fluid distributions in schizophrenic patients, their siblings, and controls. Arch Gen Psychiatry 55:1084–1091, 1998

36. Buchsbaum MS, Hazlett EA: Positron emission tomography studies of abnormal glucose metabolism in schizophrenia. Schizophr Bull 24:343–364, 1998

37. Velakoulis D, Pantelis C: What have we learned from functional imaging studies in schizophrenia? The role of frontal, striatal and temporal areas. Aust N Z J Psychiatry 30:195–209, 1996

38. Weinberger DR, Berman KF, Zec RF: Physiologic dysfunction of dorsolateral prefrontal cortex in schizophrenia, I: regional cerebral blood flow evidence. Arch Gen Psychiatry 43:114–124, 1986

39. Baddeley A: Recent developments in working memory. Curr Opin Neurobiol 8:234–238, 1998

40. Goldman-Rakic PS, Selemon LD: Functional and anatomical aspects of prefrontal pathology in schizophrenia. Schizophr Bull 23:437–458, 1997

41. Smith EE, Jonides J: Working memory: a view from neuroimaging. Cognit Psychol 33:5–42, 1997

42. Weinberger DR, Gallhofer B: Cognitive function in schizophrenia. Int Clin Psychopharmacol 12 (suppl 4):S29–S36, 1997

43. Callicott JH, Mattay VS, Bertolino A, et al: Physiological characteristics of capacity constraints in working memory as revealed by functional MRI. Cereb Cortex 9:20–26, 1999

44. Weinberger DR, Berman KF: Prefrontal function in schizophrenia: confounds and controversies. Philos Trans R Soc Lond B Biol Sci 351:1495–1503, 1996

45. Fletcher PC, McKenna PJ, Frith CD, et al: Brain activations in schizophrenia during a graded memory task studied with functional neuroimaging. Arch Gen Psychiatry 55:1001–1008, 1998

46. Berman KF, Torrey EF, Daniel DG, et al: Regional cerebral blood flow in monozygotic twins discordant and concordant for schizophrenia. Arch Gen Psychiatry 48:625–632, 1991

47. Crespo-Facorro B, Paradiso S, Andreasen NC, et al: Recalling word lists reveals "cognitive dysmetria" in schizophrenia: a positron emission tomography study. Am J Psychiatry 156:386–392, 1999

48. Parellada E, Catafau AM, Bernardo M, et al: The resting and activation issue of hypofrontality: a single photon emission computed tomography study in neuroleptic-naive and neuroleptic-free schizophrenic female patients. Biol Psychiatry 44:787–790, 1998

49. Ragland JD, Gur RC, Glahn DC, et al: Frontotemporal cerebral blood flow change during executive and declarative memory tasks in schizophrenia: a positron emission tomography study. Neuropsychology 12:399–413, 1998

50. Scottish Schizophrenia Research Group: Regional cerebral blood flow in first-episode schizophrenia patients before and after antipsychotic drug treatment. Acta Psychiatr Scand 97:440–449, 1998

51. Gracia Marco R, Aguilar Garcia-Iturrospe EJ, Fernandez Lopez L, et al: Hypofrontality in schizophrenia: influence of normalization methods. Prog Neuropsychopharmacol Biol Psychiatry 21:1239–1256, 1997

52. McGuire PK, Quested DJ, Spence SA, et al: Pathophysiology of "positive" thought disorder in schizophrenia. Br J Psychiatry 173:231–235, 1998

53. Mellers JD, Adachi N, Takei N, et al: SPECT study of verbal fluency in schizophrenia and epilepsy. Br J Psychiatry 173:69–74, 1998

54. Kindermann SS, Karimi A, Symonds L, et al: Review of functional magnetic resonance imaging in schizophrenia. Schizophr Res 27:143–156, 1997

55. Weinberger DR, Mattay V, Callicott J, et al: fMRI applications in schizophrenia research. Neuroimage 4 (3 pt 3):S1118–S1126, 1996

56. Stevens AA, Goldman-Rakic PS, Gore JC, et al: Cortical dysfunction in schizophrenia during auditory word and tone working memory demonstrated by functional magnetic resonance imaging. Arch Gen Psychiatry 55:1097–1103, 1998

57. Callicott JH, Ramsey NF, Tallent K, et al: Functional magnetic resonance imaging brain mapping in psychiatry: methodological issues illustrated in a study of working memory in schizophrenia. Neuropsychopharmacology 18:186–196, 1998

58. Curtis VA, Bullmore ET, Brammer MJ, et al: Attenuated frontal activation during a verbal fluency task in patients with schizophrenia. Am J Psychiatry 155:1056–1063, 1998

59. Volz HP, Gaser C, Hager F, et al: Brain activation during cognitive stimulation with the Wisconsin Card Sorting Test—a functional MRI study on healthy volunteers and schizophrenics. Psychiatry Res 75:145–157, 1997

60. Yurgelun-Todd DA, Waternaux CM, Cohen BM, et al: Functional magnetic resonance imaging of schizophrenic patients and comparison subjects during word production. Am J Psychiatry 153:200–205, 1996

61. Mattay VS, Callicott JH, Bertolino A, et al: Abnormal functional lateralization of the sensorimotor cortex in patients with schizophrenia. Neuroreport 8:2977–2984, 1997

62. Bertolino A, Callicott JH, Elman I, et al: Regionally specific neuronal pathology in untreated patients with schizophrenia: a proton magnetic resonance spectroscopic imaging study. Biol Psychiatry 43:641–648, 1998

63. Bertolino A, Kumra S, Callicott JH, et al: Common pattern of cortical pathology in childhood-onset and adult-onset schizophrenia as identified by proton magnetic resonance spectroscopic imaging. Am J Psychiatry 155:1376–1383, 1998

64. Brooks WM, Hodde-Vargas J, Vargas LA, et al: Frontal lobe of children with schizophrenia spectrum disorders: a proton magnetic resonance spectroscopic study. Biol Psychiatry 43:263–269, 1998

65. Thomas MA, Ke Y, Levitt J, et al: Preliminary study of frontal lobe 1H MR spectroscopy in childhood-onset schizophrenia. J Magn Reson Imaging 8:841–846, 1998

66. Cecil KM, Lenkinski RE, Gur RE, et al: Proton magnetic resonance spectroscopy in the frontal and temporal lobes of neuroleptic naive patients with schizophrenia. Neuropsychopharmacology 20:131–140, 1999

66A. Bertolino A, Esposito G, Callicott JH, et al: Specific relationship between prefrontal neuronal *N*-acetylaspartate and activation of the working memory cortical network in schizophrenia. Am J Psychiatry 157:26–33, 2000

67. Gerez M, Tello A: Selected quantitative EEG (QEEG) and event-related potential (ERP) variables as discriminators for positive and negative schizophrenia. Biol Psychiatry 38:34–49, 1995

68. Tauscher J, Fischer P, Neumeister A, et al: Low frontal electroencephalographic coherence in neuroleptic-free schizophrenic patients. Biol Psychiatry 44:438–447, 1998

69. Weickert CS, Kleinman JE: The neuroanatomy and neurochemistry of schizophrenia. Psychiatr Clin North Am 21:57–75, 1998

70. Carlsson A, Hansson LO, Waters N, et al: Neurotransmitter aberrations in schizophrenia: new perspectives and therapeutic implications. Life Sci 61:75–94, 1997

71. Knable MB, Weinberger DR: Dopamine, the prefrontal cortex and schizophrenia. J Psychopharmacol 11:123–131, 1997

72. Byne W, Davis KL: The role of prefrontal cortex in the dopaminergic dysregulation of schizophrenia. Biol Psychiatry 45:657–659, 1999

73. Wilkinson LS, Dias R, Thomas KL, et al: Contrasting effects of excitotoxic lesions of the prefrontal cortex on the behavioural response to D-amphetamine and presynaptic and postsynaptic measures of striatal dopamine function in monkeys. Neuroscience 80:717–730, 1997

74. Weinberger DR, Berman KF, Illowsky BP: Physiological dysfunction of dorsolateral prefrontal cortex in schizophrenia, III: a new cohort and evidence for a monoaminergic mechanism. Arch Gen Psychiatry 45:609–615, 1988

75. Davis KL, Kahn RS, Ko G, et al: Dopamine in schizophrenia: a review and reconceptualization. Am J Psychiatry 148:1474–1486, 1991

76. Laruelle M: Imaging dopamine transmission in schizophrenia: a review and meta-analysis. Q J Nucl Med 42:211–221, 1998

77. Volkow ND, Fowler JS, Gatley SJ, et al: PET evaluation of the dopamine system of the human brain. J Nucl Med 37:1242–1256, 1996

78. Laruelle M, Abi-Dargham A, van Dyck CH, et al: Single photon emission computerized tomography imaging of amphetamine-induced dopamine release in drug-free schizophrenic subjects. Proc Natl Acad Sci U S A 93:9235–9240, 1996

79. Breier A, Su TP, Saunders R, et al: Schizophrenia is associated with elevated amphetamine-induced synaptic dopamine concentrations: evidence from a novel positron emission tomography method. Proc Natl Acad Sci U S A 94:2569–2574, 1997

80. Stefanis NC, Bresnick JN, Kerwin RW, et al: Elevation of D4 dopamine receptor mRNA in postmortem schizophrenic brain. Brain Res Mol Brain Res 53:112–119, 1998

81. Dean B, Hussain T, Hayes W, et al: Changes in serotonin2A and GABA(A) receptors in schizophrenia: studies on the human dorsolateral prefrontal cortex. J Neurochem 72:1593–1599, 1999

82. Bertolino A, Knable MB, Saunders RC, et al: The relationship between dorsolateral prefrontal N-acetylaspartate measures and striatal dopamine activity in schizophrenia. Biol Psychiatry 45:660–667, 1999

83. Kapur S: A new framework for investigating antipsychotic action in humans: lessons from PET imaging. Mol Psychiatry 3:135–140, 1998

84. Lieberman JA, Mailman RB, Duncan G, et al: Serotonergic basis of antipsychotic drug effects in schizophrenia. Biol Psychiatry 44:1099–1117, 1998

85. Lewis R, Kapur S, Jones C, et al: Serotonin 5-HT2 receptors in schizophrenia: a PET study using [18F]setoperone in neuroleptic-naive patients and normal subjects. Am J Psychiatry 156:72–78, 1999

86. Kouzmenko AP, Scaffidi A, Pereira AM, et al: No correlation between A(-1438)G polymorphism in 5-HT2A receptor gene promoter and the density of frontal cortical 5-HT2A receptors in schizophrenia. Hum Hered 49:103–105, 1999

87. Tamminga CA: Schizophrenia and glutamatergic transmission. Crit Rev Neurobiol 12:21–36, 1998

88. Weinberger DR: The biological basis of schizophrenia: new directions. J Clin Psychiatry 58 (suppl 10):22–27, 1997

89. Coyle JT: The glutamatergic dysfunction hypothesis for schizophrenia. Harv Rev Psychiatry 3:241–253, 1996

90. Benes FM, Vincent SL, Marie A, et al: Up-regulation of GABAA receptor binding on neurons of the prefrontal cortex in schizophrenic subjects. Neuroscience 75:1021–1031, 1996

91. Sokolov BP: Expression of NMDAR1, GluR1, GluR7, and KA1 glutamate receptor mRNAs is decreased in frontal cortex of "neuroleptic-free" schizophrenics: evidence on reversible up-regulation by typical neuroleptics. J Neurochem 71:2454–2464, 1998

92. Simpson MD, Slater P, Deakin JF: Comparison of glutamate and gamma-aminobutyric acid uptake binding sites in frontal and temporal lobes in schizophrenia. Biol Psychiatry 44:423–427, 1998

93. Kegeles LS, Humaran TJ, Mann JJ: In vivo neurochemistry of the brain in schizophrenia as revealed by magnetic resonance spectroscopy. Biol Psychiatry 44:382–398, 1998

94. Breier A, Adler CM, Weisenfeld N, et al: Effects of NMDA antagonism on striatal dopamine release in healthy subjects: application of a novel PET approach. Synapse 29:142–147, 1998

95. Volz HP, Rzanny R, Rossger G, et al: Decreased energy demanding processes in the frontal lobes of schizophrenics due to neuroleptics? A 31P-magneto-resonance spectroscopic study. Psychiatry Res 76:123–129, 1997

96. Jope RS, Song L, Grimes CA, et al: Selective increases in phosphoinositide signaling activity and G protein levels in postmortem brain from subjects with schizophrenia or alcohol dependence. J Neurochem 70:763–771, 1998

97. Shimon H, Sobolev Y, Davidson M, et al: Inositol levels are decreased in postmortem brain of schizophrenic patients. Biol Psychiatry 44:428–432, 1998

98. Raedler TJ, Knable MB, Weinberger DR: Schizophrenia as a developmental disorder of the cerebral cortex. Curr Opin Neurobiol 8:157–161, 1998

99. Saunders RC, Kolachana BS, Bachevalier J, et al: Neonatal lesions of the medial temporal lobe disrupt prefrontal cortical regulation of striatal dopamine. Nature 393:169–171, 1998

100. Bertolino A, Saunders RC, Mattay VS, et al: Altered development of prefrontal neurons in rhesus monkeys with neonatal mesial temporo-limbic lesions: a proton magnetic resonance spectroscopic imaging study. Cereb Cortex 7:740–748, 1997

101. Callicott JH, Egan MF, Bertolino A, et al: Hippocampal N-acetyl aspartate in unaffected siblings of patients with schizophrenia: a possible intermediate neurobiological phenotype. Biol Psychiatry 44:941–950, 1998

102. Poland RE, Cloak C, Lutchmansingh PJ, et al: Brain N-acetyl aspartate concentrations measured by H MRS are reduced in adult male rats subjected to perinatal stress: preliminary observations and hypothetical implications for neurodevelopmental disorders. J Psychiatr Res 33:41–51, 1999

103. Deutsch SI, Mastropaolo J, Rosse RB: Neurodevelopmental consequences of early exposure to phencyclidine and related drugs. Clin Neuropharmacol 21:320–332, 1998

104. Bullmore ET, Woodruff PW, Wright IC, et al: Does dysplasia cause anatomical dysconnectivity in schizophrenia? Schizophr Res 30:127–135, 1998

105. Frith CD: Functional brain imaging and the neuropathology of schizophrenia. Schizophr Bull 23:525–527, 1997

106. Mallet L, Mazoyer B, Martinot JL: Functional connectivity in depressive, obsessive-compulsive, and schizophrenic disorders: an explorative correlational analysis of regional cerebral metabolism. Psychiatry Res 82:83–93, 1998

107. Friston KJ, Frith CD: Schizophrenia: a disconnection syndrome? Clin Neurosci 3:89–97, 1995

108. Jennings JM, McIntosh AR, Kapur S, et al: Functional network differences in schizophrenia: a rCBF study of semantic processing. Neuroreport 9:1697–1700, 1998

109. Norman RM, Malla AK, Williamson PC, et al: EEG coherence and syndromes in schizophrenia. Br J Psychiatry 170:411–415, 1997

110. Friston KJ: The disconnection hypothesis. Schizophr Res 30:115–125, 1998

111. Andreasen NC, Paradiso S, O'Leary DS: "Cognitive dysmetria" as an integrative theory of schizophrenia: a dysfunction in cortical-subcortical-cerebellar circuitry? Schizophr Bull 24:203–218, 1998

112. Wiser AK, Andreasen NC, O'Leary DS, et al: Dysfunctional cortico-cerebellar circuits cause "cognitive dysmetria" in schizophrenia. Neuroreport 9:1895–1899, 1998

113. Martin P, Albers M: Cerebellum and schizophrenia: a selective review. Schizophr Bull 21:241–250, 1995

114. Katsetos CD, Hyde TM, Herman MM: Neuropathology of the cerebellum in schizophrenia—an update: 1996 and future directions. Biol Psychiatry 42:213–224, 1997

115. Jones EG: Cortical development and thalamic pathology in schizophrenia. Schizophr Bull 23:483–501, 1997

116. Andreasen NC: The role of the thalamus in schizophrenia. Can J Psychiatry 42:27–33, 1997

14

The Frontal Lobes and Traumatic Brain Injury

Marilyn F. Kraus, M.D., Harvey S. Levin, Ph.D.

The involvement of the frontal lobes in closed head injury (CHI) is supported by both neuropathological and neuroimaging studies that show that this region is the most common site of focal brain lesions.

VULNERABILITY OF THE FRONTAL LOBES TO CLOSED HEAD INJURY

Pathophysiology and Neuroimaging Evidence

The proximity of the orbitofrontal and anterior temporal regions to bony protrusions and cavities contributes to their vulnerability to injury, particularly when rotational acceleration is imparted to the freely moving head.[1] Acceleration-deceleration forces can cause the brain to be forced up against these bony surfaces, causing both coup and contrecoup injury. Of the mechanisms of diffuse injury in CHI, diffuse axonal injury is of particular significance because it produces profound shearing and stretching of axons throughout

the brain and brain stem, as well as focal lesions in the corpus callosum.[2] This white matter damage can be diffuse and may not be detectable on structural imaging. Perhaps the most unequivocal evidence for the vulnerability of the frontal lobes after CHI was obtained in Glasgow by J.H. Adams and his co-workers,[1] who developed a contusion index based on the size and depth of contusions in fatal injuries. Adams et al. found that the contusion index was greatest in the frontal lobes, followed closely by the anterior temporal region.

Neuroimaging studies have extended the findings of frontal lobe vulnerability to less severe CHI. In a magnetic resonance imaging (MRI) study of mild to moderate head injuries, Levin et al.[3] reported the results of serially scanning 50 consecutive admissions. As shown in Figure 14–1, the frontal lobes were the most common site of focal lesion, that is, abnormal signal on MRI. Figure 14–2 depicts the resolution of abnormal signal over the first 1–3 months after mild to

Research by H.S.L. was supported by grant NS21889 from the National Institute of Neurological Disorders and Stroke.

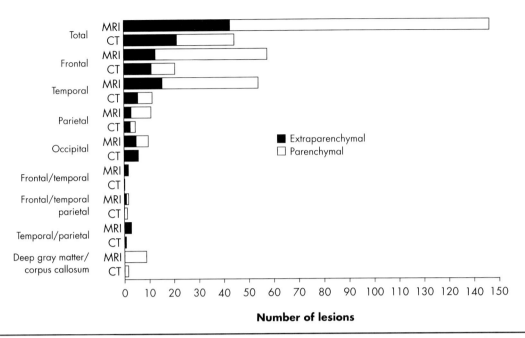

FIGURE 14–1.   Frequency and neuroanatomical site of parenchymal and extraparenchymal lesions seen on magnetic resonance imaging (MRI) and computed tomography (CT) during the initial hospitalization for mild to moderate closed head injury (*N*=50).
Source.   Reproduced from Levin H, Williams D, Eisenberg H, et al: "Serial Magnetic Resonance Imaging and Neurobehavioral Findings After Mild to Moderate Closed Head Injury." *Journal of Neurology, Neurosurgery and Psychiatry* 55:255–262, 1992. Used with permission.

moderate CHI, which was paralleled by recovery of neurobehavioral functioning.

The issue also arises of apparent frontal lobe injury that, although it is suggested by the biomechanics of the injury, neuropsychological testing, and neurobehavioral disorder, eludes currently available structural neuroimaging.[4] Preliminary evidence suggests that the substrate of deficits that clinicians and investigators attribute to frontal lobe dysfunction in head-injured patients could be elucidated by functional imaging.[5,6]

Neuropsychological Evidence

The vulnerability of the frontal lobes to damage in CHI has been invoked to explain the frequent disruption of executive control functions involving mood, behavior, and aspects of cognition.[7] The functional heterogeneity of the orbitofrontal and dorsolateral regions has received support from experimental investigation of nonhuman primates[8] and case reports of patients with focal frontal lesions.[7] Goldman[8] showed a dissociation between the effects of dorsolateral and orbitofrontal lesions on delayed response performance in monkeys; this dissociation depended on their age at the time of ablation and when they were tested. Thus,

the clinical picture in frontal lobe damage is variable and depends on several factors, including not only the characteristics of the injury itself but also the premorbid functioning and age of the individual.

Clinical descriptions of patients who have sustained severe head injury often include features that are associated with frontal lobe injury, such as poor impulse control, decreased flexibility, impaired attention, perseveration, and diminished divergent thinking, particularly on measures of verbal fluency and figural fluency. Often, however, these neurobehavioral features demonstrated on testing are not associated with firm evidence of frontal lobe damage from structural brain imaging. The neuropsychological evidence for frontal lobe dysfunction after CHI is derived from several studies, including the work by Stuss and colleagues. The study reported by Stuss et al.[4] in 1985 was quite provocative because it included patients who were thought to have attained a good recovery yet showed impairments on tasks that are widely used to assess frontal lobe functions, such as interference effects on the Stroop Test, difficulties with attention, and vulnerability to interference on memory tests. Stuss et al. found that patients who had relatively preserved performance on the Wechsler Adult Intelli-

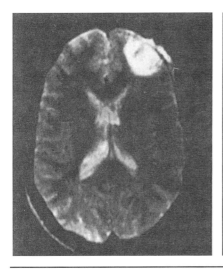 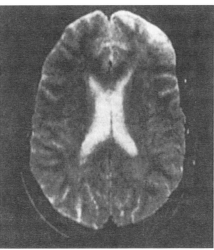 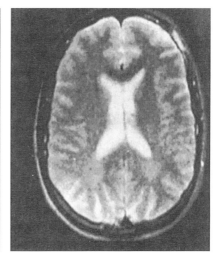

FIGURE 14–2. Magnetic resonance image (MRI) obtained 3 days after injury for a 27-year-old man whose initial Glasgow Coma Scale score was 14 when he was admitted to the hospital after being struck by a tow line under high tension.

The area of left frontal lobe increased signal (33 ccs) was interpreted as a contusion. Follow-up MRI showed resolution of the lesion at 1 month (*center*) and at 3 months (*right*).

gence Scale (WAIS) nevertheless had difficulty with shifting and maintaining responses on the Wisconsin Card Sorting Test (WCST). The study by Stuss et al. matched a healthy control group (on age, education, and the WAIS) with the survivors of head injuries who were thought to have attained a good recovery. Stuss et al. found that the head-injured patients showed an impairment on interference memory tests, that is, on the Brown-Peterson task, in which a series of three consonants or vowels is presented and the patient is then asked to count backward as an interference test. After a variable delay, the patient is asked to recall the three syllables. Stuss et al. found that the CHI patients had difficulty in recalling the series of letters after a delay filled by the distractor interference task. Taken together, the pattern of neuropsychological findings reported by Stuss et al. implicated frontal lobe dysfunction. However, this study lacked neuroimaging to provide clinicopathological correlation with the cognitive testing.

NEUROBEHAVIORAL SEQUELAE OF FRONTAL LOBE INJURY IN ADULTS AND CHILDREN

Current evidence indicates that although maturation of the frontal lobes extends at least into adolescence,[9,10] developmental changes in performance on a

task similar to delayed response have been documented even in human infants.[11] In adults who experience a CHI involving the frontal lobes, already established functions are disrupted. An understanding of the component parts of this so-called syndrome can allow for more effective evaluation and intervention. Case reports of frontal lobe injury sustained during childhood and during adulthood have documented the development of cognitive deficit and aberrant behavior, as illustrated below.

Early Frontal Lobe Injury

Price et al.[12] described a young woman who was referred for evaluation because of alleged child neglect. History revealed that at age 4, Ms. A had sustained a head injury when she was struck by a car. An MRI scan showed bilateral frontal lobe damage that involved the right hemisphere to a greater extent than the left. Neuropsychological assessment disclosed a low normal intellectual level (WAIS Verbal IQ=78; Performance IQ=83). The patient showed a marked susceptibility to interference on the Stroop Interference Task, in which one has to overcome the dominant tendency to read the names of color words rather than to specify the color of the print in which the word appears. In addition, Ms. A had difficulty in performing Trail Making B, in which she was asked to alternate between numeric and alphabetic sequences. What was even more striking about this patient than her cognitive deficits was that she showed very poor judgment and also, over the years following her injury, became progressively more irritable, assaultive, and sexually disinhibited. The investigators devised an innovative cognitive task in which Ms. A was asked to identify, from a multichoice display, the key variable that was essential for a plant to thrive (such as water or food). She had a great deal of difficulty with the inferential reasoning required to perform this task.

Frontal Lobe Lesions Shown by MRI in a Patient With "Diffuse" Brain Injury

We reported the case of Ms. B, the first CHI patient we studied by using MRI.[13] This young woman had sustained a severe head injury 5 years earlier and was in a coma for nearly a month. We selected this particular patient because her neuropsychological findings (such as decreased verbal fluency and perseverative invention of designs) were compatible with presumed frontal lobe dysfunction despite computed tomography (CT) scans that consistently failed to show a structural frontal lobe lesion. However, MRI disclosed bilateral parasagittal frontal lobe lesions, particularly involving, but not restricted to, the white matter (Figure 14–3).

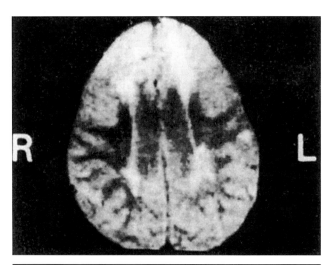

FIGURE 14–3. Magnetic resonance image (MRI) 5 years after severe "diffuse" head injury disclosed increased signal intensities in parasagittal regions of both frontal lobes, greater on the left than on the right. The frontal lobe white matter was primarily affected, but gray matter also was involved on the left superior frontal gyrus, and intensity was increased in the left postcentral gyrus. Deep white matter lesions in each occipital lobe, greater on the left than on the right, also were present on other slices, as was white matter injury extending across the splenium.
Source. Reproduced from Levin H, Handel S, Goldman A, et al: "Magnetic Resonance Imaging After 'Diffuse' Nonmissile Head Injury." *Archives of Neurology* 42:963–968, 1985. Used with permission.

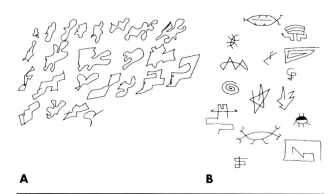

A	B

FIGURE 14–4. **A:** Perseverative productions on the figural fluency task by Ms. B, whose magnetic resonance image disclosed bilateral parasagittal frontal lesions 5 years after a severe head injury that had been interpreted as diffuse insult according to computed tomography scan findings. **B:** Figures created by a control subject matched for age and education to Ms. B.

Figure 14–4 illustrates Ms. B's perseverative productions on the figural fluency task, in which she was given 4 minutes to invent novel designs. In contrast to the creative productions (B) by a programmer in our laboratory who had a similar educational level and age, Ms. B tended to repeat the same basic designs (A) despite reminders by the examiner to draw unique figures. Ms. B had a marked perseverative tendency in figural fluency and reduced word finding, despite recovery to an average intellectual level.

OTHER COGNITIVE TASKS SENSITIVE TO FRONTAL LOBE DYSFUNCTION

We have investigated several cognitive tasks to assess frontal dysfunction in group studies of head-injured patients.

Memory

One test that has been used in the neuropsychological literature to study cognitive impairment presumably related to frontal lobe injury is Release From Proactive Inhibition,[14] which involves an element of interference. This task involves recall of a series of words, typically three per series, belonging to the same semantic category (e.g., animals) over multiple trials. The patient is given a distractor task to perform between presentation and the examiner's signal for recall. The task consists of two conditions involving either a shift to a new semantic category or a nonshift condition, in which words from the same semantic category are presented.[14] Nonimpaired adults show a decrement in recall efficiency over trials, a process that is attributed to a build-up or interference involving words from the same category. The enhanced recall (release from proactive inhibition) shown by the nonimpaired subjects under the shift condition has been interpreted as evidence for sensitivity to semantic features and the functional integrity of the prefrontal region. Patients with Korsakoff's psychosis, a memory disorder that has been linked to secondary frontal lobe damage, do not have the release from proactive inhibition associated with a semantic shift. This barrier to release from proactive inhibition has been interpreted as indirect evidence for frontal lobe dysfunction in Korsakoff's patients.

In view of a case report by Zatorre and McEntee[15] of a head-injured patient who sustained frontal lobe lesions and failed to show release from proactive inhibition, our group used the Release From Proactive Inhibition task in 14 young adults who had sustained a severe head injury at least 1 year earlier.[16] Figure 14–5 shows enhanced recall in both the CHI and the noninjured groups following the shift condition, a finding

consistent with preserved release from proactive inhibition. On the basis of MRI scan results, Goldstein and Levin[16] divided the CHI patients into three small subgroups: patients with frontal lesions, those with extrafrontal lesions, and those with diffuse injury (i.e., no areas of abnormal signal). As shown in Figure 14–5, release from proactive inhibition was preserved irrespective of the localization of abnormal signal on MRI. Although our findings failed to support a relation between localization of lesion and release from proactive inhibition, caution is advised in drawing firm conclusions from these small samples.

Metamemory

The dysexecutive syndrome of Baddeley and Wilson[17] is characterized by poor attentional control, diminished speed of information processing, and a breakdown of boundaries between different memory domains for various categories of information that results in confabulation, intrusions, faulty retrieval, or semantic memory deficits. The dysexecutive syndrome also involves lack of organization and poor planning, so that the patient is unable to set goals and carry them out.

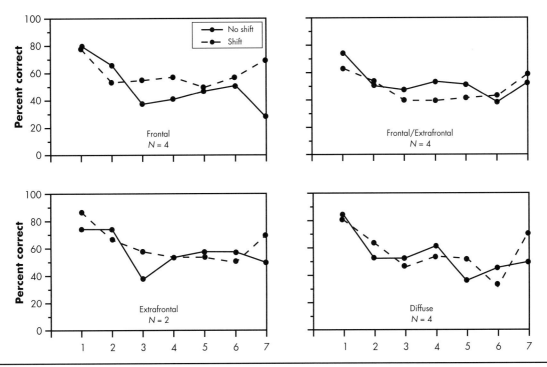

FIGURE 14–5. Mean percent recall as a function of shift and no-shift conditions on the Release From Proactive Inhibition task for head-injured patients with frontal lobe lesions (frontal), frontal lobe lesions in addition to extrafrontal lesions (frontal/extrafrontal), lesions outside the frontal lobes (extrafrontal), and the absence of lesions (diffuse), as seen by magnetic resonance imaging.

Metamemory refers to the knowledge and skills related to the effective use of memory. Hirst and Volpe[18] studied metamemory in a group of patients who had confirmed or suspected frontal lobe damage, including three head-injured patients and two patients who had ruptured the anterior communicating artery. These individuals had poor knowledge of how memory worked, as reflected by their responses to a questionnaire about the effects of delay on memory. Interestingly, the patients with frontal lobe damage had normal recall of unrelated words. However, when they were given a list of words that could be grouped into semantic categories, these patients did not cluster them when recalling the word list. In contrast, nonimpaired control subjects tended to exhaust their recall of words in a category before recalling words in a different category.

Our group was interested in the semantic organization of memory because of its implications for rehabilitation. Levin and Goldstein[19] used a similar task in which words belonging to specific categories, such as fruits, parts of a house, and animals, were presented in a random order. We were interested in whether the CHI patients would organize their recall by first clustering the words into semantic categories. In comparison with control subjects without CHI, chronic survivors of severe CHI clustered a smaller proportion of the words across trials, even after correcting for the absolute level of recall. As shown in Figure 14–6, across trials the control subjects progressively increased the proportion of words that they clustered according to semantic category. Although a similar pattern is seen in the recall by head-injured patients, they used this strategy at a much lower level than did the noninjured control subjects.

Problem Solving

Our research has included other tasks that we postulate are dependent on the integrity of the frontal lobes, including a game that many have played as children called "Twenty Questions."[20] The Twenty Questions task requires the ability to reflect on the conceptual nature of items that are shown on a display of 42 pictures. Groups of items scattered in different locations on the Twenty Questions display share common attributes (e.g., living things). The goal for the patient is to guess the item that the examiner has in mind by using the fewest questions. Denney and Denney[20] reported a developmental trend with regard to the type of question that was posed. As children mature from approximately age 6 through age 12, they tend more

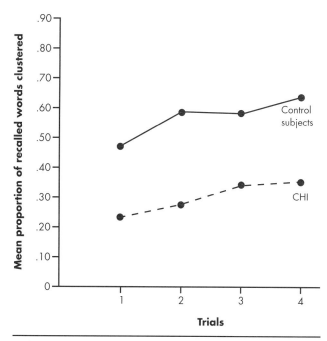

FIGURE 14–6. Proportion of clustering and recall by patients with closed head injury (CHI) as compared with noninjured control subjects, plotted across trials. The proportion of words clustered has been corrected for the absolute number of words recalled.

frequently to ask constraint-type questions ("Is it a living thing?"), which eliminate several items, whereas they ask a decreasing proportion of hypothesis-type questions ("Is it a tree?"), which eliminate only a single item.[20] A third type of question, known as "pseudoconstraint" ("Does it bark?") is a variant of the hypothesis question. Our group postulated that this conceptual shift in child development from hypothesis to constraint questions reflects maturation of the frontal lobes.

Goldstein and Levin[16] administered the Twenty Questions Test to young adults who had sustained a severe head injury at least 1 year previously. Figure 14–7 shows the proportions of the questions asked that conform to the three types: the hypothesis, the constraint, and the pseudoconstraint. The "condition" indicated refers to the three items the patients were asked to guess, corresponding to the three trials of this task. The histogram indicates that CHI patients asked a higher proportion of hypothesis questions, whereas noninjured control subjects asked a higher proportion of constraint questions. The head-injured patients also asked a higher proportion of pseudoconstraint questions. Goldstein and Levin suggested that the Twenty Questions and similar tasks may have a role in the

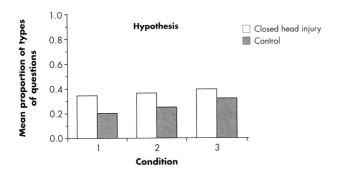

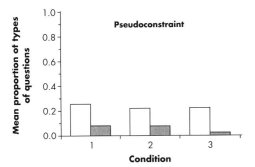

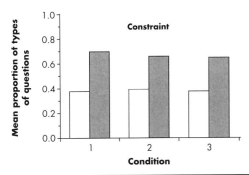

FIGURE 14–7. Histogram displaying the types of questions asked by head-injured patients as compared with noninjured control subjects on three trials of the Twenty Questions task.

In contrast to noninjured control subjects, who asked constraint-type questions that eliminated several alternatives, head-injured patients tended to ask questions that were pertinent to only a single item in the display (hypothesis- or pseudoconstraint-type questions).

Source. Reproduced from Goldstein F, Levin H: "Question-Asking Strategies After Severe Closed Head Injury." *Brain and Cognition* 17:23–30, 1991. Used with permission.

clinical evaluation of head-injured patients, particularly in a rehabilitation context.

Initiation and Inhibition

Fluency measures, which involve initiation of a response sequence, are also known to be highly sensitive to frontal lobe lesions in humans.[21] Inhibitory control has been studied extensively in both animals and humans,[22] including tasks such as the go/no-go (making a positive response to a particular signal and inhibiting the response to a negative signal). A related task used in human studies is a competitive or conflictual motor performance,[23] in which the patient is asked to perform a motor response opposite to that of the examiner.

Planning

Clinicians and investigators have ascribed planning to the frontal lobes. In animal research, maze learning has been used to study planning ability, whereas in human studies, investigators have used the Porteus Mazes Test to study the sequelae of frontal lobectomy and frontal lobotomy.[24]

Shallice[25] developed the Tower of London to investigate impairment of sequential planning. This task is performed by rearranging beads on three vertical rods to match a model, using as few moves as possible. This task has been postulated to engage working memory to concurrently accomplish subgoals (intermediate moves) while maintaining the goal solution in memory. In a study designed to investigate the relation of frontal lobe lesions to Tower of London performance, Levin et al.[26] administered the task to 134 pediatric CHI patients, including 94 in the 6- to 10-year age range and 40 who were 11 to 16 years old at the time of testing. The patients were subdivided into those with severe and those with mild or moderate head injury (Glasgow Coma Scale score ≤ 8 vs. > 8) within each age range. The percentage of Tower of London problems solved within the limit of three trials decreased and the number of broken rules (such as picking up more than one bead at a time) increased as a function of severity of head injury. Figure 14–8 shows that the number of broken rules increased markedly as a function of severity of head injury in the 6- to 10-year-olds but not in the 11- to 16-year group. Consistent with the impression of more marked effects of severity of head injury in the younger children, the interaction of age with severity of head injury was significant.

To investigate the relation of frontal lobe lesions to solving the Tower of London problems, Levin et al.[26] measured the volume of areas of abnormal signal in the frontal and extrafrontal regions. These investigators used a hierarchical multiple regression analysis to determine whether the size of the frontal lobe lesion incremented the prediction of Tower of London performance that was based on severity of injury and the

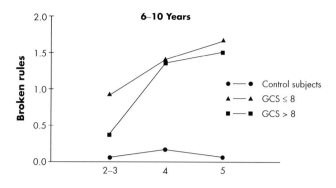

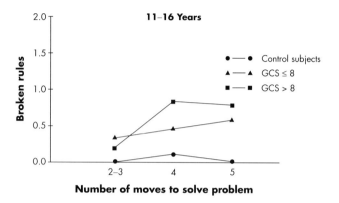

FIGURE 14–8.   Number of broken rules incurred as a function of the complexity of the Tower of London problems for head-injured and control children in the age groups 6–10 (*top*) and 11–16 years (*bottom*).

In general, head-injured children broke the rules more frequently than did the control subjects, a pattern that was more pronounced in the younger children. GCS=Glasgow Coma Scale.

Source.   Reproduced from Levin H, Mendelsohn D, Lilly M, et al: "Tower of London performance in relation to magnetic resonance imaging following closed head injury in children." *Neuropsychology* 8:171–179, 1994. Used with permission.

interaction of severity with age. As shown in Figure 14–9 (top left), the incremental multiple correlation provided by the addition of total frontal lobe lesion size reached significance for the number of broken rules but not for the percentage of problems solved on trial 1 or the initial planning time, which was defined as the latency from the beginning of the trial until the child initiated a move. Figure 14–9 (bottom) indicates that the contribution of total prefrontal lesion size to predicting Tower of London performance was confirmed for orbital lesions (broken rules), dorsolateral lesions (percentage who solved trial 1), and white matter lesions (broken rules) situated in the frontal lobes. As reflected in Figure 14–9 (top right), the incremental

squared multiple correlations provided by the addition of focal extrafrontal lesions were nonsignificant. These findings indicate that both the severity of injury and the volume of frontal lobe lesions contribute to impaired planning as measured by the Tower of London.

Delayed Response, Temporal Discrimination, Temporal Organization, and Frequency Monitoring

Temporal discrimination or temporal organization of behavior is one of the functions that have been shown to be important in nonhuman primate models of frontal lobe function.[8] In the animal model, this temporal function could take the form of a fixed interval conditioning or delayed response. In the animal model of frontal lobe lesions, delayed response and delayed alternation are examples of working memory tasks that assess the capacity to guide behavior by an internal representation. Delayed-response tasks have been used in clinical studies with varying results.[3,27] Although Oscar-Berman et al.[27] found that the delayed response was impaired in patients with alcoholic Korsakoff's psychosis (who presumably have frontal lobe involvement), Levin et al.[3] were unable to find delayed-response deficits in children and adolescents who had sustained moderate to severe CHI.

Cognitive tasks that involve temporal organization, monitoring frequency and recency, have been used in both animal and human studies. Milner et al.[28] showed that frequency monitoring (e.g., judging which of two words was more frequently presented) was sensitive to frontal lobectomy. Depending on whether the material was verbal or nonverbal, frequency monitoring was sensitive to either left frontal or right frontal lobectomy in patients with intractable seizures. We studied monitoring of word frequency by head-injured patients.[29] Words were presented in random order at varied frequencies (0–7) over trials to patients who were then tested on forced-choice and frequency estimation tasks. After being presented with the words at varying frequencies on the forced-choice task, the patients were asked to circle the word in each pair that they judged to have been presented more frequently. The second task (absolute frequency estimation) asked the patient to estimate how frequently each word had been presented. Figure 14–10, which plots the mean judged frequency against the actual frequency of presentation, shows that noninjured control subjects matched on age and education to the survivors of severe head injury accurately estimated the word fre-

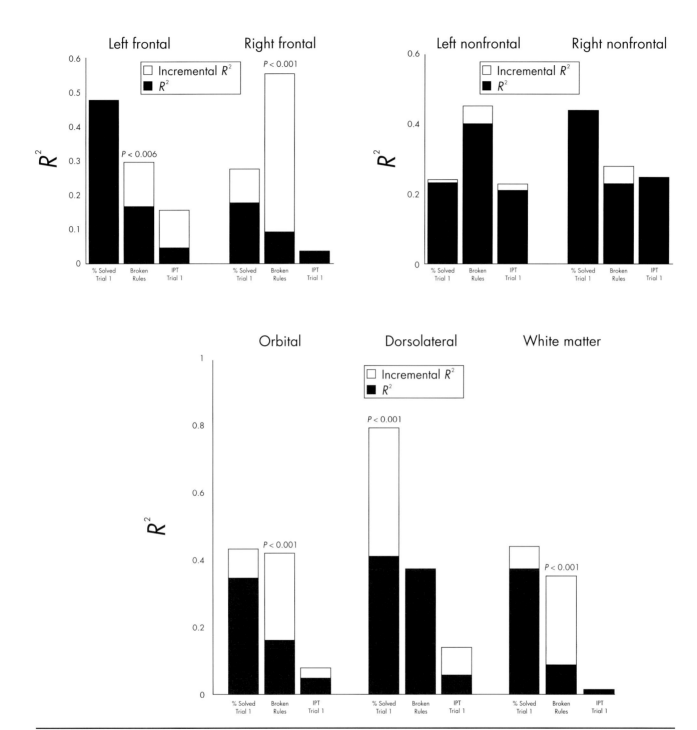

FIGURE 14–9.   Histograms depicting squared multiple correlations obtained in multiple regressions.

The incremental R^2 indicates the additional information provided by lesion size for predicting Tower of London performance. The results are shown for the total area of abnormal signal, exclusively or predominantly in the left or right frontal lobes (*top*), the extrafrontal region (*middle*), and subregions of the frontal lobes (*bottom*). IPT=initial planning time.

Source.   Reproduced from Levin H, Mendelsohn D, Lilly M, et al: "Tower of London performance in relation to magnetic resonance imaging following closed head injury in children." *Neuropsychology* 8:171–179, 1994. Used with permission.

quency, whereas frequency judgment by the CHI patients deviated progressively with the presentation frequency. Whether this impairment in frequency judgment is related to structural or metabolic imaging of frontal lobe lesions is a question for future research. Although we did not use either type of neuroimaging in this study, the pattern of findings bears a resemblance to the results in patients with frontal lobectomy.

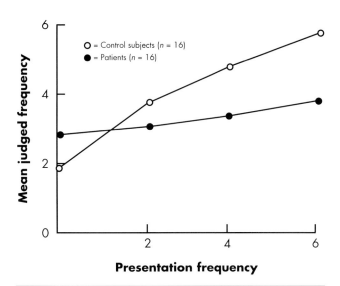

FIGURE 14–10.   Mean judged frequency of word presentation plotted against the actual frequency of presentation for head-injured patients and noninjured control subjects.

In contrast to the linear relationship of the estimated frequency to actual frequency of presentation for noninjured control subjects, the deviation in the frequency judgment by head-injured patients increased with the actual frequency of the words.

Source.   Reproduced from Levin H, Goldstein F, High WM Jr, et al: "Automatic and Effortful Processing After Severe Closed Head Injury." *Brain and Cognition* 7:283–297, 1988. Used with permission.

NEUROPSYCHIATRIC SEQUELAE OF CLOSED HEAD INJURY

Although the frontal and temporal lobes are commonly involved, CHI can cause a heterogeneous group of neuropsychiatric symptoms because the injuries tend to be diffuse, rarely limited to one discrete brain region or functional system. Dysfunction can occur in aspects of cognition, mood, and behavior. A rather loosely defined diagnosis of postconcussional syndrome is often used, although it is not well qualified or quantified. Features can include headache, dizziness, fatigue, disrupted sleep, restlessness, photophobia and phonophobia, mood disturbances, disorganized thinking, apathy, disinhibition/impulsivity, memory impairment, and attention/concentration deficits. Seizures can follow different severities of CHI and most commonly are partial complex. This also adds to the risk of neuropsychiatric sequelae. Although relatively uncommon, and usually seen only with more severe injuries, psychotic symptoms can occur or even devel-

op over time. CHI of different severities may result in any combination and quality of these symptoms. Generally, the symptoms of postconcussional syndrome are self-limited in mild, uncomplicated injuries, as shown in a multicenter trial.[30] But a subgroup of patients with mild CHI continue to have persistent deficits. Many have difficulty returning to work, home, or school after CHI. For all severities of injury, providing a comprehensive evaluation that addresses the patient's deficits and educates the family about the sequelae of CHI is essential to developing an effective treatment plan.

In many cases, frontal lobe dysfunction contributes to a broad range of symptoms and deficits.[31] Clinicians should become familiar with the signs and symptoms of the various disorders of mood, behavior, and cognition, such as the prefrontal syndromes, that can be seen after CHI. Appreciating the neurological antecedent to these sequelae is important so that treatment is appropriate and rational. The prefrontal syndromes have been reviewed in detail elsewhere[32,33] and in Chapters 3 and 8 in this book. In the remainder of this chapter, we provide an overview of common problems and pharmacological treatment options.

Mood disturbance is common after CHI.[34,35] True depression or mania may develop, but mood lability is probably the most frequent mood-related complaint after CHI. Robinson et al.[36] and others[37] have reported that mood disturbance may be lateralized following CHI, with mania more common after right frontal injury and depression more likely to follow left frontal trauma. Family members often report that patients have lost their ambition or, alternatively, that they seem "wired" and cannot control their behavior. Differentiating depression from apathy and hypomania from disinhibition (both common in prefrontal dysfunction) may be difficult in some patients. If neuropsychological evaluation and knowledge of the pathology point to prefrontal dysfunction, it is rational to direct treatment accordingly.

Cognitive problems following CHI range from decreased attention and concentration to prominent amnesia and disorganized thinking. Some patients appear to have developed attention-deficit disorder; they may become easily distracted and restless and may feel overstimulated. Restlessness and difficulty in processing multiple stimuli are often significant problems. Mentation may slow down, and cognitive flexibility may decrease. The ability to carry out activities that require sequencing and multiple steps may become impaired. Diminished insight can cause patients to insist on returning to their preinjury responsibilities despite their new cognitive limitations. In more advanced cases, cognitive dysfunction may cause patients to rely on others to oversee their activities of daily living (see Salloway, Chapter 10, "Case 6: Traumatic Brain Injury," in this volume).

The difficulty that many CHI patients experience in adapting to novel environments may lead to repeated failures in new and challenging work settings. These failures, when seen in conjunction with apathy (associated with mesial frontal pathology), are often interpreted as indicative of a personality disorder.

Dyscontrol syndromes may predominate when the injury involves the orbitofrontal surface of the frontal lobes.[38] Patients with these syndromes may appear jocular, impulsive, shallow, and insensitive and can lose the capacity to monitor and regulate their behavior. Milder cases may be limited to increased irritability, a "short fuse," and verbal hostility toward friends or family. At the more extreme end, physical violence, impulsive self-destructive behavior, or sexual disinhibition may be apparent. These patients may meet criteria for antisocial personality disorder and have been called "pseudopsychopathic."[38] Clinically, traumatically brain injured patients tend to have diffuse injury to the prefrontal cortex, with resulting variability in deficits and symptoms.

Milder CHIs can magnify preexisting negative personality traits.[39] At the other extreme, caregivers may hardly recognize the patient's personality. The patient may alienate family members at a time when support is critical. The patient may try to return to work, only to find the workplace overwhelming and distracting.[40] Conflicts may develop with co-workers and superiors. The patient may use loud and inappropriate language to express frustration. The loss of productivity and decrease in occupational and family status can have a highly negative effect on the patient's self-esteem.

PHARMACOLOGICAL TREATMENT

Historically, pharmacological intervention with brain-injured patients has been based chiefly on experience involving primary psychiatric disorders, developmental disorders, and clinical experience. Treatment can be aimed at observable symptoms, based on hypotheses about the underlying neurochemical dysfunction, or both. To date, there have been few published reports of controlled trials.[41] Only a brief overview of current pharmacological interventions is presented here; the reader is referred to the listed references for more detail.

With frontal pathology, mood dysregulation is common, ranging from depression to lability. Antidepressant medications, carbamazepine, or sodium valproate may help to stabilize mood after CHI.[42] The anticonvulsants carbamazepine and valproate, as well as the newer agents such as gabapentin, can be useful not only for mood stabilization but also for irritability and aggression. Gabapentin is showing promise as a treatment for chronic pain, and we have found it very useful for chronic headaches following CHI.[43] Choice of agent, dosage, and side effects should be carefully monitored because patients with CHI tend to be more sensitive to psychoactive agents than are patients with primary mood disorders. The serotonergic antidepressants are often well tolerated and effective. In the setting of frontal lobe dysfunction, dopaminergic agents such as amantadine or levodopa/carbidopa can stabilize mood.[44,45]

Treatment of cognitive dysfunction begins with modifying the patient's environment to prevent overstimulation. Structure and routine are especially important when the frontal lobes are impaired. Clinical evidence, primarily from case reports, indicates that certain cognitive deficits can improve with pharmacological interventions. Case reports and small case series support the use of the psychostimulants in patients with head injury.[46–50] Methylphenidate and dextroamphetamine enhance dopaminergic and noradrenergic transmission,[51] which may partly explain their effectiveness. Many of the symptoms experienced by these patients resemble those of attention-deficit disorder, so these agents represent a logical choice. They are often very effective for symptoms of distractibility, impaired attention span, impulsivity, and irritability. They also can be useful for organic mood disorders such as depression in medically or neurologically ill patients, and they are very well tolerated in the dosages used.[52–56] Clinically, negative effects on seizure threshold are not common. Animal studies suggest that these agents can be beneficial in enhancing cortical recovery.[57] Controlled studies are under way in human subjects, and a preliminary report by Plenger et al.[58] is encouraging.

Dopaminergic agents such as amantadine, levodopa/carbidopa, and bromocriptine also have shown clinical usefulness in patients with head injury.[44,45,59,60] Anderson et al.[61] described positive results on visual attention, speed of information processing, attention span, learning capacity, and alertness in two patients with traumatic brain injury who were given amantadine, 200–400 mg/day. Amantadine has been used in other populations, such as in Alzheimer's dementia patients, for a variety of symptoms. A controlled study in which amantadine was used for mild dementia found augmented P300 amplitude, suggesting improved cognitive processing.[62] Apathetic or disinhibited and impulsive patients may respond to treatment with dopamine agonists with minimal side effects. In a published case series, Kraus and Maki[44] assessed the effectiveness of amantadine hydrochloride. It improved several measures of cognitive function significantly and behavior problems associated with frontal lobe dysfunction, such as apathy, impulsivity, and disinhibition, in a series of seven patients whose original injury occurred at least several years earlier. Following up on these preliminary clinical data, Kraus et al.[63] reported on an open trial of amantadine hydrochloride in 23 subjects with traumatic brain injury that had occurred at least 6 months ago. Significant improvement was found for several tasks representing frontal lobe function, attention, and motor speed. On clinical assessment, 11 subjects reported improvement in all three areas assessed—cognition, mood, and behavior. Nine reported improvement in only one or two areas; three denied any response, although one subject showed areas of improvement on repeat testing.

Clinically, in our experience, the addition of a second dopaminergic agent such as levodopa/carbidopa may enhance response but needs to be done carefully because of increased risk of side effects.[45] Not all patients improve, however, and side effects such as increased agitation, gastrointestinal symptoms, decreased appetite, and, rarely, psychosis may occur.[42] An agent originally developed for Alzheimer's dementia is showing promise as a cognitive treatment for traumatic brain injury. We have used the cholinesterase inhibitor donepezil with some success in improving memory and cognition in some of our patients, often in combination with other treatments such as a dopaminergic agent. At present, only case reports are available,[64] and larger controlled studies must be done.

In the first published pilot report on the use of amantadine in recovery from experimental traumatic brain injury, Dixon et al.[65] assessed the effect of daily amantadine treatment on functional recovery (motor and spatial memory performance) following traumatic brain injury in rats based on a controlled cortical impact model. Amantadine-treated rats improved signif-

icantly during a 5-day water maze task. Daily administration of amantadine significantly enhanced recovery of spatial memory performance deficits but not motor deficits following traumatic brain injury. Investigation is under way to assess this potential effect on recovery in traumatic brain injury patients.

The efficacy of amantadine in traumatic brain injury may be attributable to its effect on dopamine transmission, its role as an N-methyl-D-aspartate antagonist, its effects on the balance among different neurotransmitter systems, or a combination of these attributes.

In general, anticholinergic agents should be avoided, if at all possible, because of the potential for aggravating cognitive deficits and for lowering the seizure threshold in brain-injured patients. Neuroleptics should be reserved to use as a treatment of last resort. They not only can aggravate symptomatology but also may be deleterious to cortical recovery.[57]

Treatment of frontal lobe dysfunction can be difficult. Along with a good psychosocial assessment, information about alcohol and drug use should be obtained because substance abuse may exacerbate problems of self-control. In addition to the dopaminergic agents, the selective serotonin reuptake inhibitors, buspirone, trazodone, β-adrenergic receptor blockers, and anticonvulsant medications have been used to treat aggression, disinhibition, and dyscontrol.[59,66] Prescribing multiple medications is often unavoidable. For example, our experience suggests that combining dopaminergics with serotonergic agents (e.g., sertraline) or carbamazepine can have an additive or possibly a synergistic effect in brain-injured patients with a range of symptoms and deficits. Obviously, more controlled studies are needed.

Nonspecific symptoms, such as headache and sleep disturbance, also are common following injury. Alone, these symptoms can affect mood and cognition adversely. Following CHI, they can significantly interfere with recovery and rehabilitation. These symptoms are sometimes self-limited or may respond secondarily to treatment aimed at other symptoms, such as mood disorders.

Posttraumatic headache has not been well studied but tends to have a mixed tension-vascular quality. Stress, overstimulation, and exposure to noise and bright light bring on a headache for many patients. The treatment of posttraumatic headache is essentially the treatment of chronic headache. Current guidelines for the treatment of migraine or tension headache can be used.[67] However, caution should be used to avoid agents, such as anticholinergics or narcotics, that could be problematic in head-injured patients. Current wisdom cautions against the chronic use of non-steroidal anti-inflammatory drugs, which can actually worsen the problem.[68] Instead, long-term prophylaxis with agents such as antidepressants, calcium channel blockers, valproate, or β-blockers can be instituted.[67] The serotonergic antidepressants, including fluoxetine and sertraline, may be useful. If anticholinergic side effects develop with use of low-dose amitriptyline, nortriptyline may be a more reasonable choice.

Sleep disturbances also aggravate other symptoms and interfere with recovery. Again, care should be taken in choosing pharmacological treatment. Often, headache and sleep disturbance occur together; in this case, we find that nortriptyline can be very helpful if tolerated. A low dose of trazodone also can be effective, along with education about sleep hygiene. A regular schedule is important because disrupted sleep-wake cycles are common and aggravate other symptomatology.

CONCLUSIONS

The frontal lobes are frequently involved in CHI. Although injury to the brain is often diffuse, specific cognitive, behavioral, and mood disorders can reasonably be attributed to frontal lobe damage, directly or indirectly. Treatment and rehabilitation require a multidisciplinary approach. Educating the patient and family about the sequelae of CHI is essential. Modifying the patient's home and work environments often leads to a significant improvement in the patient's level of functioning. Pharmacological interventions can be effective in certain cases and can enhance rehabilitation efforts.

REFERENCES

1. Adams JH, Graham DI, Scott G, et al: Brain damage in fatal non-missile head injury. J Clin Pathol 33:1132–1145, 1980
2. Blumbergs P, Jones N, North J: Diffuse axonal injury in head trauma. J Neurol Neurosurg Psychiatry 52:938–941, 1989
3. Levin H, Williams D, Eisenberg H, et al: Serial magnetic resonance imaging and neurobehavioral findings after mild to moderate closed head injury. J Neurol Neurosurg Psychiatry 55:255–262, 1992
4. Stuss D, Hugenholtz H, Richard M, et al: Subtle neuropsychological deficits in patients with good recovery after closed head injury. Neurosurgery 17:41–47, 1985
5. Prayer L, Wimberger D, Oder W, et al: Cranial MR imaging and cerebral ^{99m}Tc HM-PAO-SPECT in patients with subacute or chronic severe closed head injury and normal CT examinations. Acta Radiol 34:593–599, 1993
6. Ichise M, Chung D, Wang P, et al: Technetium-99m-HM-PAO SPECT, CT and MRI in the evaluation of patients with chronic traumatic brain injury: a correlation with neuropsychological performance. J Nucl Med 35:217–226, 1994
7. Damasio H, Grabowski T, Frank R, et al: The return of Phineas Gage: clues about the brain from the skull of a famous patient. Science 264:1102–1105, 1994
8. Goldman P: Functional development of the prefrontal cortex in early life and the problem of neuronal plasticity. Exp Neurol 32:366–387, 1971
9. Chugani H, Phelps M: Imaging human brain development with positron emission tomography. J Nucl Med 32:23–26, 1991
10. Passler M, Isaac W, Hynd G: Neuropsychological development of behavior attributed to frontal lobe functioning in children. Dev Neuropsychol 1:349–370, 1985
11. Diamond A, Zola-Morgan S, Squire L: Successful performance by monkeys with lesions of the hippocampal formation on AB and object retrieval, two tasks that mark developmental changes in human infants. Behav Neurosci 103:526–537, 1989
12. Price B, Daffner K, Stowe R, et al: The comportmental learning disabilities of early frontal lobe damage. Brain 113:1383–1393, 1990
13. Levin H, Handel S, Goldman A, et al: Magnetic resonance imaging after "diffuse" nonmissile head injury. Arch Neurol 42:963–968, 1985
14. Wickens D: Encoding categories of words: an empirical approach to meaning. Psychol Rev 77:1–15, 1970
15. Zatorre R, McEntee W: Semantic encoding deficits in a case of traumatic amnesia. Brain Cogn 2:331–345, 1983
16. Goldstein F, Levin H: Question-asking strategies after severe closed head injury. Brain Cogn 17:23–30, 1991
17. Baddeley A, Wilson B: Frontal amnesia and the dysexecutive syndrome. Brain Cogn 7:212–230, 1988
18. Hirst W, Volpe BT: Memory strategies with brain damage. Brain Cogn 8:379–408, 1988
19. Levin H, Goldstein F: Organization of verbal memory after severe closed-head injury. J Clin Exp Neuropsychol 8:643–656, 1986
20. Denney D, Denney N: The use of classification for problem-solving: a comparison of middle and old age. Dev Psychol 9:275–278, 1973
21. Benton A: Differential behavioral effects in frontal lobe disease. Neuropsychologia 6:53–60, 1968
22. Drewe E: Go-no go learning after frontal lobe lesions in humans. Cortex 11:8–16, 1975
23. Luria A, Haigh B: Restoration of Function After Brain Injury. New York, Macmillan, 1963

24. Porteus S, Diamond A: Porteus Maze changes after psychosurgery. Journal of Mental Science 108:53–58, 1962

25. Shallice T: Specific impairments in planning. Philos Trans R Soc Lond B Biol Sci 298:199–209, 1982

26. Levin H, Mendelsohn D, Lilly M, et al: Tower of London performance in relation to magnetic resonance imaging following closed head injury in children. Neuropsychology 8:171–179, 1994

27. Oscar-Berman M, McNamara P, Freedman M: Delayed-response tasks: parallels between experimental ablation studies and findings in patients with frontal lesions, in Frontal Lobe Function and Dysfunction. Edited by Levin H, Eisenberg H, Benton A. New York, Oxford University Press, 1991, pp 230–255

28. Milner B, Petrides M, Smith M: Frontal lobes and the temporal organization of memory. Human Neurobiology 4:137–142, 1985

29. Levin H, Goldstein F, High WM Jr, et al: Automatic and effortful processing after severe closed head injury. Brain Cogn 7:283–297, 1988

30. Levin H, Mattis S, Ruff R, et al: Neurobehavioral outcome following minor head injury: a three-center study. J Neurosurg 66:234–243, 1987

31. Campbell J, Duffy J, Salloway S: Treatment strategies for patients with prefrontal syndromes. J Neuropsychiatry Clin Neurosci 6:411–418, 1994

32. Mega M, Cummings J: Frontal-subcortical circuits and neuropsychiatric disorders. J Neuropsychiatry Clin Neurosci 6:358–370, 1994

33. Duffy J, Campbell J: The regional prefrontal syndromes: a theoretical and clinical overview. J Neuropsychiatry Clin Neurosci 6:379–387, 1994

34. Fedoroff J, Starkstein S, Forrester A, et al: Depression in patients with acute traumatic brain injury. Am J Psychiatry 149:918–923, 1992

35. Jorge R, Robinson R, Arndt S, et al: Comparison between acute- and delayed-onset depression following traumatic brain injury. J Neuropsychiatry Clin Neurosci 5:43–49, 1993

36. Robinson R, Boston J, Starkstein S, et al: Comparison of mania with depression following brain injury: causal factors. Am J Psychiatry 145:172–178, 1988

37. Shukla S, Cook B, Mukherjee S, et al: Mania following head trauma. Am J Psychiatry 144:93–96, 1987

38. Blumer D, Benson D: Personality changes with frontal and temporal lobe lesions, in Psychiatric Aspects of Neurologic Disease. Edited by Benson D, Blumer D. New York, Grune & Stratton, 1975, pp 151–170

39. Prigatano G: Personality disturbances associated with traumatic brain injury. J Consult Clin Psychol 60:360–368, 1992

40. Ota Y: Psychiatric studies on civilian head injuries, in The Late Effects of Head Injury. Edited by Walker A, Caveness W, Critchley M. Springfield, IL, Charles C Thomas, 1969, pp 110–119

41. Kraus MF: The neuropsychiatry of traumatic brain injury: an overview of assessment and pharmacologic interventions, in Traumatic Brain Injury. Edited by Marion D. New York, Thieme, 1999, pp 173–185

42. Gualtieri C: Pharmacotherapy and the neurobehavioral sequelae of traumatic brain injury. Brain Inj 2:101–129, 1988

43. Merren MD: Gabapentin for pain and tremor: a large case series. South Med J 91:739–744, 1998

44. Kraus MF, Maki PM: The effect of amantadine hydrochloride on neuropsychiatric sequelae of brain injury: case studies and review. J Neuropsychiatry Clin Neurosci 9:1–9, 1997

45. Kraus MF, Maki PM: The combined use of amantadine and L-dopa/carbidopa in the treatment of chronic brain injury. Brain Inj 11:455–459, 1997

46. Gualtieri C, Evans R: Stimulant treatment for the neurobehavioral sequelae of traumatic brain injury. Brain Inj 2:273–290, 1988

47. Evans R, Gualtieri C, Patterson D: Treatment of chronic closed head injury with psychostimulant drugs: a controlled case study and appropriate evaluation procedure. J Nerv Ment Dis 162:366–371, 1987

48. Lipper S, Tuchman M: Treatment of chronic post-traumatic organic brain syndrome with dextroamphetamine: first reported case. J Nerv Ment Dis 162:366–371, 1976

49. Speech T, Rao S, Osmon D, et al: A double blind controlled study of methylphenidate in closed head injury. Brain Inj 7:333–338, 1993

50. Bleiberg J, Garmoe W, Cedarquist J, et al: Effects of dexedrine on performance consistency following brain injury. Neuropsychiatry Neuropsychol Behav Neurol 6:245–248, 1993

51. Kuczenski R: Biochemical actions of amphetamines and other stimulants, in Stimulants: Neurochemical, Behavioral and Clinical Perspectives. Edited by Creese I. New York, Raven, 1983, pp 31–53

52. Kraus M, Burch E: Methylphenidate hydrochloride as an antidepressant: controversy, case studies, and review. South Med J 85:985–991, 1992

53. Kaufman M, Cassem N, Murray G, et al: Use of psychostimulants in medically ill patients with neurologic disease and major depression. Can J Psychiatry 29:46–49, 1984

54. Woods S, Tesar G, Murray G, et al: Psychostimulant treatment of depressive disorders secondary to medical illness. J Clin Psychiatry 47:12–15, 1986

55. Lingam V, Lazarus L, Groves L, et al: Methylphenidate in treating post-stroke depression. J Clin Psychiatry 49:151–153, 1988

56. Lazarus L, Winemiller D, Lingam V, et al: Efficacy and side effects of methylphenidate for post stroke depression. J Clin Psychiatry 53:447–449, 1992

57. Feeney D, Gonzales A, Law W: Amphetamine, haloperidol and experience interact to affect rate of recovery after motor cortex injury. Science 217:855–857, 1982

58. Plenger P, Dixon CE, Castillo R, et al: Subacute methylphenidate treatment for moderate to moderately severe traumatic brain injury: a preliminary double-blind placebo-controlled study. Arch Phys Med Rehabil 77:536–540, 1996

59. Gualtieri C (ed): Neuropsychiatry and Behavioral Pharmacology. New York, Springer-Verlag, 1991

60. Parks RW, Crockett DJ, Manji HK, et al: Assessment of bromocriptine intervention for the treatment of frontal lobe syndrome: a case study. J Neuropsychiatry Clin Neurosci 4:109–111, 1992

61. Anderson S, Berstad J, Finset A, et al: Amantadine in cognitive failure in patients with traumatic head injuries. Tidsskr Nor Laegeforen 112:2070–2072, 1992

62. Semlitsch H, Anderer P, Saletu B: Topographic mapping of long latency "cognitive" event-related potentials (P300): a double-blind, placebo controlled study with amantadine in mild dementia. J Neural Transm 4:319–336, 1992

63. Kraus M, Dixon CE, Smith G, et al: A PET study utilizing [11C]raclopride and [18F]FDG to assess a trial of amantadine hydrochloride in traumatic brain injury. Poster presented at the annual meeting of the Society of Biological Psychiatry, May 15, 1999

64. Taverni JP, Seliger G, Lichtman SW: Donepezil medicated memory improvement in traumatic brain injury during post acute rehabilitation. Brain Inj 12:77–80, 1998

65. Dixon CE, Kraus MF, Ma X, et al: Amantadine improves water maze performance following traumatic brain injury in rats. Restorative Neurology and Neuroscience 14:285–294, 1999

66. Silver J, Yudofsky S: Psychopharmacology, in Neuropsychiatry of Traumatic Brain Injury. Edited by Silver J, Yudofsky S, Hales R. Washington, DC, American Psychiatric Press, 1994, pp 631–670

67. Schulman EA, Silberstein SD: Symptomatic and prophylactic treatment of migraine and tension type headache. Neurology 42:16–21, 1992

68. Sheftell FD: Chronic daily headache. Neurology 42:32–36, 1992

15

The Frontal Lobes and Content-Specific Delusions

Emily D. Richardson, Ph.D., Paul F. Malloy, Ph.D.

Delusions are defined as false beliefs based on incorrect inference about external reality and firmly sustained in spite of the opinions of others or contrary evidence.[1] Although psychological factors can be important in the production of delusions, contemporary research has shown that delusions also can result from identifiable neurological disease. Delusions have been reported in association with virtually every major class of neurological insult, from generalized disturbances such as toxic-metabolic disorders to focal lesions such as tumor and stroke.[2] Delusions are quite common in some neurological disorders, such as degenerative or cerebrovascular dementia.[3–6]

The recent neuropsychiatric literature has contained increasing numbers of cases of monosymptomatic or content-specific delusions (CSDs)—delusions that have a specific theme or topic. There appears to be a particularly strong relation between CSDs and neurological disease, especially neurological lesions affecting the frontal lobes and right hemisphere. In this chapter, we argue that a diagnostic distinction of CSDs from other delusions appears to be justified on the basis of different phenomenology, treatment response, and prognosis. Most important, CSDs are etiologically distinct, in that they are frequently caused by identifiable neurological insult or disease.

OVERVIEW OF CONTENT-SPECIFIC DELUSIONS

Types of Content-Specific Delusions

Various CSDs involving the reduplication of elements of the environment have been identified. These can include delusions that a place has been duplicated (*reduplicative paramnesia*) or a variety of delusions concerning duplication of persons (*'s syndrome and its variants*). Delusions involving sexual themes also have been described as occurring in a monosymptomatic form. The sexual delusions most often encountered in the literature involve delusions of infidelity by a loved one (*Othello syndrome* or *delusional jealousy*) and the delusion of being involved in an amorous relationship (*de Clérambault syndrome* or *erotomania*). Content-specific somatic delusions have ranged from delusional illness (e.g., *delusional infestation*), to distortions of the body (e.g., *lycanthropy*), to the belief that one is dying or is dead (e.g., *Cotard's syndrome*).

Reduplicative paramnesia is the delusion that a place familiar to the patient exists in two or more physical locations simultaneously. The earliest description of reduplicative paramnesia was by Pick,[7] who described a patient who claimed that Pick's clinic in Prague had a duplicate in another city. A variant of the syndrome occurs when a place is thought to exist in an impossible location, often sharing characteristics with that setting. For example, Benson et al.[8] described a patient who believed that the Boston Veteran's Affairs Hospital was located in a spare bedroom in his home. This variant has been termed *disorientation for place* by some writers.[9] A third variant often seen in individuals with dementia is the belief that a familiar place, usually one's home, is a strange place. These disorders can involve erroneous under- or overidentification of a place.

Capgras's syndrome is a type of reduplicative delusion involving the belief that persons well known to the patient, such as family members, have doubles or are imposters.[10] The double or imposter is sometimes perceived as differing slightly in some physical characteristic from the "genuine" person, but the patient may have difficulty verbalizing the precise nature of this difference. Several variations of this syndrome have been identified. *Doppelganger* or *subjective doubles* is the belief that the patient himself or herself has a double or impersonator.[11] *Fregoli syndrome* is the belief that a person is capable of taking on the appearance of others while retaining his or her own psychological identity.[12] *Intermetamorphosis* is the belief that a person is changing in both physical and psychological identity to become another person.[13]

One type of content-specific sexual delusion is Othello syndrome (also known as delusional jealousy or morbid jealousy), the belief that a loved one is involved in a sexual or amorous relationship with another person. The term refers, of course, to the tragic Shakespearean character who was convinced by the evil Iago that his wife, Ophelia, was unfaithful. Usually, the supposed lover is someone known to the patient, such as a friend or neighbor. Delusional jealousy can be difficult to diagnose because of the reluctance of patients to discuss the subject, the difficulty of verifying the fidelity of the spouse, and the fact that a patient may be delusional even when the spouse has in fact been unfaithful at some point.[14] However, the delusional nature of the belief is usually apparent when the patient begins to read undue meaning into mundane events. For example, we have described a happily married patient who developed delusional jealousy after a cerebral infarct. This man found evidence of imagined illicit visits by a lover in tracks in the snow near the house, a window left partly open, and innocuous remarks made by the wife about the neighbor (the supposed lover) who was 40 years her junior.[15]

A second type of sexual delusion is de Clérambault syndrome (or erotomania), the belief that one is involved in an amorous relationship. Often the purported lover is a famous person, such as a movie actor or rock star, or someone in a prestigious occupation such as a doctor.[16] Erotomania is usually recognized quite easily by the complaints of the target of the delusion and the unfortunate fact that many patients with the disorder engage in behavior that is blatantly inappropriate or actually criminal. Many examples of this syndrome have been reported in the media. Perhaps the best-known case is the attempted assassination of President Reagan by John Hinckley as an expression of his love for actress Jodie Foster. Other examples include a woman who stalked the home and purloined the credit cards of comedian David Letterman, claiming to be his wife. Another woman repeatedly invaded the property of singer Michael Jackson, claiming to be the inspiration for his song "Billy Jean."

Delusions confined to somatic distortions include delusions of disease or infestation, delusions involving distortion of the body, and the delusion that one is dead or dying. One common somatic or hypochondriacal delusion is the belief that one is infested with parasites or other macroscopic organisms. Various terms have been used to describe this delusion, including *delusional parasitosis, delusional infestation, parasitophobia, dermatophobia, acarophobia,* and *Ekbom syndrome.* Delusions of parasitosis can exist as an isolated psychosis or as part of a more complicated medical and/or psychiatric illness. Clinical signs include self-inflicted wounds from efforts to extricate parasites and the collection of bottles and jars purported to contain samples of the parasites.[17] This disorder is commonly seen in dermatological settings. Most dermatologists report having seen at least one such case in the previous 5 years.[18] The delusion has been reported to occur primarily in older individuals (older than 50 years) and can be precipitated by an actual dermatological condition.[19] Related to delusions of infestation are the hypochondriacal delusions of contagion or disease (such as the delusion of having acquired immunodeficiency syndrome [AIDS]).[20,21] Several cases have been reported in which the patient believed that one or more parts of his or her body were distorted. For example, Walter[22] reported a case in which a 55-year-old electrician inserted a knitting needle into his urethra because of a persistent belief that he had a urethral stricture. Similarly, Wang and Lee[23] described a 66-year-old man who repeatedly and severely damaged his forehead, creating a brain abscess, because he believed that a "toxic root" was lodged there. Other somatic delusions reported in the literature include delusions of body odor,[24,25] lycanthropy[26] (the belief that one has become a werewolf), and supernumerary delusions (belief that one has extra limbs).[27–29]

Cotard's syndrome, koro, and dhat represent the ultimate in dysmorphic delusions, involving the belief that one is about to die or is already dead. In Cotard's syndrome, the patient believes that he or she is dead, despite the contrary evidence that he or she remains animate and that vital signs are present. In koro, the sensation of penile retraction is coupled with an intense fear that death will occur once the retraction is complete. Koro has been reported mainly in Southeast Asia, and it occurs in both epidemic and sporadic forms.[30] Similar to koro is dhat syndrome, a neurosis purportedly seen only in India. In dhat, the belief that semen is being discharged in the urine is coupled with a religiously based belief that a vital life fluid is being drained from the body.[31]

Content-Specific Delusions Compared With Perceptual or Transient Disorders

Specific delusions must be distinguished from purely perceptual or hallucinatory disturbances and from generalized disturbance of cognition. That is, to be properly and convincingly diagnosed as a delusion, the disturbance must involve a mistaken belief (not merely a misperception) and must be persistent (not a transitory effect of confusion). For example, in *autoscopy,* the patient experiences a second self, as in the subjective doubles variant of Capgras's syndrome. However, the phenomena differ in that a person with autoscopy seems to actually see the double rather than believing the double to be active elsewhere, as in subjective doubles. Hence, autoscopy is properly grouped with illusions or perceptual disturbances rather than delusional beliefs. A second example is *prosopagnosia,* or the inability to discriminate faces. The prosopagnosic person may fail to recognize his wife, whereas the Capgras patient will insist that the present person is an imposter and that the "real" wife is somewhere else. Capgras's syndrome can occur with prosopagnosia, but the perceptual disturbance and the delusional belief are dissociable.[32] Intermetamorphosis includes a perceptual distortion, in that people change their appearances, but we have grouped it with delusional syndromes because of the prominent belief that the imposter's psyche inhabits these changed persons. Other visual agnosias, such as *simultanagnosia,* can im-

pair recognition of persons or objects. These can again be distinguished from delusions by the absence of an associated erroneous belief and by the involvement of other objects in the misperception.

Delusions also must be reasonably persistent. Many patients who are in confusional states express strange beliefs, but the beliefs typically change from hour to hour and do not persist once the confusion resolves. Patients with dementia also may momentarily mistake one family member for another, but they respond to correction readily. These transitory phenomena clearly do not qualify as delusions.

Although these conceptual distinctions are reasonably clear, in clinical practice these various disorders can become intertwined. A patient may first experience a perceptual change, which can become elaborated into a delusional belief. For example, the demented patient with cataracts may mistake inanimate objects in a dark room for persons and then come to believe that deceased relatives are present in the home. Berrios[19] pointed out that in some cases of delusional parasitosis in elderly patients with dementia, the individual first developed a pruritus that later became elaborated into the infestation delusion. Such beliefs may become entrenched and reach the magnitude of a delusion by the time the patient is examined by a professional.

Content-Specific Delusions Compared With Primary Delusional (Paranoid) Disorder

CSDs differ clinically in several ways from the more common delusions found in association with primary psychiatric disorder. For example, patients with primary paranoid disorders are usually guarded and suspicious. When their delusions are challenged, patients typically will escalate their defenses and often will incorporate the examiner into the delusion ("You must be working for the CIA, too!"). In paranoid schizophrenia, the delusions are often accompanied by hallucinations and thought disorder.

In contrast, patients with CSDs usually are described as forthcoming and cooperative. Although they insist that their delusional beliefs are true, they often admit to puzzlement or bemusement regarding aspects of the delusion. Rather than escalate their defenses by becoming hostile, they are more likely to confabulate an explanation. For example, a patient with a delusion of duplication[33] was asked how she could have two sets of children with identical names. She appeared momentarily puzzled and then stated,

"My husband was in the navy, and we moved around a lot; it was hard to keep that straight." Patients with CSDs also have other characteristically "frontal lobe" behavioral features, including unconcern about their condition and decreased foresight.

PREVALENCE OF CONTENT-SPECIFIC DELUSIONS

CSDs are thought to be relatively rare disorders, with prevalence estimates ranging from less than 1% to 5.3% in psychiatric settings.[34,35] However, these studies were limited to retrospective chart reviews, which can be influenced by the examiner's lack of thoroughness in assessing delusional thoughts or by failure to recognize CSDs because of unfamiliarity with the syndromes. When interviewers have specifically assessed such syndromes, the estimates have been considerably higher. For example, Dohn and Crews[36] observed that Capgras's syndrome was frequently overlooked in psychiatric patients and found that the delusion actually had a 15% prevalence in their sample of adult inpatients with previous diagnoses of schizophrenia. Kirov et al.[37] reported a prevalence of 4.1% among consecutive admissions to a psychiatric hospital, but they excluded all patients with evidence of a neurological basis for the delusions and those with gross cognitive deficits. Hakim et al.[38] found that when specific inquiries were made, 8% of the patients admitted for alcohol abuse reported specific delusions regarding duplication of place.

CSDs also may be more common in certain neurological populations. For example, several researchers[6,39] found that about 25% of patients with Alzheimer's disease have CSDs concerning misidentification of people. Geller[40] found that the prevalence of delusional jealousy was highest in organic psychoses (7.0%), paranoid disorders (6.7%), alcohol psychosis (5.6%), and schizophrenia (2.5%), whereas in affective disorder, delusions of jealousy could be found in only 0.1%. Similarly, el Gaddal[41] found high rates of de Clérambault syndrome in association with organic disorders (21.3%); 35% of the patients with the erotomanic delusion had schizophrenia, paranoia, or paraphrenia; 22.5% had affective disorder; and 10% had neurotic disorder.

Setting also can have an important effect on observed prevalence. Certain CSDs, such as de Clérambault syndrome, occur at higher rates in forensic settings because of the propensity of these patients to act violently toward the object of the delusion.[42] Somatic delusions of infestation are seen more frequently in general medical than in psychiatric settings because of the physical complaints associated with the delusion.[43] CSDs have even been found in epidemic proportions in certain cultures or historical periods; the delusion of possession by evil spirits is found in up to 20% of Japanese psychiatric patients.[44]

LITERATURE REVIEW

In this section, we review the English-language literature through 1999 regarding neurological causes of CSD. A limitation of the literature to date is that most descriptions of CSDs have been single case studies or small series. It is therefore necessary to review multiple reports in order to draw conclusions about etiology and localization of cerebral dysfunction. Unfortunately, many modern reports fail to include neurological workup, despite the clear association between many CSDs and neurological disease. We subdivided cases into those in which 1) a generalized or systemic disorder (e.g., hypothyroidism) related to the genesis of the delusion was documented or 2) focal lesions were associated with the development of the delusion, and significant neurodiagnostic information was provided (including, at minimum, some form of neuroimaging). Finally, detailed reviews were conducted on the focal cases to determine whether particular lesion locations were associated with the development and maintenance of the delusion.

Reduplicative Paramnesia

Forstl and colleagues[45] reviewed 260 case reports of misidentification syndromes, reporting 17 with reduplicative paramnesia. The patients with reduplicative paramnesia more frequently had head trauma or cerebral infarction and showed more evidence of right hemisphere lesions on computed tomography (CT) scan or neuropsychological testing than did the patients with other misidentification syndromes. However, details of the individual cases were not presented in this review.

Table 15–1 presents detailed data from 25 cases of reduplicative paramnesia with neurological workups appearing in the literature to date (1976–1999). Benson and colleagues[8] were the first to posit a specific mechanism for reduplicative paramnesia; they described a head-injured young man with reduplicative paramnesia who believed that the hospital was located in a dis-

TABLE 15–1. Neurodiagnostic findings in reduplicative paramnesia

Reference	Etiology	CT/MRI	EEG	Neurological examination	Neuropsychological testing
Alexander et al.[68]	Head trauma	BI frontal and R temporal	WNL	Mild R facial weakness, L hemiparesis, poor tandem gait	VS, NVM, FL deficits
Benson et al.[8]					
Case 1	Head trauma	BI frontal, R>L	BI frontal, R>L	R anosmia	VIQ=127, PIQ=96, MQ=137
Case 2	Head trauma	Angiography: R mass lesion	NR	L hemiparesis, L ankle clonus, L Hoffman, L visual neglect	VIQ=85, PIQ=44, MQ=59
Filley and Jarvis[128]	Head trauma	R hygroma	WNL	L hemiparesis, L sensory loss, diffuse hyperreflexia	VIQ=118, PIQ=104; VS, VM, NVM, FL deficits
Fisher[9]	Infarct	R parietal-occipital	NR	L hemiparesis, L sensory loss, L field defect, L neglect	NR
Hakim et al.[38]					
Case 1	Alcoholic only	WNL	NR	NR	VIQ=100, PIQ=85, MQ=94; FL deficits
Case 2	Alcoholic and infarct	R hemisphere	NR	NR	NR
Case 3	Alcoholic and contusion	R hemisphere	NR	NR	VIQ=78, PIQ=72, MQ=62; FL deficits
Case 4	Alcoholic and infarct	R hemisphere	NR	NR	VIQ=85, PIQ=70, MQ=105; FL deficits
Joseph[139]					
Case 1	NR	WNL	Nonlateralized slowing	WNL	"BI parietal and frontal lobe dysfunction...diffuse R hemisphere dysfunction"
Kapur et al.[47]	Hemorrhage	R frontal	NR	WNL	VIQ=78, PIQ=78; NVM, FL deficits; L neglect, confabulation
Lewis[140]	Hemorrhage, seizures, overdose	BI frontal and occipitotemporal	BI occipitotemporal slowing, R>L	L divergent squint, poor color vision, isolated scotoma	VIQ=72, PIQ=61; naming, memory, and especially VS deficits (FL not reported)
Metcalfe et al.[46]	Infarct	L occipitoparietal	NR	Dense R homonymous hemianopia	NR

(continued)

TABLE 15–1. Neurodiagnostic findings in reduplicative paramnesia (*continued*)

Reference	Etiology	CT/MRI	EEG	Neurological examination	Neuropsychological testing
Murai et al.[69]					
Case 1	Ruptured aneurysm R ACA	R frontal, frontal subcortical	NR	L hemiparesis	VIQ=76, PIQ=51; VM, NVM, FL deficits
Case 2	Head trauma	Bl frontal, R>L	NR	Mild diplegia	VIQ=79, PIQ=70; VM, FL deficits
Case 3	Infarct	R frontal	NR	NR	NR
Case 4	Infarct	R subcortical (putamen)	NR	L neglect	NR
Case 5	Infarcts	R subcortical (thalamus), L frontal	"R hemisphere suppression"	"Aphasia and amnestic syndrome"	NR
Ruff and Volpe[127]					
Case 1	Tumor	R parietofrontal	NR	L hemiparesis, L inferior quadrantanopsia, L extinction	VIQ=115, PIQ=80; VS, NVM, FL deficits
Case 2	Hematoma, AVM	R frontoparietal	NR	L hemiparesis, L extinction	VS, NVM deficits; FL not tested
Case 3	Tumor and hemorrhage	R frontoparietal	NR	L hemiparesis, L extinction	VIQ=110, PIQ=76; VS, NVM, FL deficits
Case 4	Subdural hematoma	R frontal			VIQ=80, PIQ=56; VS, NVM>VM, FL deficits
Sellal et al.[141]	Viral encephalitis	R temporal and anterior temporal, R septal nucleus, hippocampus, parahippocampal gyrus, Bl cingulate, orbital, rectus gyrus, insula	NR	Grasp reflex, perseverations, confabulations, utilization behavior, apathy	VIQ=102, PIQ=70; VS, NVM, FL deficits
Staton et al.[122]	Head trauma	R temporal, Bl frontal	R temporal slowing	L hyperreflexia, + Babinski, and central facial palsy	PIQ<VIQ: VS, NVM>VM, "problem-solving" deficits
Vighetto et al.[142]	Infarct	R temporoparietal, Bl frontal	NR	NR	VIQ=119, PIQ=106; VS, NVM deficits; FL not reported

Note. ACA=anterior communicating artery; AVM=arteriovenous malformation; Bl=bilateral; CT=computed tomography; EEG=electroencephalography; FL=frontal lobe; L=left; MQ=Memory Quotient from Wechsler scales; MRI=magnetic resonance imaging; NR=not reported; NVM=nonverbal memory; PIQ=Performance Intelligence Quotient from Wechsler scales; R=right; VIQ=Verbal Intelligence Quotient from Wechsler scales; VM=verbal memory; VS=visuospatial; WNL=within normal limits.

tant army base where he had been stationed in the past. CT scan identified bilateral frontal lesions (right worse than left), and the patient had marked deficits on neuropsychological testing of frontal or executive functions. Subsequent case studies have shown neuroimaging evidence of either right frontal or bilateral frontal involvement in most cases, with some having right posterior lesions (either alone or in combination with frontal damage), and electroencephalography (EEG) and neurological examination data tend to support right hemisphere involvement in the production of reduplicative paramnesia. Only one case has been found in the literature that indicates a focal left-sided posterior lesion in the production of reduplicative paramnesia,[46] although additional neurodiagnostic testing (EEG, neuropsychological testing) was not conducted on the patient to rule out more diffuse dysfunction. Kapur et al.[47] reported one case with demonstrable damage limited to the right frontal region, suggesting frontal damage alone may be sufficient to produce reduplicative paramnesia. Across these 25 cases, traumatic and vascular etiologies predominated.

Capgras's Syndrome

About 58% of the patients with Capgras's syndrome who receive adequate neurodiagnostic workups are found to have primary psychiatric disorder, uncomplicated by demonstrable neurological disease.[33] The most common diagnosis in these cases is paranoid schizophrenia, followed by affective disorder with psychotic features.[45]

Capgras's syndrome and its variants also have been reported in association with a variety of systemic diseases and diffuse neurological disorders. Systemic etiologies have included metabolic disturbances such as myxedema,[48,49] pseudohypoparathyroidism,[50,51] anemia,[52] hepatic dysfunction,[53] and vitamin B$_{12}$ deficiency[54]; intoxication and reactions to drugs, including cocaine,[55] chloroquine,[56] disulfiram,[57] digoxin,[58] and lithium[59]; cerebral infections such as encephalitis[60,61] and AIDS[62]; subarachnoid hemorrhage[63]; migraine[64]; post–electroconvulsive therapy confusion[65]; minor head trauma[66]; and degenerative dementia.[67]

Alexander and colleagues[68] were the first to report a Capgras delusion clearly related to a specific neurological structural lesion, involving the right hemisphere with predominantly frontal and temporal lobe damage. This localization was confirmed in a detailed review of the literature on Capgras's syndrome,[33] which we summarize here. Table 15–2 reproduces a

TABLE 15–2. Summary of neurodiagnostic findings in 58 cases of Capgras delusions with neurological workups

Etiology	66% neurologically abnormal (38/58)
	26% trauma (10/38)
	21% degenerative (8/38)
	34% vascular (13/38)
	8% seizures (3/38)
	11% tumor (4/38)
Neuroimaging	59% abnormal (33/56)
	45% right hemisphere (15/33)
	12% left hemisphere (4/33)
	42% bilateral (14/33)
	52% frontal lobe (17/33)
	45% temporal (15/33)
	6% subcortical (2/33)
Electroencephalography	69% abnormal (22/32)
	64% right predominance (14/22)
	5% left predominance (1/22)
	32% diffuse (7/22)
Neurological examination	31% abnormal (15/48)
	87% left-sided abnormalities (13/15)
	13% right-sided abnormalities (2/15)
Neuropsychological tests	85% abnormal (34/40)
	Executive, visuospatial, memory

summary describing the findings in Capgras cases with neurodiagnostic information based on the pertinent portion of our previous review and including an update of case reports published since that first article (1990–1999).[69–81]

Right hemisphere or bilateral lesions were invariably found on neuroimaging, with few exclusively left hemisphere lesions. EEG and neurological examination findings also implicated right hemisphere pathology. In terms of specific localization, 72% of the cases with CT or magnetic resonance imaging (MRI) scans had right frontal, temporal, or frontotemporal involvement. Neuropsychological testing documented spatial, executive, and nonverbal memory problems, consistent with the right frontotemporal localization on neuroimaging studies.

SEXUAL DELUSIONS

Sexual delusions are found in primary psychiatric disorders, including schizophrenia, delusional (paranoid) disorder, and affective disorder.[82] As noted earlier in this chapter, when these delusions occur in primary psychiatric disorder, they are usually accompanied by hallucinations, other bizarre thinking, or prominent mood disturbance. Delusional jealousy is a relatively rare symptom in primary psychiatric patients, with an estimated prevalence of fewer than 1% of inpatients.[83]

Sexual delusions occur in higher numbers in association with several diffuse neurological illnesses, particularly alcoholism.[84] In a review of the prevalence of the disorder in 8,134 psychiatric inpatients, for example, Soyka et al.[14] found that delusional jealousy occurred in 5.6% of the patients with alcohol psychosis and 7.0% of the patients with other organic psychosis. In a presentation of 81 cases of delusional jealousy, Shepard[82] reported that 7% were related to chronic alcohol abuse. Sexual delusions also have been found in conjunction with metabolic disturbances such as adrenocortical suppression[85] and hyperthyroidism[86]; degenerative dementias such as Alzheimer's,[82] Huntington's,[3] and Parkinson's disease[87]; and diffuse head injury.[88,89]

Unfortunately, a review of the English-language literature of delusional jealousy in the last 20 years found that 35 of the 45 cases did not report formal neurological workups. Of these cases, 9 were nonetheless reported to have an associated organic condition, including chronic alcohol abuse[82] and toxicity to medication.[87] Only 9 of the 45 published cases of delusional jealousy reported relatively complete neurological workups.[15,85,90–94] In 7 of these, the patients were found to have neurological abnormalities, and another patient's delusion was ascribed to amphetamine abuse, although neurological deficits were not evident. Thus, at least 38% (17 of 45) of the cases reported in the recent literature most likely had a neurological basis for their delusion of infidelity.

Only a few cases have been reported on delusional jealousy associated with documented focal neurological impairment. In the three cases reported by Shepard[82] in which the patients had neurological disease, the dysfunction or lesions were primarily right hemisphere or right frontal as determined by EEG and/or autopsy. Richardson and colleagues[15] reported the case of a previously happily married elderly man who developed the delusion that his wife was unfaithful shortly after recovery from a large right middle cerebral artery infarction, and Westlake and Weeks[94] recently described a case of delusional jealousy associated with an infarction in the frontal and deep

parietal areas on the right. These cases are consistent with the above literature review, which implicates right hemisphere and frontal systems pathology in CSDs. A more recent report, however, described a case in which an Othello delusion emerged in association with bifrontal pathology with no evidence of right posterior dysfunction,[90] and another case report suggested that the delusion was associated with a cerebellar lesion producing diffuse cerebral changes, including edema and ventricular dilatation.[92] As was discussed with reduplicative paramnesia in an earlier subsection, right frontal dysfunction may be sufficient to produce Othello delusions, but this conclusion must be viewed as tentative given the dearth of published cases with adequate workups.

Many recent cases of de Clérambault syndrome (erotomanic delusions) also have been reported without information about neurological status. Of the 235 case reports culled from the English-language literature in the past 20 years, only 19 (8%) reported partial workups, including some combination of CT scans, EEGs, neurological examinations, and/or neuropsychological examinations.[41,88,89,95–103] Of the cases with abnormal neurological findings, etiologies have included head injury,[88] posttraumatic seizures,[89] meningioma,[95] Alzheimer's disease,[96] aneurysm rupture,[100] resection of tumor,[102] or arteriovenous malformation[41] and radiation necrosis.[103] Given the paucity of material, a relation between focal neurological dysfunction and erotomania remains to be shown.

SOMATIC DELUSIONS

Somatic delusions have been reported to occur in conjunction with several medical conditions affecting brain functions, including metabolic disorders,[104] cannabis intoxication,[105] and medication reactions.[26,106] Diffuse neurological diseases causing somatic delusions have included degenerative dementias,[107] metastatic lymphoma,[19] generalized seizure disorder,[26] and "organic brain syndrome."[108]

Cases of somatic delusions with more focal brain lesions also have been reported and are included in Table 15–3. Flynn et al.[109] described a case of delusional infestation in association with focal cerebrovascular disease. A 67-year-old man with no psychiatric history presented with the complaint of crawling sensations beneath the skin on the left side of his head, which he attributed to "worms." As is characteristic of patients with secondary delusions, he had no other delusions,

TABLE 15–3. Neurodiagnostic findings in somatic delusions

Reference	Etiology	CT/MRI/SPECT	EEG	Neurological examination	Neuropsychological testing
Adunsky[143] (delusional infestation)					
Case 1	Infarction	R frontal lobe	NR	L hemiparesis	"No cognitive deficits"; MMSE=29/30
Case 2	Infarction	R temporoparietal	NR	Mild residual hemiparesis	"Cognitively preserved"
Berrios[19] (delusional infestation)					
Case 3	Infarction of pituitary tumor	Enlarged pituitary fossa with destruction of inferior dorsum sella	NR	NR	NR
Flynn et al.[109] (delusional infestation)	Infarct	Bl periventricular, R frontal, R splenium	WNL	Mild fine motor deficit, bradykinesia, diffuse increased tone, DTR	NR
May and Terpenning[144] (delusional infestation)					
Case 5	Tumor	Pituitary fossa tumor	NR	NR	"Mildly cognitively impaired"
Murthy et al.[145] (delusional infestation)	Tumor	Presurgery: R FL extending to L paracalcarine region; 8-month follow-up: large bifrontal tumor, hyperdensity in R occipital horn	NR	WNL	NR
Drake[115] (Cotard's syndrome)					
Case 1	Tumor	R frontal	R temporal delta and seizure activity	L hemiparesis	NR
Case 2	Head trauma	R temporal atrophy, R frontal encephalomalacia	R frontotemporal delta and seizure activity	NR	NR
Case 3	Infarct	R frontal	R temporal sharp and slow waves	NR	Average IQ, "mild deficits consistent with anterior R cerebral dysfunction"

(continued)

TABLE 15–3. Neurodiagnostic findings in somatic delusions (*continued*)

Reference	Etiology	CT/MRI/SPECT	EEG	Neurological examination	Neuropsychological testing
Joseph and O'Leary[114] (Cotard's syndrome)	NR	Bl frontal and temporal atrophy	NR	WNL	"Diffuse cortical and subcortical organic dysfunction with bifrontal and anterior R hemisphere predominance"
Petracca et al.[146] (Cotard's syndrome)	NA	CT/MRI WNL; pre-ECT SPECT: hypoperfusion FL, frontosubcortical; post-ECT: increased perfusion in all areas	WNL	WNL	Pre-ECT: MMSE=5; 1-month post-ECT: MMSE=27
Young et al.[147] (Cotard's syndrome)	Head injury	R temporoparietal, internal capsule; Bl frontal atrophy; R temporoparietal hypoperfusion	NR	L hemiparesis, L hemianopia	NVM, VS abnormal
Kourany and Williams[110] (dysmorphic: excessive hair)	NR	WNL	WNL	WNL	NR
Kulick et al.[26] (lycanthropy)	Seizures	WNL	R temporal sharp waves	NR	NR
Dalby et al.[148] (dysmorphic: L eye)	Head trauma	L temporoparietal	L temporal sharp waves and spikes	R hemiplegia, possible R field defect, aphasia	VIQ=107, PIQ=87; VM, VS, BI motor speed, mild language deficits
Signer and Benson[149] Case 1 (dysmorphic)	NA	WNL	WNL	Neuroleptic-induced buccal, appendicular dyskinesia	"Cognitive exam WNL"
Halligan et al.[27] (dysmorphic: extra limb)	Hematoma	R basal ganglia hematoma, blood in R lateral, 3rd, 4th ventricles	NR	L hemiplegia, L sensory loss, L hemianopia, L neglect	VIQ=116, attention, NVM, construction deficits; VM WNL
Rogers and Franzen[28] (dysmorphic: extra limb)	Head injury	R lateral ventricle effacement/hemorrhage, R subcortical edema	NR	NR	FL, NVM deficits; VM, "parietal tests" WNL
Vuilleumier et al.[29] (dysmorphic: extra limbs)	Tumor removal, infarct	R predominant parasagittal parietal	NR	Bl lower limb severe weakness/proprioceptive sensory loss, R worse than L	Marked VS deficits

TABLE 15–3. Neurodiagnostic findings in somatic delusions (*continued*)

Reference	Etiology	CT/MRI/SPECT	EEG	Neurological examination	Neuropsychological testing
Signer et al.[111] (pseudocyesis)					
Case 1	NA	WNL	BI slowing	NR	VIQ=53, PIQ=72
Case 3	Infarct	R basal ganglia, anterior limb of internal capsule, FL	NR	L visual extinction, L facial weakness, L decreased upgaze/saccades, L increased tone	FL, VM, NVM, VS deficits
Case 4	Anoxia	NR	NR	L optokinetic nystagmus, L decreased strength, L increased tone	NVM, VM, FL deficits
Case 5	Early developmental defects	Diffuse atrophy	Diffuse slowing	L hyperreflexia, frontal release signs	"Mild mental retardation"
Case 6	NA	FL, brain stem multiple small infarcts	NR	WNL	FSIQ=83
Jibiki et al.[24] (delusion of odor)	NR	BI frontal atrophy; SPECT BI frontal hypoperfusion	WNL	WNL	VIQ=98, PIQ=87; FL deficits
Takeuchi et al.[25] (delusion of odor)	Ruptured suprasellar dermoid cyst	Suprasellar cyst	WNL	WNL	NR

Note. BI=bilateral; CT=computed tomography; DTR=deep tendon reflexes; ECT=electroconvulsive therapy; EEG=electroencephalography; FL=frontal lobe; FSIQ=full scale intelligence quotient from Wechsler scales; L=left; MMSE=Mini-Mental State Exam; MRI=magnetic resonance imaging; NA=not applicable; NR=not reported; NVM=nonverbal memory; PIQ=Performance Intelligence Quotient from Wechsler scales; R=right; SPECT=single photon emission computed tomography; VIQ=Verbal Intelligence Quotient from Wechsler scales; VM=verbal memory; VS=visuospatial; WNL=within normal limits.

hallucinations, thought disorder, or mood disturbance. MRI scan showed hyperintensities in the right subcortical frontal, right splenial, and bilateral periventricular areas.

Keck et al.[105] reported on 12 cases of lycanthropy (werewolfism), of which 3 had abnormal EEG findings. One of these 3 was the patient later described in full by Kulick et al.,[26] a second case had left temporal spike and waves on EEG, and a third had generalized slowing. The remaining 9 patients had normal EEG and neurological examination results. Kulick et al. also described a case in which a patient's delusion of being a cat persisted for 15 years despite attempts at treating his epilepsy. EEG demonstrated right temporal sharp waves, but his CT scan had normal results.

Other somatic delusions involving body distortion (dysmorphic delusions) also have been reported in association with neurological deficits and include delusions of body odor,[24,25] excessive hair,[110] extra limbs (supernumerary delusion),[27–29] and pregnancy (pseudocyesis).[111] In the cases of the supernumerary delusion and pseudocyesis, in which neurological deficits were present, the evidence suggests a predominance of right hemisphere pathology (see Table 15–3).

The somatic delusions of impending death or of being dead also have been shown to emerge in the context of neurological disease. Joseph[112] originally reported two cases of koro in which CT scan and brain electrical activity mapping data indicated that koro may be a form of right temporoparietal or bitemporoparietal dysfunction similar to sexual epilepsy. Joseph[113] described another patient with a number of delusions, including Cotard's syndrome. CT scan revealed bilateral frontal and temporal atrophy. Neuropsychological evaluation indicated diffuse dysfunction with bifrontal and anterior right predominance. Joseph and O'Leary[114] further investigated localization in Cotard's syndrome by blindly comparing the CT scans of eight patients who had the syndrome with those of eight control subjects matched as closely as possible for age, sex, race, and principal psychiatric diagnosis. Compared with control subjects, patients with Cotard's syndrome had more brain atrophy in general and more median frontal lobe atrophy in particular. Parietal disease did not discriminate between the index and control groups. They concluded that Cotard's syndrome may be associated with multifocal brain atrophy and medial frontal lobe disease. Drake[115] reported on three patients with Cotard's syndrome. One had chronic seizure disorder, and EEG showed epileptiform activity in the right temporal region. A right

posteroinferior frontal astrocytoma was detected on MRI and confirmed with biopsy. The second patient developed Cotard's delusion after a closed head injury. CT scan revealed right temporal lobe atrophy and right frontal encephalomalacia. The third patient developed adult-onset seizure disorder, with right temporal slowing on EEG. CT and MRI showed right frontal infarct.

In summary, the case report literature is inadequate to justify any statements regarding localization of neurological dysfunction in the development of the somatic delusions of infestation or lycanthropy. However, some support exists for the hypothesis that right hemisphere dysfunction contributes to the development of the somatic delusions of extra limbs, pseudocyesis, and Cotard's syndrome, with most reported cases having right temporal or frontal abnormalities.

A NEUROPSYCHOLOGICAL MODEL OF MONOSYMPTOMATIC DELUSIONS

Role of the Right Hemisphere

Weinstein and colleagues[116] were the first to note the importance of right hemisphere pathology in CSDs when they observed an association between right brain damage and reduplication delusions. Levine and Grek[117] later reported that delusions frequently arose in patients in whom right hemisphere stroke was superimposed on generalized cerebral atrophy.

The specific site within the right hemisphere may determine the particular nature of the delusional distortion. Thus, right posterior temporoparietal lesions may produce a sense of unfamiliarity concerning place,[8] right inferior temporal lesions may produce disorders in recognition or sense of familiarity of persons,[68] and anterior parietal lesions may produce dysmorphic distortions. These misperceptions then may be elaborated into delusions—respectively, reduplicative paramnesia, Capgras's syndrome, and somatic types. Although this model has the advantage of being testable, the lack of localization data in many of these disorders makes it impossible to confirm these hypotheses at this time.

Role of the Temporal Lobes

Reduplicative paramnesia and Capgras's syndrome and its variants represent either under- or overidentification of the object of the delusion.[118] On the one hand, in Capgras's syndrome, the patient mistakenly perceives the person as unfamiliar by underidentification. In Fregoli syndrome, on the other hand, the patient misperceives diverse persons as the same person by overidentification.

Feinberg and Shapiro[119] emphasized the importance of the right temporal lobe in producing the misidentification delusions. They reviewed the evidence from stimulation and seizure studies indicating that the right temporal lobe plays an important role in producing the experience of familiarity. Patients with temporal lobe epilepsy, for example, have an irritative lesion that results in frequent feelings of déjà vu, or an erroneous experience of familiarity. Destructive lesions in the right temporal lobe in secondary Capgras's syndrome may logically result in the feeling of unfamiliarity. Cutting[120] has put forth a similar argument regarding the role of the right hemisphere in identification.

Role of the Frontal Lobes

Crucial factors in the persistence of delusions may be the length of time the perceptual distortion continues and the ability of the patient to correct the misperception on the basis of new information. Frontal lesions may affect the latter self-corrective function, making it impossible to resolve conflicting information. The patient may show unconcern and confabulation when confronted with these conflicts.[121]

Staton et al.[122] suggested such an explanation for reduplicative paramnesia. They hypothesized that damage to the right temporal lobe and posterior tertiary association areas caused a disconnection of premorbid memory stores from new memory registration. Frontal lobe indifference was thought to facilitate the continued misinterpretation and inability to integrate new information with past experience but not to be essential for its genesis. Thus, a pattern of right hemisphere damage superimposed on dysfunctional frontal systems may be a necessary component to the development of fixed delusions. Hakim and colleagues[38] put forth a similar model, noting that most reduplicative paramnesia cases involve an acute right hemisphere lesion superimposed on diffuse orbitofrontal disease.

Alexander et al.[68] noted the importance of frontal damage in Capgras's syndrome, in terms of both the inability to resolve conflicts and confabulation of a second persona. Jeste et al.[5] found that Alzheimer's disease patients with delusions had poorer perfor-

mance on tests of frontal lobe function than nondelusional demented patients or age-matched control subjects. Joseph et al.[123] found that schizophrenic patients with Capgras delusions had significantly more frontal atrophy than did nondelusional patients.

Role of Psychological Factors

Psychological or functional interpretations for the development of delusions are not incompatible with this neuropsychological explanation. For example, in the Othello case described by Richardson et al.,[15] the patient was preoccupied with the impotence that followed his stroke. His sexual dysfunction had resulted in exaggerated and frustrating attempts at sexual intimacy that predated the development of his delusion that his wife was unfaithful. Sexual dysfunction is common in both males and females after stroke, particularly with right hemisphere damage.[124] Similarly, hypogonadism and impotence are common problems in alcoholic patients, and preoccupation with these problems may contribute to the relatively high incidence of delusional jealousy in this population.[40]

PROGNOSIS AND TREATMENT OF CONTENT-SPECIFIC DELUSIONS

In degenerative dementia, delusions are usually transitory phenomena, occurring in the early to middle stages and disappearing when cognitive deficits become severe.[6,96] In other etiologies such as cerebrovascular disease, they often occur acutely and persist for many months or years.[125] Prognosis appears to vary with the type of delusion and the underlying etiology.

Many underlying systemic causes (e.g., infections, toxic reactions, metabolic disturbances) of CSDs are readily treated, resulting in elimination of the delusion. For example, Santiago et al.[48] reported resolution of Capgras's syndrome following treatment of underlying thyroid disease. Shimizu et al.[126] reported that a Capgras delusion waxed and waned with control of underlying diabetes mellitus but was resistant to concurrent neuroleptic treatment. Aizenberg et al.[106] described a woman who developed delusional parasitosis when taking phenelzine, with complete remission when the medication was discontinued.

Reduplicative paramnesia often remits spontaneously, albeit after a long period of rehabilitation and daily reorientation.[8,47,127] Filley and Jarvis[128] described a case of reduplicative paramnesia that responded to low doses of haloperidol. Staton and colleagues[122] reported successful treatment of persistent reduplicative paramnesia with fluphenazine hydrochloride in a patient who had previously failed trials of haloperidol and trifluoperazine.

Spontaneous resolution of Capgras delusions also has been reported.[127] However, Joseph[129] described a patient whose chronic psychosis and intermittent psychotic misidentification of the Capgras and intermetamorphosis types were refractory to neuroleptic treatment. On administration of a trial of clorazepate, complete remission of psychotic symptoms was achieved for the first time in 19 years, but these symptoms recurred when the patient discontinued her clorazepate.

Delusional parasitosis has been reported to respond well to haloperidol[130] or pimozide[17,18,107,131–135] in numerous case reports. Pseudocyesis (delusion of pregnancy) also has been reported to respond to pimozide.[136] Successful treatment of combined Capgras and dysmorphic delusions with haloperidol has been reported as well.[110] Other somatic delusions such as lycanthropy sometimes have been refractory to treatment.[26]

Thus, monosymptomatic delusions have been successfully treated with neuroleptics such as haloperidol,[110] and newer medications such as pimozide show promise in treating diverse CSDs.[137] However, there has been no systematic treatment follow-up research,[33] and data are limited to uncontrolled case studies.

The effectiveness of psychological interventions may vary with the type of delusion and the degree to which neurological factors are involved. For example, psychotherapy or placebo treatment alone has been notably ineffective in delusional parasitosis.[17] However, sex therapy and marital counseling are essential adjuncts to medication in treating delusional jealousy when the patient has related sexual dysfunction.

Untreated monosymptomatic delusions can be significant barriers to recovery from substance abuse and stroke and may result in more restrictive placement of elderly patients. Even if the delusion is not treatable, its appropriate diagnosis can be useful in explanations to family, who may blame the patient for his or her inappropriate behavior. Professionals are not immune from these biases. Morriss et al.[138] found that 21% of 125 patients newly admitted to nursing homes had delusions that were frequently undiagnosed. Delusional patients were more behaviorally disturbed before admission than nondelusional patients. These behavior problems were often the reason for admission, and delusions persisted after admission. Nursing home staff members infrequently identified and often inappropriately treated delusional patients.

CONCLUSIONS

Misinterpretation of events is common in brain disease, especially with diffuse or multifocal disorders such as encephalopathy, delirium, or degenerative disease. However, delusions associated with toxic-metabolic disease are usually simple (e.g., persecutory, ideas of reference) and often resolve with treatment of the underlying disturbance, whereas those associated with degenerative dementia tend to remit as the disease progresses.

More focal damage may result in CSDs, with the content determined by a combination of the site of cortical lesion and the premorbid personality of the patient. The right hemisphere and the frontal lobes appear to play an important role in the genesis and maintenance of delusions. CSDs appear to be persistent, and effective treatments have yet to be identified in controlled clinical trials. However, neuroleptics in combination with psychotherapy and behavioral interventions have been effective in many cases.

REFERENCES

1. American Psychiatric Association: Diagnostic and Statistical Manual of Mental Disorders, 4th Edition. Washington, DC, American Psychiatric Association, 1994
2. Cummings JL: Organic delusions: phenomenology, anatomical correlations, and review. Br J Psychiatry 146:184–197, 1985
3. Cummings JL, Victoroff JI: Noncognitive neuropsychiatric syndromes in Alzheimer's disease. Neuropsychiatry Neuropsychol Behav Neurol 3:140–158, 1990
4. Mendez MF, Martin RJ, Smyth KA, et al: Psychiatric symptoms associated with Alzheimer's disease. J Neuropsychiatry Clin Neurosci 2:28–33, 1990
5. Jeste DV, Wragg RE, Salmon DP, et al: Cognitive deficits of patients with Alzheimer's disease with and without delusions. Am J Psychiatry 149:184–189, 1992
6. Rubin EH: Delusions as part of Alzheimer's disease. Neuropsychiatry Neuropsychol Behav Neurol 5:108–113, 1992
7. Pick A: On reduplicative paramnesia. Brain 26:242–267, 1903
8. Benson DF, Gardner H, Meadows JC: Reduplicative paramnesia. Neurology 26:147–161, 1976

9. Fisher CM: Disorientation for place. Arch Neurol 39:33–37, 1982

10. Capgras J, Reboul-Lachaux J: L'illusion des "sosies" dans un délire systematisé chronique. Bulletin de la Société Clinique de Médecine Mentale 2:6–16, 1923

11. Christodoulou GN: Syndrome of subjective doubles. Am J Psychiatry 135:249–251, 1978

12. Courbon P, Fail G: Syndrome "d'illusion de Fregoli" et schizophrénie. Bulletin de la Société Clinique de Médecine Mentale 15:121–124, 1927

13. Courbon P, Tusques J: L'illusion de intermétamorphose et de charme. Ann Med Psychol 90:401–406, 1932

14. Soyka M, Naber G, Volcker A: Prevalence of delusional jealousy in different psychiatric disorders: an analysis of 93 cases. Br J Psychiatry 158:549–553, 1991

15. Richardson E, Malloy P, Grace J: Othello syndrome secondary to right cerebrovascular infarction. J Geriatr Psychiatry Neurol 4:160–165, 1991

16. Leong GB, Silva JA: The physician as erotomanic object. West J Med 156:77–78, 1992

17. Wykoff RF: Delusions of parasitosis: a review. Rev Infect Dis 9:433–437, 1987

18. Reilly TM, Batchelor DH: Presentation and treatment of delusional parasitosis: a dermatological perspective. Int Clin Psychopharmacol 1:340–353, 1986

19. Berrios GE: Delusional parasitosis and physical disease. Compr Psychiatry 26:395–403, 1985

20. Colenda CC, Kryzanowski L, Klinger R: Major depression in late life with AIDS delusions: a case report and review. Gen Hosp Psychiatry 12:207–209, 1990

21. Mahorney SL, Cavenar JJ: A new and timely delusion: the complaint of having AIDS. Am J Psychiatry 145:1130–1132, 1988

22. Walter G: An unusual monosymptomatic hypochondriacal delusion presenting as self-insertion of a foreign body into the urethra. Br J Psychiatry 159:283–284, 1991

23. Wang C-K, Lee JY-Y: Monosymptomatic hypochondriacal psychosis complicated by self-inflicted skin ulceration, skull defect and brain abscess. Br J Dermatol 137:299–302, 1997

24. Jibiki I, Kagara Y, Kishizawa S, et al: Case study of monosymptomatic delusion of unpleasant body odor with structural frontal abnormality. Neuropsychobiology 30:7–10, 1994

25. Takeuchi H, Kubota T, Kabuto M, et al: Ruptured suprasellar dermoid cyst presenting olfactory delusion. Neurosurgery 33:97–99, 1993

26. Kulick AR, Pope HJ, Keck PJ: Lycanthropy and self-identification. J Nerv Ment Dis 178:134–137, 1990

27. Halligan PW, Marshall JC, Wade DT: Three arms: a case study of supernumerary phantom limb after right hemisphere stroke. J Neurol Neurosurg Psychiatry 56:159–166, 1993

28. Rogers MJ, Franzen MD: Delusional reduplication following closed-head injury. Brain Inj 6:469–476, 1992

29. Vuilleumier P, Reverdin A, Landis T: Four legs: illusory reduplication of the lower limbs after bilateral parietal lobe damage. Arch Neurol 54:1543–1547, 1997

30. Bernstein RL, Gaw AC: Koro: proposed classification for DSM-IV. Am J Psychiatry 147:1670–1674, 1990

31. Chadda RK, Jain BK: An unusual case of Capgras' syndrome. Am J Psychiatry 147:369–370, 1990

32. Synodinou C, Christodoulou GN: Capgras' syndrome and prosopagnosia. Br J Psychiatry 132:413–416, 1977

33. Malloy P, Cimino C, Westlake R: Differential diagnosis of primary and secondary Capgras delusions. Neuropsychiatry Neuropsychol Behav Neurol 5:83–96, 1992

34. Fishbain DA: The frequency of Capgras delusions in a psychiatric emergency service. Psychopathology 20:42–47, 1987

35. Retterstol N: Paranoid psychoses with hypochondriac delusions as the main delusion. Acta Psychiatr Scand 44:334–353, 1968

36. Dohn HH, Crews EL: Capgras syndrome: a literature review and case series. Hillside J Clin Psychiatry 8:56–74, 1986

37. Kirov G, Jones P, Lewis SW: Prevalence of delusional misidentification syndromes. Psychopathology 27:148–149, 1994

38. Hakim H, Verma NP, Greiffenstein MF: Pathogenesis of reduplicative paramnesia. J Neurol Neurosurg Psychiatry 51:839–841, 1988

39. Mendez MF, Martin RJ, Smyth KA, et al: Disturbances of person identification in Alzheimer's disease: a retrospective study. J Nerv Ment Dis 180:94–96, 1992

40. Geller JL: Prevalence of delusional jealousy in different psychiatric disorders: an analysis of 93 cases. Br J Psychiatry 158:549–553, 1991

41. el Gaddal YY: De Clerembault's syndrome (erotomania) in organic delusional syndrome. Br J Psychiatry 154:714–716, 1989

42. DePauw DG, Szulecka TK: Dangerous delusions: violence and the misidentification syndrome. Br J Psychiatry 152:91–96, 1988

43. Morris M: Ekbom's syndrome. Psychiatric Bulletin 51, 1989

44. Iida J: The current situation in regard to the delusion of possession in Japan. Jpn J Psychiatry Neurol 43:19–27, 1989

45. Forstl H, Almeida OP, Owen AM, et al: Psychiatric, neurological and medical aspects of misidentification syndromes: a review of 260 cases. Psychol Med 21:905–910, 1991

46. Metcalfe RA, Neary D, Northern B: Reduplicative paramnesia associated with a left occipito-parietal hematoma (abstract). J Neurol Neurosurg Psychiatry 54:474, 1991

47. Kapur N, Turner A, King C: Reduplicative paramnesia: possible anatomical and neuropsychological mechanisms. J Neurol Neurosurg Psychiatry 51:579–581, 1988

48. Santiago JM, Stoker DL, Beigel A, et al: Capgras' syndrome in a myxedema patient. Hosp Community Psychiatry 38:199–201, 1987

49. Madakusira S, Hall TBI: Capgras syndrome in a patient with myxedema. Am J Psychiatry 138:1506–1508, 1981

50. Preskorn SH, Reveley A: Pseudohypoparathyroidism and Capgras syndrome. Br J Psychiatry 133:34–37, 1978

51. Hay GG, Jolley DJ, Jones RG: A case of the Capgras syndrome in association with pseudo-hypoparathyroidism. Acta Psychiatr Scand 50:73–77, 1974

52. MacCallum WG: Capgras syndrome with an organic basis. Br J Psychiatry 123:639–642, 1973

53. Pies R: Capgras phenomenon, delirium, and transient hepatic dysfunction. Hosp Community Psychiatry 33:382–383, 1982

54. Zucker DK, Livingston RL, Nakra R, et al: B$_{12}$ deficiency and psychiatric disorders: case report and literature review. Biol Psychiatry 16:197–205, 1981

55. Chen E: Delusions and hallucinations of cocaine abusers and paranoid schizophrenics: a comparative study. J Psychol 125:301–310, 1991

56. Bhatia MS, Dhar NK, Singhal PK: Capgras' syndrome in chloroquine induced psychosis (letter). Indian Pediatr 25:905–906, 1988

57. Daniel DG, Swallows A, Wolff F: Capgras delusion and seizures in association with therapeutic dosages of disulfiram. South Med J 80:1577–1579, 1987

58. Quinn D: The Capgras syndrome: two case reports and a review. Can J Psychiatry 26:126–129, 1981

59. Canagasabey B, Katona CL: Capgras syndrome in association with lithium toxicity. Br J Psychiatry 159:879–881, 1991

60. Nikolovski OT, Fernandez JV: Capgras syndrome as an aftermath of chickenpox encephalitis. Psychiatric Opinion 15:30–44, 1978

61. Weiss HS: An organic etiology for Capgras syndrome? Am J Psychiatry 141:615–617, 1984

62. Crichton P, Lewis S: Delusional misidentification, AIDS and the right hemisphere. Br J Psychiatry 157:608–610, 1990

63. Forstl H: Capgras' delusion: an example of coalescent psychodynamic and organic factors. Compr Psychiatry 31:447–449, 1990

64. Bhatia MS: Capgras syndrome in a patient with migraine. Br J Psychiatry 157:917–918, 1990

65. Hay GG: Electroconvulsive therapy as a contributor to the production of delusional misidentification. Br J Psychiatry 148:667–669, 1986

66. Bienenfeld D, Brott T: Capgras' syndrome following minor head trauma. J Clin Psychiatry 50:68–69, 1989

67. Forstl H, Burns A, Jacoby R, et al: Neuroanatomical correlates of clinical misidentification and misperception in senile dementia of the Alzheimer type. J Clin Psychiatry 52:268–271, 1991

68. Alexander M, Stuss DT, Benson DF: Capgras syndrome: a reduplicative phenomenon. Neurology 29:334–339, 1979

69. Murai T, Toichi M, Sengoku A, et al: Reduplicative paramnesia in patients with focal brain damage. Neuropsychiatry Neuropsychol Behav Neurol 10:190–196, 1997

70. Absher JR, Oberg G, Benson DF: Capgras' syndrome with focal frontal lobe patients (abstract). Neurology 42 (suppl 3):224, 1992

71. Christodoulou GN, Margariti MM, Malliaras DE, et al: Shared delusions of doubles. J Neurol Neurosurg Psychiatry 58:499–501, 1995

72. DePauw KW: Fregoli and infarction. J Nerv Ment Dis 175:433–438, 1987

73. Durani SK, Ford R, Sajjad SHA: Capgras syndrome associated with a frontal lobe tumour. Irish Journal of Psychological Medicine 8:135–136, 1991

74. Hayman MA, Abrams R: Capgras' syndrome and cerebral dysfunction. Br J Psychiatry 130:68–71, 1977

75. Lebert F, Pasquier F, Steinling M, et al: SPECT data in a case of secondary Capgras delusion. Psychopathology 27:211–214, 1994

76. Mace CJ, Trimble MR: Psychosis following temporal lobe surgery: a report of six cases. J Neurol Neurosurg Psychiatry 54:639–644, 1991

77. Paill'ere-Martinot ML, Dao-Castellana MH, Masure MC, et al: Delusional misidentification: a clinical, neuropsychological and brain imaging case study. Psychopathology 27:200–210, 1994

78. Silva JA, Leong GB, Garza-Trevino ES, et al: A cognitive model of dangerous delusional misidentification syndromes. J Forensic Sci 39:1455–1467, 1994

79. Silva JA, Leong GB, Lesser IM, et al: Bilateral cerebral pathology and the genesis of delusional misidentification. Can J Psychiatry 40:498–499, 1995

80. Silva JA, Leong GB, Wine DB: Misidentification delusions, facial misrecognition, and right brain injury [see comments]. Can J Psychiatry 38:239–241, 1993

81. Silva JA, Tekell JL, Leong GB, et al: Delusional misidentification of the self associated with nondominant cerebral pathology (letter). J Clin Psychiatry 56:171, 1995

82. Shepard M: Morbid jealousy: some clinical and social aspects of a psychiatric symptom. Journal of Mental Science 107:687–753, 1961

83. Crowe RR, Clarkson C, Tsai M, et al: Delusional disorder: jealous and nonjealous types. European Archives of Psychiatry and Neurological Sciences 237:179–183, 1988

84. Shrestha K, Ress DW, Rix KJB, et al: Sexual jealousy in alcoholics. Acta Psychiatr Scand 72:283–290, 1985

85. Hassanyeh F, Murray RB, Rodgers H: Adrenocortical suppression presenting with agitated depression, morbid jealousy, and a dementia-like state. Br J Psychiatry 159:870–872, 1991

86. Hodgson RE, Murray D, Woods MR: Othello's syndrome and hyperthyroidism. J Nerv Ment Dis 180:663–664, 1992

87. McNamara P, Durso R: Reversible pathologic jealousy (Othello syndrome) associated with amantadine. J Geriatr Psychiatry Neurol 4:157–159, 1991

88. Barnhill LJ, Gualtieri CT: Two cases of late-onset psychosis after closed head injury. Neuropsychiatry Neuropsychol Behav Neurol 2:211–217, 1989

89. Signer SF, Cummings JL: De Clerambault's syndrome in organic affective disorder: two cases. Br J Psychiatry 151:404–407, 1987

90. Silva JA, Leong GB: A case of organic Othello syndrome (letter). J Clin Psychiatry 54:277, 1993

91. Pollock BG: Successful treatment of pathological jealousy with pimozide. Can J Psychiatry 27:86–87, 1982

92. Leong GB, Silva JA, Garza-Trevino ES, et al: The dangerousness of persons with the Othello syndrome. J Forensic Sci 39:1445–1454, 1994

93. Soyka M: Delusional jealousy and localized cerebral pathology (letter). J Neuropsychiatry Clin Neurosci 10: 472, 1998

94. Westlake RJ, Weeks SM: Pathological jealousy appearing after cerebrovascular infarction in a 25-year-old woman. Aust N Z J Psychiatry 33:105–107, 1999

95. Doust JW, Christie H: The pathology of love: some clinical variants of de Clerambault's syndrome. Soc Sci Med 12:99–106, 1978

96. Drevets WC, Rubin EH: Erotomania and senile dementia of Alzheimer type. Br J Psychiatry 151:400–402, 1987

97. el Assra A: Erotomania in a Saudi woman. Br J Psychiatry 155:553–555, 1989

98. Munro A, O'Brien JV, Ross D: Two cases of "pure" or "primary" erotomania successfully treated with pimozide. Can J Psychiatry 30:619–622, 1985

99. O'Dwyer JM: Coexistence of the Capgras and de Clerambault's syndromes. Br J Psychiatry 156:575–577, 1990

100. Anderson CA, Camp J, Filley CM: Erotomania after aneurysmal subarachnoid hemorrhage: case report and literature review. J Neuropsychiatry Clin Neurosci 10:330–337, 1998

101. Fujii DE, Ahmed I, Takeshita J: Neuropsychologic implications in erotomania: two case studies. Neuropsychiatry Neuropsychol Behav Neurol 12:110–116, 1999

102. John S, Ovsiew F: Erotomania in a brain-damaged male. J Intellect Disabil Res 40:279–283, 1996

103. Wijeratne C, Hickie I, Schwartz R: Erotomania associated with temporal lobe abnormalities following radiotherapy. Aust N Z J Psychiatry 31:765–768, 1997

104. Pope FM: Parasitophobia as the presenting symptom in vitamin B_{12} deficiency. Practitioner 204:421–422, 1970

105. Keck PE, Pope HG, Hudson JI, et al: Lycanthropy: alive and well in the twentieth century. Psychol Med 18:113–120, 1988

106. Aizenberg D, Schwartz B, Zemishlany Z: Delusional parasitosis associated with phenelzine. Br J Psychiatry 159:716–717, 1991

107. Renvoize EB, Kent J, Klar HM: Delusional infestation and dementia: a case report. Br J Psychiatry 150:403–405, 1987

108. Surawicz FG, Banta R: Lycanthropy revisited. Canadian Psychiatric Association Journal 20:537–542, 1975

109. Flynn FG, Cummings JL, Scheibel J, et al: Monosymptomatic delusions of parasitosis associated with ischemic cerebrovascular disease. J Geriatr Psychiatry Neurol 2:134–139, 1989

110. Kourany RF, Williams BV: Capgras' syndrome with dysmorphic delusion in an adolescent. Psychosomatics 25:715–717, 1984

111. Signer SF, Weinstein RP, Munoz RA, et al: Pseudocyesis in organic mood disorders: six cases. Psychosomatics 33:316–323, 1992

112. Joseph AB: Koro: computed tomography and brain electrical activity mapping in two patients. J Clin Psychiatry 47:430–432, 1986

113. Joseph AB: Cotard's syndrome in a patient with coexistent Capgras' syndrome, syndrome of subjective doubles, and palinopsia. J Clin Psychiatry 47:605–606, 1986

114. Joseph AB, O'Leary DH: Brain atrophy and interhemispheric fissure enlargement in Cotard's syndrome. J Clin Psychiatry 47:518–520, 1986

115. Drake ME: Cotard's syndrome and temporal lobe epilepsy. Psychiatric Journal of the University of Ottawa 13:36–39, 1988

116. Weinstein EA, Kahn RL, Sugarman LA: Phenomenon of reduplication. Archives of Neurology and Psychiatry 67:808–814, 1952

117. Levine DN, Grek A: The anatomic basis for delusions after right cerebral infarction. Neurology 34:577–582, 1984

118. Vie J: Un trouble de l'identification des personnes: l'illusion des sosies. Annals of Medical Psychology 88:214–237, 1930

119. Feinberg TE, Shapiro RM: Misidentification-reduplication and the right hemisphere. Neuropsychiatry Neuropsychol Behav Neurol 2:39–48, 1989

120. Cutting J: Delusional misidentification and the role of the right hemisphere in the appreciation of identity. Br J Psychiatry 14 (suppl):70–75, 1991

121. Joseph R: Confabulation and delusional denial: frontal lobe and lateralized influences. J Clin Psychol 42:507–520, 1986

122. Staton RD, Brumback RA, Wilson H: Reduplicative paramnesia: a disconnection syndrome of memory. Cortex 18:23–36, 1982

123. Joseph AB, O'Leary DH, Wheeler HG: Bilateral atrophy of the frontal and temporal lobes in schizophrenic patients with Capgras syndrome: a case-control study using computed tomography. J Clin Psychiatry 51:322–325, 1990

124. Coslett HB, Heilman KM: Male sexual function: impairment after right hemisphere stroke. Arch Neurol 43:1036–1039, 1986

125. LaMancusa JC, Cole AR: Visual manifestations of occipital lobe infarction in three patients on a geriatric psychiatric unit. J Geriatr Psychiatry Neurol 1:231–234, 1988

126. Shimizu T, Inami Y, Sugita Y, et al: Delusions of substitution and diabetes mellitus. Int J Psychiatry Med 21:105–112, 1991

127. Ruff RL, Volpe BT: Environmental reduplication associated with right frontal and parietal lobe injury. J Neurol Neurosurg Psychiatry 44:382–386, 1981

128. Filley CM, Jarvis PE: Delayed reduplicative paramnesia. Neurology 37:701–703, 1987

129. Joseph AB: Delusional misidentification of the Capgras and intermetamorphosis types responding to clorazepate: a case report. Acta Psychiatr Scand 75:330–332, 1987

130. Andrews E, Bellard J, Walter RW: Monosymptomatic hypochondriacal psychosis manifesting as delusions of infestation: case studies of treatment with haloperidol. J Clin Psychiatry 47:188–190, 1986

131. Bond WS: Delusions of parasitosis: a case report and management guidelines. DICP 23:304–306, 1989

132. Damiani JT, Flowers FP, Pierce DK: Pimozide in delusions of parasitosis. J Am Acad Dermatol 22:312–313, 1990

133. Mitchell C: Successful treatment of chronic delusional parasitosis. Br J Psychiatry 155:556–557, 1989

134. Driscoll MS, Rothe MJ, Grant-Kels JM, et al: Delusional parasitosis: a dermatologic, psychiatric, and pharmacologic approach. J Am Acad Dermatol 29:1023–1033, 1993

135. Ungvari G, Vladar K: Pimozide treatment for delusion of infestation. Activitas Nervosa Superior 28:103–107, 1986

136. DePauw KW: Three thousand days of pregnancy: a case of monosymptomatic delusional pseudocyesis responding to pimozide. Br J Psychiatry 157:924–928, 1990

137. Munro A: Excellent response of pathologic jealousy to pimozide. Canadian Medical Association Journal 131:852–853, 1984

138. Morriss RK, Rovner BW, Folstein MF, et al: Delusions in newly admitted residents of nursing homes. Am J Psychiatry 147:299–302, 1990

139. Joseph AB: Capgras syndrome. Br J Psychiatry 148:749–750, 1986

140. Lewis SW: Brain imaging in a case of Capgras' syndrome. Br J Psychiatry 150:117–121, 1987

141. Sellal F, Fontaine SF, Van Der Linden M, et al: To be or not to be at home? A neuropsychological approach to delusion for place. J Clin Exp Neuropsychol 18:234–248, 1996

142. Vighetto A, Aimard G, Confavreux C, et al: Une observation anatomo-clinique de fabulation (ou délire) topograpigue. Cortex 16:501–507, 1980

143. Adunsky A: Early post-stroke parasitic delusions (letter; comment). Age Ageing 26:238–239, 1997

144. May WW, Terpenning MS: Delusional parasitosis in geriatric patients. Psychosomatics 32:88–94, 1991

145. Murthy P, Jayakumar PN, Sampat S: Of insects and eggs: a case report. J Neurol Neurosurg Psychiatry 63:522–523, 1997

146. Petracca G, Migliorelli R, Vazquez S, et al: SPECT findings before and after ECT in a patient with major depression and Cotard's syndrome. J Neuropsychiatry Clin Neurosci 7:505–507, 1995

147. Young AW, Robertson IH, Hellawell DJ, et al: Cotard delusion after brain injury. Psychol Med 22:799–804, 1992

148. Dalby JT, Arboleda-Florez J, Seland TP: Somatic delusions following left parietal lobe injury. Neuropsychiatry Neuropsychol Behav Neurol 2:306–311, 1989

149. Signer SF, Benson DF: Two cases of Capgras symptom with dysmorphic (somatic) delusions. Psychosomatics 28:327–328, 1987

16

Neurosurgical Treatment for Refractory Obsessive-Compulsive Disorder

Implications for Understanding Frontal Lobe Function

Per Mindus, M.D, Ph.D., Steven A. Rasmussen, M.D., Christer Lindquist, M.D., Ph.D., George Noren, M.D.

Neurosurgical treatment for otherwise refractory obsessive-compulsive and related disorders has been the focus of several recent reviews.[1–6] In this chapter, we review recent work—and new views on earlier findings—relevant to neurosurgical treatment for obsessive-compulsive disorder (OCD). We then discuss the implications of OCD and its neurosurgical treatment for understanding frontal lobe function and its connections with ventral medial subcortical structures.

REASONS THAT SURGERY IS USED FOR OBSESSIVE-COMPULSIVE DISORDER

Over the years, neurosurgery has been kept in the psychiatric treatment armamentarium for OCD for

two main reasons. First, it is recognized that a minority of OCDs have a chronic disabling course [7–11] refractory to modern pharmacological[10,11] and psychological treatment.[2,12,13] No systematic information on the percentage of OCD patients who develop such malignant cases is available, but our own estimate is that about 10% of the patients do so. Many of these individuals may be candidates for neurosurgical treatment. Second, extensive, but uncontrolled, evidence suggests that such cases may respond to stereotactic neurosurgical lesions that interrupt frontal subcortical connections, such as capsulotomy,[1–5,14] cingulotomy,[6,15–17] subcaudate tractotomy,[18–21] and limbic leukotomy.[1–5,21–23] A limited number of such operations are performed today, both in the Western world and elsewhere.[5] To date, more than 300 cases treated neu-

Drs. E-O Backlund, L. Kihlström, L. Leksell, and B. A. Meyerson were also involved in the treatment of the patients. The work was supported, in part, by grants from Karolinska Institute, Karolinska Hospital, and Swedish Medical Research Council (K94-21P-11025-01A and B95-21X-11250-01A).

rosurgically for refractory OCD have been reported.[2,4] This is undoubtedly an underestimate of the true rate because at some sites patients are treated on a routine clinical basis and are not reported in the scientific literature.[2–4] It has been estimated that fewer than one-third of the patients referred for surgery will ultimately undergo it (Malizia, personal communication, June 1992; Mindus et al., unpublished data, May 1996).

Neurosurgical treatment for mental illness, or psychosurgery, may be defined as the destruction of apparently normal brain tissue with the objective of alleviating incapacitating mental symptoms that prove refractory to conventional, nonsurgical treatment. *Psychosurgery* is an obvious misnomer because it is the psychiatric patient—not the psyche—that is operated on. More important, the term tends to be associated with primitive procedures of the past that differ from today's interventions in several important respects. Contemporary neurosurgical treatment of mental illness has more refined indications, contraindications, targets, and surgical techniques.[2–5] Consequently, the efficacy and risk profile of today's procedures are far superior to those of earlier procedures; these operations are analogous to modern neurosurgery for uncontrollable epileptic seizures, medically refractory parkinsonism, and certain pain conditions. For these reasons, the term *psychosurgery* should be dropped in favor of *neurosurgical treatment* of OCD.

EARLY NEUROSURGICAL TREATMENTS

In its severe form, OCD can be one of the most disabling major psychiatric disorders. For this reason, and in the absence of therapeutic alternatives, lobotomy and other forms of extensive neurosurgical intervention were occasionally offered to severely ill OCD patients in the 1930s and 1940s.[24] According to a few case series, many patients obtained symptom relief. The unacceptable side effects of lobotomy led researchers to carefully review the evidence derived from animal experimentation and from the operations. They concluded that the efficacy of the operations resulted from interference of connections between the orbitomedial frontal cortex or the cingulate gyri and deeper subcortical structures. Untoward intellectual and personality changes were believed to arise from the unnecessary extension of the lesions into the dorsolateral cortex or its projections.[2,24,25] The findings of Meyer and Beck[25] gave further impetus to

the work to refine the surgical technique. In 1954, they reported findings from autopsies of patients previously treated with lobotomy or related procedures. With regard to the efficacy of the procedures, the authors noted, "it is striking that in the unimproved, the ventro-medial sector [of the frontal lobes] was involved in none and the cingulate only rarely" (p. 15).[25] They also speculated that a "circumscribed lesion at or just in front of the tip of the anterior horn will sever connections to anterior areas of the frontal region" (p. 6). Subsequently, a number of neurosurgeons used stereotactic techniques to create discrete lesions via electrocoagulation in these target areas for the treatment of a wide variety of psychiatric illnesses, schizophrenia being the main indication.

The French neurosurgeon Talairach and co-workers[26] were the first to make selective lesions in the anterior limb of the internal capsules. They were unimpressed by the results in schizophrenia, but they reported satisfactory results in patients with "névroses anxieuses" (not otherwise specified). A few years later, the Swedish neurosurgeon Leksell[27] used his stereotactic system to produce bilateral radiofrequency heat lesions in the anterior limb of the internal capsule. He termed his procedure *bilateral anterior capsulotomy*. The first 116 patients operated on by Leksell for various mental disorders were followed up prospectively by a psychiatrist, Herner,[28] who published his observations in a detailed monograph in 1961. Again, the results in schizophrenic patients were disappointing; at follow-up after 24–80 months, only 9 (14%) of 64 were judged as having a "satisfactory response." The best results, however, were obtained in 18 patients with obsessional neurosis, 9 of whom (50%) were rated as having a satisfactory response. Subsequently, several European groups took up capsulotomy as a treatment for refractory OCD and other forms of anxiety disorders.[2,4,14,29,30]

Meanwhile, a somewhat different approach was used in the United States; the lesions were placed in the cingulate bundle, and the procedure was later termed *cingulotomy*. With regard to the perceived rationale for cingulotomy, the work of Papez,[31] Maclean,[32] Fulton and Jacobsen,[33] and Nauta[34] was important. Maclean[32] noted: "The medial forebrain bundle and its continuation as the cingulum may be considered to be to the limbic system what the internal capsule is to the [cortex] of the brain (p. 614)." This evidence, together with the promising results of cingulotomy reported by others,[35,36] gave the immediate stimulus for Ballantine et al.[37] to initiate, in 1962, a study of the safety and efficacy of stereotactic cingulotomy for the treatment of severe forms of mental disorders.

In the United Kingdom, Knight[38] concentrated on lesions in the orbitomedial quadrant of the frontal lobe, just under the head of the caudate nucleus, in the substantia innominata. Knight termed his approach *subcaudate tractotomy.* Kelly[23,39] and associates, also working in the United Kingdom, extended the subcaudate tractotomy lesions and included multiple lesions in the cingulum. They termed their multitarget procedure *limbic leukotomy.* The current neurosurgical procedures being used in the treatment of OCD and their target areas are shown in Table 16–1.

SELECTION GUIDELINES FOR SURGICAL TREATMENT

OCD patients who are considered for neurosurgical intervention have an extreme form of the disorder and are not representative of the general OCD population.[40] This difference is to some extent reflected in the inclusion criteria for surgery and must be borne in mind when discussing the relation between neurosurgical treatment, OCD, and frontal lobe function. The current criteria are described here.

The evaluation procedure for neurosurgical treatment has been developed in collaboration between centers over many years. Because the patients referred for these procedures almost invariably have complex histories with multiple Axis I and Axis II diagnoses, multidisciplinary committees have been established to evaluate potential candidates for surgical intervention. The difficult clinical judgments to be made regarding candidacy require expertise in general psychiatry, neuropsychiatry, neuropsychology, neurology, and neurosurgery. Although indications for surgery may vary slightly between centers, they usually include the following:

1. The patient is an adult who meets current diagnostic criteria for OCD.
2. The duration of illness exceeds 5 years.
3. The disorder is causing substantial suffering, as evidenced by a current score on the Yale-Brown Obsessive-Compulsive Scale (Y-BOCS) of at least 26.
4. The disorder is causing substantial reduction in the patient's psychosocial functioning, as evidenced by a score of 50 or lower on the Global Assessment of Functioning (GAF) scale.

TABLE 16–1. Common neurosurgical procedures indicated in otherwise intractable obsessive-compulsive disorder

Procedure	Reference	Target area
Cingulotomy	Ballantine et al. 1987[16]	Rostral cingulum
Subcaudate tractotomy	Göktepe et al. 1975[19]	Substantia innominata
Limbic leukotomy	Kelly 1980[23]	Rostral cingulum and substantia innominata
Capsulotomy	Mindus and Meyerson 1994[4]	Anterior limb of the internal capsule

5. All currently accepted pharmacological and behavior therapy treatments tried systematically alone or in combination for at least 5 years have been without appreciable effect on the symptoms or have been discontinued because of intolerable side effects.
6. If a comorbid psychiatric condition is present, this disorder has been thoroughly addressed with appropriate trials of first-line treatments.
7. The prognosis, without neurosurgical intervention, is considered poor.
8. The patient gives informed consent.
9. The patient agrees to participate in the preoperative evaluation program and the postoperative rehabilitation program.
10. The referring physician is willing to acknowledge responsibility for the postoperative long-term management of the patient.

CONTRAINDICATIONS TO SURGICAL TREATMENT

Contraindications generally include the following, although they vary somewhat between centers, and some, such as upper age limit, are considered only relative:

1. The patient is younger than 20 or older than 65 years.
2. The patient has a complicating current or lifetime Axis I diagnosis, such as organic brain syndrome, schizophrenia, delusional disorder, or manifest abuse of alcohol, sedative, or illicit drugs. The term *complicating* is crucial here; for a condition to

qualify as complicating, it must substantially complicate function, treatment, or the patient's ability to comply with treatment or lead to serious adverse events such as overdose or paradoxical reactions.

3. A complicating current Axis II diagnosis from Cluster A (such as paranoid personality disorder) or Cluster B (such as antisocial or borderline personality disorder) that is a significant part of the presenting problem is regarded by many experts as a contraindication (although there are no systematic studies published to support this idea). A current Cluster C personality disorder (such as avoidant or obsessive personality disorder) need not be considered a contraindication because it may, in fact, disappear with successful treatment of the coexistent OCD.

4. The patient has a complicating current Axis III diagnosis with brain pathology, such as atrophy or tumor.

EFFICACY OF THE DIFFERENT PROCEDURES

Comparison across different reports has obvious methodological limitations, but it can provide an approximation of the outcome of the operations. The two best outcome categories (responders) may be contrasted with the two worst (nonresponders). The results are shown in Table 16–2. Although the size of the database varies across procedures, it appears that the relative efficacy of the four procedures in producing clinically meaningful symptom reduction is comparable.

TABLE 16–2. Comparison of success rates across reports of neurosurgical procedures in current use in otherwise intractable obsessive-compulsive disorder

Procedure	N	Percentage	
		Responders	Nonresponders
Cingulotomy	32	56	16
Subcaudate tractotomy	18	50	8
Limbic leukotomy	49	61	8
Capsulotomy	116	67	8

Note. The two best outcome categories (responders) were compared with the two worst outcome categories (nonresponders).

Clearly, the above method of comparing published results is methodologically inferior to prospective comparative studies. Consequently, the Swedish neurosurgeon Kullberg[41] compared 13 capsulotomy and 13 cingulotomy patients in a prospective study. She found that results were significantly better in the capsulotomy (6 of 13, or 46%) than in the cingulotomy group (3 of 13, or 23%) but that the transient postoperative "psychorganic syndrome" was "much more marked" after capsulotomy than after cingulotomy. Kullberg's findings of a superior efficacy of capsulotomy over cingulotomy in OCD were supported by Hay et al.,[42] who noted that patients with cingulotomy lesions extensive enough to involve the anterior limb of the internal capsule did well compared with those whose lesions were more restricted.

Obviously, the above data do not permit definitive conclusions about the relative efficacy and safety of the current procedures, but they indicate that the operations may produce clinically meaningful improvement in some cases of otherwise refractory OCD and that the results across studies are comparable, capsulotomy possibly being a little more effective. It may well be that capsulotomy is also slightly more disruptive in terms of frontal lobe function (see section on cognitive function). Capsulotomy has been in use in Europe for more than three decades.[2,4,5] It has recently been introduced by neurosurgeons in the United States as well, and it is the procedure most often reported in anxiety disorders including OCD. Moreover, in the other procedures in current use, the lesions involve relatively larger areas of gray matter, white matter, or both. By comparison, capsulotomy has the theoretically appealing advantage of involving discrete, circumscribed lesions in white matter of the anterior limb of the internal capsule.[5]

THERMOCAPSULOTOMY AND GAMMA CAPSULOTOMY

Two surgical techniques for capsulotomy have been described: the radiofrequency thermocapsulotomy and the radiosurgical gamma capsulotomy techniques. To indicate how frontal lobe function may be affected by this type of surgery, we briefly describe the procedures. In the thermocapsulotomy procedure,[2,5] thermistor electrodes are introduced bilaterally into the target area under the guidance of a stereotactic system and magnetic resonance imaging (MRI). The lesions are then produced by heating the uninsulated tip of the electrode to approximately 75°C for 75 seconds, creating a lesion approximately 5 mm by 15–18 mm. The patients do not report any subjective sensations while the targets are being lesioned. A week or two after capsulotomy, fatigue may be a prominent feature in some but not all cases. Also, a decrease in initiative and mental drive may be noted during the first 2–3 postoperative months. This appears to correlate with circumlesional edema, as determined with MRI, and disappears simultaneously with its resolution (Mindus et al., unpublished data, June 1996); after 3 months, initiative and mental drive usually return to preoperative levels.[2,4]

In the radiosurgical or gamma capsulotomy procedure, also developed by Leksell and co-workers in Sweden,[43–45] the lesions are produced by the cross-firing of approximately 200 narrow beams of cobalt-60 gamma irradiation from a Gamma Knife (Elekta Radiosurgery, Inc.™, Atlanta, GA). Craniotomy and shaving are unnecessary. The biological effect of each individual gamma beam is negligible. At their point of focus, however, their combined effects induce a radionecrosis. The method has been successfully used now for more than 20 years in the treatment of arteriovenous malformations, acoustic neurinomas, meningiomas, craniopharyngeomas, pituitary adenomas, and other forms of intracranial pathology.[46] No case of radiation-induced malignancy has been observed in the more than 20 years the Gamma Knife has been in use. To date, approximately 40 anxiety disorder and 50 OCD patients have undergone gamma capsulotomy; hence, there is considerably less experience with this procedure than with the thermocapsulotomy technique. Published results appear comparable, however.[2,47–49] Gamma capsulotomy can be performed on an outpatient basis. Figure 16–1 shows the lesions induced by gamma capsulotomy in the transaxial and coronal planes.

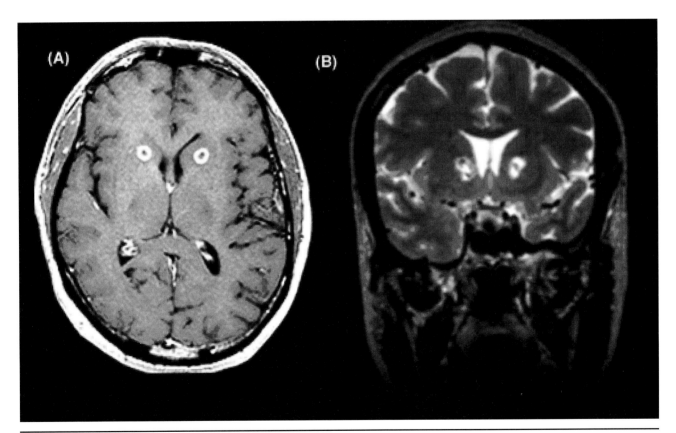

FIGURE 16–1. The gamma capsulotomy lesions in the anterior limb of the internal capsule interrupt fibers that connect orbitofrontal and cingular cortex with the dorsomedial thalamus.

Left: T_1-weighted axial magnetic resonance imaging scan at the level of the lateral ventricles, showing small bilateral low-signal areas in the base of the anterior limb of the internal capsule 4 months after Gamma Knife capsulotomy. **Right:** T_1-weighted coronal magnetic resonance imaging view at the level of the frontal horns of the lateral ventricles in the same patient 4 months after gamma capsulotomy, showing areas of decreased attenuation in the anterior limb of the internal capsule bilaterally.

In a Swedish gamma capsulotomy study, three targets in each capsule were irradiated, with the theoretically appealing purposes of creating elongated lesions similar to those produced in thermocapsulotomy and tailoring the fields of irradiation according to the individual anatomy of the capsules.[49] A highly significant reduction in target symptoms occurred over time in the five OCD patients and in two of the six patients with non-OCD anxiety disorders (agoraphobia and generalized anxiety disorder). No clinically meaningful improvement was obtained, however, in the four other cases of non-OCD anxiety disorders. At the 5-year follow-up, both the neuropsychiatric (Mindus et al., unpublished data, June 1996) and the neuroradiological[49] status of the patients appeared stable.

Unfortunately, the cumulative radiation doses used in this study were high, which increased the incidence of undesired side effects such as fatigue, apathy, disinhibition, and other symptoms indicative of the frontal lobe damage. These observations suggested that lower radiation doses to smaller target volumes should be used in future studies. Although this approach may be assumed to reduce the rate of undesired side effects, it may to some extent also reduce the chances of lesioning a crucial number of relevant fibers. In this work, however, it is preferable to err on the safe side and extend the lesions in a second intervention, if warranted clinically.

To obtain more information on the long-term efficacy and safety of gamma capsulotomy, all 34 patients treated at the Karolinska Hospital between the years 1976 and 1992 were entered into a follow-up study that was completed in 1997. Twenty-seven patients (of whom 17 had OCD) were available. Follow-up MRI showed that the lesions were sharply delineated, with no reactions or only minimal reactions in the surrounding tissues. In most cases, both the volume and the configuration of the lesions were similar between patients and across hemispheres. The site of the lesion varied, however, and one unfortunate patient had bilateral lesions in her caudates, although she had neither apparent neuropsychiatric sequelae nor attenuation of her symptoms. In this early case in the series, pneumoencephalography was used for target localization, a method clearly inferior to the MRI technique used today.

A PROSPECTIVE CAPSULOTOMY STUDY

Several methodological problems complicate the interpretation of earlier studies. Difficulties include lack of controlled evidence; insufficient information about the preoperative diagnostic workup; and problems with the methods used to establish the therapy-refractory nature of the illness, the measures used to estimate outcome, rater's bias, the duration of follow-up, and confounding factors such as treatment after surgery. These aspects have been discussed in detail elsewhere.[2–5] For the purpose of this chapter, it may be of interest, however, briefly to review data from prospective study of capsulotomy in refractory OCD that was designed to avoid some of the above methodological shortcomings.

The study comprised all consecutive Swedish-speaking OCD patients who received thermocapsulotomy at the Karolinska Hospital from 1979 through 1990 (Mindus et al., unpublished data, June 1997). All patients were selected as previously outlined and were operated on by the same neurosurgeon who used the same technique for the visualization of the targets and the production of the lesion as described elsewhere.[5] Preoperatively, the patients' symptoms were diagnosed on the basis of current diagnostic criteria, and the treatment-refractory nature of their illnesses was carefully documented. The obsessive-compulsive subscale of the Comprehensive Psychopathological Rating Scale[50] (CPRS-OC) was used as a measure of clinical morbidity. Serial ratings were made by the same rater before capsulotomy; 2, 6, 9, and 12 months after capsulotomy; and again after a mean of 8 (range=3–15) years. The patients also were examined with neuropsychological tests, a personality inventory, and neuroradiological examinations, performed at baseline and at regular intervals after capsulotomy. The preliminary findings of this study are described below.

During the study period, 24 patients underwent thermocapsulotomy for otherwise intractable OCD. Of these, 2 patients were lost to follow-up. In the remaining 22 patients, a highly significant symptom reduction was found at the 1-year follow-up compared with baseline ($t_{21}=3.69$, $P<0.001$, two-tailed). The main changes in scores were present already at the 2-month follow-up ($t_{21}=4.03$, $P<0.002$, two-tailed), with nonsignificant changes ($t_{21}=1.08$, $P=0.291$, two-tailed) at subsequent rating sessions up to the 8-year follow-up. Because the mean duration of the patients' illnesses exceeded 15 years, this rapid symptom alleviation is remarkable. On postoperative CPRS-OC scores, 5 (23%) of the patients had higher scores at the 8-year follow-up compared with baseline; that is, they had a worse outcome on this measure. Two patients (9%)

improved by 1%–25%, 5 (23%) improved by 26%–50%, 3 (14%) improved by 51%–75%, and 7 (32%) improved by 75%–100%.

These findings agree well with those of a recent study of cingulotomy in refractory OCD in which a similar design was used.[51] This made possible a comparison of the number of patients who had a reduction of 35% or greater (an outcome criterion frequently used in drug studies) on the dependent measure used in the two studies. Eight (44%) of the 18 cingulotomy patients improved by 35% or greater, and the corresponding figure for capsulotomy was 10 of 22 (45%). These findings support the contention that the results of these types of procedures are comparable and that intervention may benefit even refractory OCD patients. The strengths of the studies are their prospective, intraindividual design; careful preoperative diagnostic workup and documentation of adequacy of previous nonsurgical treatment attempts; and independent assessments of obsessive-compulsive symptomatology with reliable and validated instruments. Their weaknesses include, obviously, the absence of nonsurgical or sham control subjects.

SIDE EFFECTS

Personality

Because capsulotomy may be assumed to affect, directly or indirectly, frontal lobe function, the operation may give rise to personality changes. Is there a price, in terms of negative personality changes, that the patient may have to pay for any symptom alleviation? This important issue has been addressed by several independent groups. Of particular interest here is the work by two Swedish psychiatrists, Rylander and Bingley, pioneers in frontal lobe research. They were among the first to report personality alterations in patients undergoing lobotomy.[24,52] One of Rylander's early (1947) observations may be summarized here. The patient was a woman who was a high-ranking Salvation Army officer. During many years in the hospital, she incessantly ruminated about her sins committed against the Holy Ghost. She underwent standard lobotomy. When the operation was over, she was quite silent. Rylander[24] reported: "After the dressing had been taken off, I asked her 'How are you now? What about the Holy Ghost?' Smiling, she answered, 'Oh, the Holy Ghost; there is no Holy Ghost'" (p. 702). Unfortunately, no account of the long-term outcome of

the intervention in this case is available. Many years later, Bingley and Rylander studied prospectively patients undergoing gamma or thermocapsulotomy.[14,47] Their observation that the patients did not manifest personality changes after capsulotomy may seem all the more important because these researchers knew what to look for.

It is well known that impulsiveness is one of the most conspicuous symptoms of frontal lobe dysfunction.[53] For this reason, a method capable of detecting negative personality changes following intervention must cover impulsiveness and related features such as psychopathy, hostility, and aggressiveness. One such instrument is the Karolinska Scales of Personality (KSP), developed by Schalling et al.[54] It contains scales measuring traits related to frontal lobe function and scales reflecting different dimensions of anxiety proneness. Numerous studies have been performed by independent investigators who have shown the KSP to differentiate between diagnostic subgroups and to correlate significantly with biological markers for vulnerability to certain psychopathological conditions.[54]

Mindus and Edman (unpublished data, June 1994) gave the KSP to the 22 OCD patients described in the previous section. Before surgery, abnormally high mean scores (+1 SD to +2 SD) were found on 4 of the 15 scales, 3 of which reflect anxiety proneness and 1 of which reflects psychasthenic traits. At the 1-year follow-up, the scores remained at the same level on all scales, with two exceptions (Indirect Aggressiveness and Guilt), which changed in the direction of normality. In particular, the scores on the KSP related to impulsiveness, psychopathy, hostility, and aggressiveness were within the normal range. The findings agree with those reported after capsulotomy in mixed groups of OCD and non-OCD anxiety disorder patients, obtained both with the same instruments[55] and with different instruments.[14,29,56,57]

With regard to impulsiveness, it is interesting to note that patients whose scores on the CPRS-OC at follow-up were significantly reduced (responders) had significantly lower preoperative scores on the KSP related to impulsiveness than those who were rated as nonresponders. The preoperative scores of both groups were, however, within normal limits (±1 SD). Also, a significant change in impulsiveness occurred over time in both subgroups but in different directions: the responders, who were lower on this measure before capsulotomy, had higher postoperative scores, whereas the scores of the nonresponders showed the opposite pattern (Mindus and Edman, unpublished data, June

1994). These findings may be interpreted as suggesting that a favorable outcome of capsulotomy is related to the preoperative level of impulsiveness. Satisfactory results may be associated with a slight increase in impulsiveness. One possibility that deserves further study is whether too low a level of impulsiveness at baseline, as measured by the KSP, may serve as a marker of unresponsiveness to this form of treatment.

These observations may permit the conclusion that negative personality changes are not likely to occur after capsulotomy. It must be remembered that this conclusion is based on observations made on groups of patients and does not preclude the possibility that negative changes may occur in individual patients. In particular, it may be assumed that increased lesion volume may increase the risk of adverse personality changes, at least in vulnerable individuals.[5,49]

COGNITIVE FUNCTIONS

Is there a price in terms of cognitive dysfunction that the capsulotomy patient may have to pay for symptom alleviation? This issue also has been addressed by several investigators,[14,28,29,56] who used a restricted range of psychometric tests in a total of approximately 200 capsulotomy patients. No evidence was found of reduced intellectual function after capsulotomy. Of course, as has been pointed out,[2,56] these findings do not exclude the possibility that more specific tests could reveal dysfunction in systems involving the frontal lobes. The main basis for raising this possibility is that although the targets of capsulotomy are not located within the frontal lobes proper, but in some of their connections with other parts of the brain, the operation may nonetheless be expected to affect frontal lobe function.

There are several additional reasons to study the neuropsychology of these patients. First, neuropsychological hypotheses concerning a brain basis for OCD have focused on frontolimbic circuits. Second, neuropsychological knowledge relies heavily on observations following different types of brain trauma or disease, and in such cases, lesions tend to involve relatively wide areas of the brain. By comparison, capsulotomy involves well-defined areas. Finally, unlike individuals who become neuropsychologically impaired because of brain trauma or disease, capsulotomy patients can be studied prospectively.

For these reasons, Nyman and Mindus[58] administered a comprehensive neuropsychological test battery to 10 patients before and at 1 year after thermocapsulotomy. The Wisconsin Card Sorting Test[59] (WCST) was included in the test battery to further elucidate frontal lobe function. Five of the patients had a principal diagnosis of OCD, and five had a non-OCD anxiety disorder such as agoraphobia or generalized anxiety disorder. Although extremely disabled by their illness before surgery, the patients performed within the normal range on most tests. At 1 year after capsulotomy, measures of clinical morbidity and of psychosocial functioning improved significantly, and the general neuropsychological performance remained remarkably intact. In five patients, three of whom had OCD, the postoperative performance on the WCST had deteriorated, however. In this subgroup, but not in the remaining patients, perseverative responses were more common after the operation than before it, reflecting impairment of abstract conceptualization and of the ability to use feedback to modify behavior. Unfortunately, the investigators were unable to find particular neuropsychological or clinical features, including outcome, that distinguished these five patients from those who did well on the WCST after capsulotomy. This may be interpreted as suggesting that the individual may have to pay a cognitive price, even in the absence of symptom alleviation (i.e., regardless of the response to the operation).

It should be noted that poorer postoperative performance on the WCST does not appear to be specific to capsulotomy; poorer WCST performance also was reported in OCD patients after cingulotomy[42] and subcaudate tractotomy.[60] Obviously, a common denominator for these observations may be that all three procedures affect frontal lobe function.

Although admittedly sparse, these data may be interpreted as suggesting that in vulnerable individuals, capsulotomy as well as other procedures in current use may give rise to increased perseverative behavior in the laboratory and in the real world. This risk must be weighed against the potential clinical benefit of neurosurgery in this extremely disabled, sometimes suicidal patient population.

FEATURES OF OCD RELATED TO FRONTAL LOBE FUNCTION

Certain core features of OCD symptoms may be intuitively linked to frontal lobe function. Pathological doubt is one of the central manifestations of this illness. The person goes to the door, shuts it, locks it, feels that it is locked, knows that it is locked, turns around, and walks away. All of a sudden, he or she feels that it is absolutely necessary to go back and check. It appears clinically that the memory of the action of locking the door is insufficient. This phenomenon could be related to a deficit in working memory (see Goldman-Rakic, Chapter 5, in this volume). Recent positron-emission tomography (PET) data suggest that obsessive-compulsive patients have reduced metabolic activity in the striatum while performing implicit memory tasks compared with control subjects.[61,62]

Another important core feature of OCD that may be related to frontal lobe function is abnormal risk assessment. From a clinical perspective, it appears that the anticipatory function of the frontal lobes is overactive in OCD. Patients may incessantly ruminate about the risk of being contaminated with, say HIV, and shun public bathrooms, although they admit knowing that the actual risk is negligible.

A third core feature is the phenomenon that may be called incompleteness; the patient needs to carry out a motor action in a particular way, or a particular number of times, until he or she has a feeling of completeness, that the action has been done just right. For example, one OCD patient, when entering his physician's office, felt that his shoulders must be equidistant from the door frames; he may have had to go in and out 50 times before he felt that he succeeded, at last relieved of this torturing feeling of incompleteness.

NEUROSURGERY IN OBSESSIVE-COMPULSIVE DISORDER AND FRONTAL LOBE INVOLVEMENT

It is well known that there are extensive interconnections between the frontal lobes, the basal ganglia, and limbic and paralimbic structures. Consequently, neurosurgically induced lesions placed in different brain targets may ameliorate OCD symptoms by exerting their effects on the same frontal lobe region. Indeed, evidence suggests that this may be the case. For example, intervention in the orbitofrontal area, as in subcaudate tractotomy, or in the orbitofrontal-thalamic tract, as in capsulotomy, or in the midline thalamic nuclei, as in certain forms of thalamotomy,[63] all have been associated with improvement in OCD. In other words, although different neurosurgical interventions

have different stereotactic targets, they may have the same functional target; that is, they may be assumed to affect, directly or indirectly, the same brain circuits. Moreover, surgically induced lesions in one brain region may affect other regions, proximal or distal to the lesion. For example, it has been shown in humans that lesions in the substantia innominata after subcaudate tractotomy caused extensive degeneration in the ventral portion of the internal capsule[64]; the fiber tract degeneration could be traced back to the dorsomedial nucleus of the thalamus, which has extensive interconnections with the limbic system, including the orbitomedial frontal region.[53,65–68]

In neurobiological models of OCD, neural circuits involving the basal ganglia, limbic system, and frontal lobes have been implicated in the pathophysiology of the disorder. Baxter[69] proposed that hyperactivity in the orbitofrontal region and caudate nucleus leads to decreased thalamic inhibition and thalamic excitation, causing OCD symptoms. It is noteworthy that the targets of current neurosurgical intervention in OCD are located within these same structures. With regard to the mechanism underlying the possible efficacy of capsulotomy, the projections within the implicated circuit, the frontal-striatal-pallidal-thalamic-frontal loop,[65] are believed to pass through the anterior limb of the internal capsule, the target of capsulotomy. Moreover, of the entire neocortex, only the frontal lobes have direct, monosynaptic connections with subcortical regions. These fiber systems have been shown to pass through the internal capsule.[67] It has been suggested[6,23] that there may be two important components of the functional neuroanatomy of OCD: the aforementioned circuit, which mediates the obsessive-compulsive component, and a less specific anxiety component mediated through the Papez circuit, including the cingulum bundle, the target of cingulotomy. An alternative theory ascribes a more specific role to the anterior cingulate cortex in mediating obsessive-compulsive symptoms.[70]

Increased metabolic rates of glucose in the orbital gyri and in the caudate, which have been consistently reported findings and are assumed to be related to the pathophysiology of OCD, may be decreased or normalized following successful treatment with medication or behavior therapy.[68,71] It may be assumed that similar changes may follow successful neurosurgical treatment. The findings of a small study from the Karolinska Hospital give some support to this contention.[72] Serial PET examinations of five OCD patients before and at regular intervals after thermocapsulotomy showed significant reductions in absolute values of glucose metabolism at the 1-year follow-up compared with values before the operation. It was speculated that this reduction in regional brain metabolism was somehow related to the reduction in symptoms that followed capsulotomy. The surgical patients' preoperative values in the orbital gyri were lower, however, than those found in healthy control subjects, an unexpected finding. This may represent a "burnout" phenomenon in the brains of these patients, who were not only intractable but also more severely ill and had longer durations of illness than the patients scanned elsewhere.[2,72]

Ideally, a discussion of the putative therapeutic mechanisms of neurosurgery for OCD should rest on insights into the neurobiology of OCD. Granted, abnormal findings on both structural imaging (computed tomography [CT], MRI) and functional imaging (electroencephalography [EEG], PET, single photon emission computed tomography [SPECT]) have been observed in the brains of OCD patients compared with both other psychiatric patients and control subjects without psychiatric disorders. Thus far, however, no single pathognomonic structural aberration has been identified. Interestingly, in responding patients, some of the metabolic changes observed with PET were normalized after both drug and behavior treatment. Particularly, pretreatment and posttreatment correlation data between the orbital cortex and the caudate nucleus seem to indicate that there is a functional imbalance between these brain regions in OCD that may be restored with successful treatment, be it with drugs, behavior therapy,[69,71] or surgery.[72] A recent study showed that neuronal inhibition is decreased in the cerebral cortex in OCD after transcranial magnetic stimulation.[73]

In summary, the body of evidence indicates that the underlying pathophysiology of OCD may involve multiple brain regions and multiple transmitter systems and that a functional imbalance may exist between these systems in OCD. Antiobsessional treatment may be assumed to affect that functional imbalance by somehow changing the interconnectivity between the frontal lobes and other parts of the brain, including limbic and paralimbic structures. With regard to neurosurgical operations in cases of otherwise intractable OCD, both their effects and their side effects may be viewed as expressions of their influence on the functional imbalance, affecting both neuropsychiatric and neuropsychological features as well as personality traits.

FUTURE RESEARCH

There are ethical, clinical, and scientific reasons to carry out research in this field.[74] From an ethical point of view, operations that involve the irrevocable destruction of brain tissue need to be comprehensively and continuously evaluated with the most sophisticated techniques available. Clinically, it can be argued that neurosurgical treatments are potentially life-saving in some desperate cases. Scientifically, it can be argued that these procedures offer a unique opportunity to study brain-behavior relationships in patients with extreme forms of OCD before and after a defined intervention aimed at disconnecting parts of fundamental brain regions such as the frontal lobes and the limbic system.

Only a single report of a sham controlled study[75] appears in the literature. This involved four psychotic patients, none of whom improved after a sham procedure in which skin incisions and burr holes were made without the production of cerebral lesions. Considering the ethics, one official body, the Canadian Psychiatric Association, has taken a strong stand: "It is difficult to see how experimental procedures involving the use of 'placebo operations' could be ethically and acceptably undertaken" (p. 3).[76] Although obviously guided by humanitarian considerations, this position may nevertheless prove inhumane, for some clinicians refuse to refer even desolate cases for neurosurgical intervention until double-blind, controlled data have been published to show an effect; as a result, a veritable "catch-22" dilemma exists.[5]

It must be noted, however, that the above official position was taken with open surgical procedures in mind, which involved craniotomy. No craniotomy is made in gamma capsulotomy. The lesions are, instead, made by the cross-firing of the target with thin gamma rays from radioactive cobalt sources, the radiation being directed to the target through approximately 200 channels or ports in an apparatus that surrounds the patient's head. A technician can block the ports by using tungsten inserts (placebo condition), or they can be left open (active condition). By this mechanism, placebo and active conditions can be administered in a fashion that is blind even to the surgeon.

Researchers from Brown University, Harvard University, and the Karolinska Hospital are currently conducting a collaborative dose-finding study of gamma capsulotomy in treatment-intractable OCD. Fifteen patients were initially treated with a bilateral lesion in the midventral region of the anterior capsule using a 4-mm collinator and 180 Gray. Unexpectedly, at

6-month to 1-year follow-up, only 1 of the 15 patients was much or very much improved. Thirteen patients had a second stage procedure in which bilateral lesions directly ventral to the initial lesion were made in the capsule. Forty percent of the patients' symptoms were rated as much or very much improved. Fifteen additional patients received two bilateral shots of radiation (total of four). Fifty percent of these patients were much or very much improved at follow-up. As in the previous study, no significant changes in personality or other cognitive measures occurred. The fact that only 1 of the 15 patients responded to a single-stage intervention strongly argues against a significant placebo effect. A double-blind study of the procedure, currently under way at our site, should definitely confirm the efficacy of the procedure. More recently, deep brain stimulation of the capsule has been used for intractable OCD.[77,78] This procedure holds great promise because of its reversibility and the ability to turn the stimulus on and off in a controlled fashion. It also allows exploration of the question raised by Lippitz et al.[79] as to whether a right-sided unilateral lesion would be as effective as the bilateral lesion.

If such a trial lends support for the beneficial effects of these procedures, then it is hoped that dogmatism will fade, a growing percentage of appropriate candidates will be referred, and patients will be referred at an earlier phase of their illness (the mean duration of illness in most neurosurgery cohorts is 15 years!). It appears that in the heyday of lobotomy, too many were operated on too soon. Today, in contrast, it may well be that too few are operated on too late. In both situations, it is the patients who pay the price.

REFERENCES

1. Waziri R: Psychosurgery for anxiety and obsessive-compulsive disorders, in Handbook of Anxiety, Vol 4. Edited by Noyes R Jr, Roth M, Burrows GD. Amsterdam, The Netherlands, Elsevier, 1990, pp 519–535
2. Mindus P: Capsulotomy in anxiety disorders: a multidisciplinary study. Doctoral dissertation, Department of Psychiatry and Psychology, Karolinska Institute, Stockholm, Sweden, 1991
3. Mindus P, Jenike MA: Neurosurgical treatment of malignant obsessive-compulsive disorder: obsessional disorders. Psychiatr Clin North Am 4:921–938, 1992
4. Mindus P, Meyerson BA: Capsulotomy for intractable anxiety disorders, in Operative Surgical Techniques. Edited by Schmidek H, Sweet W. Philadelphia, PA, WB Saunders, 1994, pp 768–782
5. Mindus P, Rauch SL, Nyman H, et al: Capsulotomy and cingulotomy as treatments for malignant obsessive-compulsive disorder: an update, in Current Insights in Obsessive-Compulsive Disorder. Edited by Berend B, Hollander E, Marazziti M, et al. Chichester, UK, Wiley, 1994, pp 245–276
6. Jenike MA, Baer L, Ballantine HT Jr, et al: Cingulotomy for refractory obsessive-compulsive disorder: a long term follow-up of 33 patients. Arch Gen Psychiatry 48:548–555, 1991
7. Rasmussen SA, Tsuang MT: Epidemiology of obsessive-compulsive disorder: a review. J Clin Psychiatry 45:450–457, 1984
8. Noyes R Jr: The natural history of anxiety disorders, in Handbook of Anxiety, Vol 6: Clinical and Cultural Perspectives. Edited by Roth M, Noyes Jr R, Burrows GD. Amsterdam, The Netherlands, Elsevier, 1988, pp 115–133
9. Angst J, Vollrath M: The natural history of anxiety disorders. Acta Psychiatr Scand 84:446–452, 1991
10. Greist JH: Treatment of obsessive-compulsive disorder: psychotherapies, drugs, and other somatic treatment. J Clin Psychiatry 51 (suppl 8):44–50, 1990
11. Jenike MA: Approaches to the patient with treatment-refractory obsessive-compulsive disorder. J Clin Psychiatry 51 (suppl 2):15–21, 1990
12. O'Sullivan G, Marks IM: Long term outcome of phobic and obsessive-compulsive disorders after treatment, in Handbook of Anxiety, Vol 4: The Treatment of Anxiety. Edited by Noyes R Jr, Roth M, Burrows GD. Amsterdam, The Netherlands, Elsevier, 1990, pp 87–108
13. Greist JH: An integrated approach to treatment of obsessive compulsive disorder. J Clin Psychiatry 53:38–41, 1992
14. Bingley T, Leksell L, Meyerson BA, et al: Long term results of stereotactic anterior capsulotomy in chronic obsessive-compulsive neurosis, in Neurosurgical Treatment in Psychiatry, Pain and Epilepsy. Edited by Sweet WH, Obrador S, Martín-Rodríguez JG. Baltimore, MD, University Park Press, 1977, pp 287–299
15. Ballantine HT Jr: Neurosurgery for behavioral disorders, in Neurosurgery. Edited by Wilkins RH, Rengachary SS. Amsterdam, The Netherlands, Elsevier North-Holland, 1985, pp 2527–2537
16. Ballantine HT Jr, Bouckoms AJ, Thomas EK, et al: Treatment of psychiatric illness by stereotactic cingulotomy. Biol Psychiatry 22:807–819, 1987
17. Martuza RL, Chiocca EA, Jenike MA, et al: Stereotactic radiofrequency thermal cingulotomy for obsessive compulsive disorder. J Neuropsychiatry Clin Neurosci 2:331–336, 1990
18. Knight GC: Bifrontal stereotaxic tractotomy in the substantia innominata: an experience of 450 cases, in Psychosurgery. Edited by Hitchcock E, Laitinen L, Vaernet K. Springfield, IL, Charles C Thomas, 1972, pp 267–277

19. Göktepe EO, Young LB, Bridges PK: A further review of the results of stereotactic subcaudate tractotomy. Br J Psychiatry 126:270–280, 1975

20. Bartlett JR, Bridges PK: The extended subcaudate tractotomy lesion, in Neurosurgical Treatment in Psychiatry, Pain and Epilepsy. Edited by Sweet WH, Obrador S, Martín-Rodríguez JG. Baltimore, MD, University Park Press, 1977, pp 387–398

21. Richardson A: Stereotactic limbic leucotomy: surgical technique. Postgrad Med J 49:860–864, 1973

22. Mitchell-Heggs N, Kelly D, Richardson A: Stereotactic limbic leucotomy: a follow-up at 16 months. Br J Psychiatry 128:226–240, 1976

23. Kelly D: Anxiety and Emotions: Physiological Basis and Treatment. Springfield, IL, Charles C Thomas, 1980

24. Rylander G: Personality analysis before and after frontal lobotomy: the frontal lobes. Association of Researchers Into Nervous and Mental Diseases 27:691–705, 1947

25. Meyer A, Beck E: Prefrontal leucotomy and related operations: anatomical aspects of success or failure. Henderson Trust Lecture 17. Edinburgh and London, UK, Oliver & Boyd, 1954

26. Talairach J, Hecaen H, David M, et al: Recherches sur la coagulation thérapeutique des structures sous-corticales chez l'homme. Rev Neurol (Paris) 81:4–24, 1949

27. Leksell L: A stereotaxic apparatus for intracerebral surgery. Acta Chirurgica Scandinavica 99:229–233, 1949

28. Herner T: Treatment of mental disorders with frontal stereotactic thermo-lesions: a follow-up of 116 cases. Acta Psychiatr Scand Suppl 36:1–56, 1961

29. Lopez-Ibor JJ, Lopez-Ibor Alino J: Selection criteria for patients who should undergo psychiatric surgery, in Neurosurgical Treatment in Psychiatry, Pain and Epilepsy. Edited by Sweet WH, Obrador S, Martín-Rodríguez JG. Baltimore, MD, University Park Press, 1977, pp 151–162

30. Burzaco J: Stereotactic surgery in the treatment of obsessive-compulsive neurosis, in Proceedings of the 3rd World Congress of Biological Psychiatry. Edited by Perris C, Struwe G, Jansson B. Amsterdam, The Netherlands, Elsevier North-Holland, 1981, pp 1103–1109

31. Papez JW: A proposed mechanism of emotion. Archives of Neurology and Psychiatry 38:725–743, 1937

32. Maclean PD: Contrasting functions of limbic and neocortical systems of the brain and their relevance to psychophysiological aspects of medicine. Am J Med 25:611–626, 1958

33. Fulton JF, Jacobsen CF: Fonctions des lobes fronteaux; étude comparée chez l'homme, les singes et les chimpanzes. Rev Neurol (Paris) 64:552–574, 1935

34. Nauta WJH: Hippocampal projections and related neuronal pathways to the midbrain in the cat. Brain 81:319–340, 1958

35. Lewin W: Observations on selective leucotomy. J Neurol Neurosurg Psychiatry 24:37–44, 1961

36. Foltz EL, White LE: Pain "relief" by cingulotomy. J Neurosurg 19:89–100, 1962

37. Ballantine HT Jr, Cassidy WS, Flanagan NB, et al: Stereotactic anterior cingulotomy for neuropsychiatric illness and intractable pain. J Neurosurg 26:488–495, 1967

38. Knight GC: The orbital cortex as an objective in the surgical treatment of mental illness: the development of a stereotactic approach. Br J Surg 51:114–124, 1964

39. Kelly D: Physiological changes during operations on the limbic system in man. Conditioned Reflex 7:127–138, 1972

40. Rasmussen SA, Eisen JL: Treatment strategies for chronic and refractory obsessive-compulsive disorder. J Clin Psychiatry 58 (suppl 13):9–13, 1997

41. Kullberg G: Differences in effect of capsulotomy and cingulotomy, in Neurosurgical Treatment in Psychiatry, Pain and Epilepsy. Edited by Sweet WH, Obrador S, Martín-Rodríguez JG. Baltimore, MD, University Park Press, 1977, pp 301–308

42. Hay P, Sachdev P, Cumming S, et al: Treatment of obsessive-compulsive disorder by psychosurgery. Acta Psychiatr Scand 87:197–207, 1993

43. Leskell L: Stereotactic radiosurgery. J Neurol Neurosurg Psychiatry 46:797–803, 1983

44. Leksell L, Backlund E-O: Stereotactic gamma capsulotomy, in Modern Concepts in Psychiatric Surgery. Edited by Hitchcock ER, Ballantine HT Jr, Meyerson BA. Amsterdam, The Netherlands, Elsevier North-Holland, 1979, pp 213–216

45. Lindquist C, Hindmarsh T, Kihlström L, et al: MRI and CT studies of radionecrosis development in the normal human brain, in Radiosurgery: Baseline and Trends. Edited by Steiner L, Lindquist C, Forster D, et al. New York, Raven, 1992, pp 245–253

46. Steiner L, Lindquist C, Forster D, et al (eds): Radiosurgery: Baseline and Trends. New York, Raven, 1992

47. Rylander G: Stereotactic radiosurgery in anxiety and obsessive-compulsive states: psychiatric aspects, in Modern Concepts in Psychiatric Surgery. Edited by Hitchcock ER, Ballantine HT Jr, Meyerson BA. Amsterdam, The Netherlands, Elsevier North-Holland, 1979, pp 235–240

48. Mindus P, Bergström K, Levander SE, et al: Magnetic resonance images related to clinical outcome after psychosurgical intervention in severe anxiety disorder. J Neurol Neurosurg Psychiatry 50:1288–1293, 1987

49. Guo WY, Lindquist C, Kihlström P, et al: Radionecrosis created in the internal capsule for psychosurgery with the gamma knife. Doctoral dissertation, Department of Neuroradiology, Karolinska Institute, Stockholm, Sweden, 1993

50. Åsberg M, Perris C, Schalling D, et al: The CPRS: development and applications of a psychiatric rating scale. Acta Psychiatr Scand Suppl 271:1–24, 1978

51. Baer L, Rauch SL, Ballanhre HT, et al: Cingulotomy for intractable OCD. Arch Gen Psychiatry 52:384–392, 1995

52. Bingley T: On the influence on intellectual function of frontal lobotomy. Nordic Psychiatric Journal 3:49–52, 1949

53. Stuss DT, Benson DF: Personality and emotion, in The Frontal Lobes. Edited by Stuss DT, Benson DF. New York, Raven, 1986, pp 121–138

54. Schalling DS, Åsberg M, Edman G, et al: Markers for vulnerability to psychopathology: temperament traits associated with platelet MAO activity. Acta Psychiatr Scand 76:172–182, 1987

55. Mindus P, Nyman H: Normalization of personality characteristics in patients with incapacitating anxiety disorders after capsulotomy. Acta Psychiatr Scand 83:283–291, 1991

56. Mindus P, Nyman H, Rosenquist A, et al: Aspects of personality in patients with anxiety disorders undergoing capsulotomy. Acta Neurochir (Wien) 44 (suppl):138–144, 1988

57. Vasko T, Kullberg G: Results of psychological testing of cognitive functions in patients undergoing stereotactic psychiatric surgery, in Modern Concepts in Psychiatric Surgery. Edited by Hitchcock ER, Ballantine HT Jr, Meyerson BA. Amsterdam, The Netherlands, Elsevier North-Holland, 1979, pp 303–310

58. Nyman H, Mindus P: Neuropsychological correlates of intractable anxiety before and after capsulotomy. Acta Psychiatrica Scand 91:23–31, 1995

59. Heaton RK, Chelune GJ, Talley JL, et al: Wisconsin Card Sorting Test Manual, Revised and Expanded. Odessa, FL, Psychological Assessment Resources, 1993

60. Kartsounis LD, Poynton A, Bridges PK, et al: Neuropsychological correlates of stereotactic subcaudate tractotomy: a prospective study. Brain 114:2657–2673, 1991

61. Rauch SL, Savage CR, Alpert NM, et al: Probing striatal function in obsessive-compulsive disorder: a PET study of implicit sequence learning. J Neuropsychiatry Clin Neurosci 9:568–573, 1997

62. Rauch SL, Savage CR: Neuroimaging and neuropsychology of the striatum: bridging basic science and clinical practice. Psychiatr Clin North Am 20:741–768, 1997

63. Hassler R, Dieckman G: Relief of obsessive-compulsive disorders, phobias and tics by stereotactic coagulation of the rostral intralaminar and medial-thalamic nuclei, in Surgical Approaches in Psychiatry. Edited by Laitinen LV, Livingston KE. Baltimore, MD, University Park Press, 1973, pp 206–212

64. Corsellis J, Jack AB: Neuropathological observations on yttrium implants and on undercutting in the orbitofrontal areas of the brain, in Surgical Approaches in Psychiatry. Edited by Laitinen LV, Livingston KE. Baltimore, MD, University Park Press, 1973, pp 90–95

65. Modell JG, Mountz JM, Curtis GC, et al: Neurophysiologic dysfunction in basal ganglia/limbic striatal and thalamocortical circuits as a pathogenetic mechanism of obsessive-compulsive disorder. J Neuropsychiatry Clin Neurosci 1:27–36, 1989

66. Insel TR, Winslow JT: Neurobiology of obsessive-compulsive disorders. Psychiatr Clin North Am 15:813–824, 1992

67. Nauta HJW: A simplified perspective on the basal ganglia and their relation to the limbic system, in The Limbic System: Functional Organization and Clinical Disorders. Edited by Doane BK, Livingston KA. New York, Raven, 1986, pp 67–77

68. Malloy P: Frontal lobe dysfunction in OCD, in The Frontal Lobes Revisited. Edited by Perecman E. New York, Institute for Research in Behavioral Neuroscience (IRBN) Press, 1987, pp 207–223

69. Baxter LR: Neuroimaging studies of obsessive-compulsive disorder. Psychiatr Clin North Am 15:871–885, 1992

70. Rauch SL, Jenike MA: Neurobiological models of obsessive-compulsive disorder. Psychosomatics 34:20–32, 1993

71. Swedo S, Pietrini P, Leonard HL, et al: Cerebral glucose metabolism in childhood onset obsessive-compulsive disorder: revisualization during pharmacotherapy. Arch Gen Psychiatry 40:600–604, 1992

72. Mindus P, Nyman H, Mogard J, et al: Frontal lobe and basal ganglia metabolism studied with PET in patients with incapacitating obsessive-compulsive disorder undergoing capsulotomy. Nordic Journal of Psychiatry 44:309–312, 1990

73. Greenberg BD, Ziemann U, Harmon A, et al: Decreased neuronal inhibition in cerebral cortex in obsessive-compulsive disorder on transcranial magnetic stimulation. Lancet 352:881–882, 1998

74. Mathew SJ, Yudofsky SC, McCullough LB, et al: Attitudes toward neurosurgical procedures for Parkinson's disease and obsessive-compulsive disorder. J Neuropsychiatry Clin Neurosci 11:259–267, 1999

75. Livingston RE: Psychiatric Treatment. Baltimore, MD, Williams & Wilkins, 1953

76. Earp JD: Position paper: psychosurgery: the position of the Canadian Psychiatric Association. Can J Psychiatry 24:353–365, 1979

77. Greenberg BD, Murphy DL, Rasmussen SA: Neuroanatomically based approaches to OCD: neurosurgery and transcranial magnetic stimulation. Psychiatr Clin North Am 23:671–686, 2000

78. Nuttin B, Cosyns P, Demeulemeester H, et al: Electrical stimulation in anterior limbs of internal capsules in patients with obsessive-compulsive disorder. Lancet 354(9189):1526, 1999

79. Lippitz B, Mindus P, Meyerson BA, et al: Obsessive compulsive disorder and the right hemisphere: topographic analysis of lesions after anterior capsulotomy performed with thermocoagulation. Neurosurgery 44:452–458, 1999

Index

Page numbers printed in **boldface** type refer to tables or figures.

and learning in nonhuman primates, 55–56
lesions
and affect in humans, 52–53
and emotional behavior in animals, 52
and memory in humans, 56
and memory in nonhuman primates, 55
in mnemonic and higher cognitive functions, 55–56
in mood disorders, 56
in neuropsychiatric illness, 56–61
in obsessive-compulsive disorder, 21, **21,** 29, 54, 58–61, 92, 241
olfactory input to, 38, **38,** 47–49
parcellation of, 33–38
Beck's, **34**
Brodmann's, 33–34, **34**
Carmichael and Price's, 36–38, **37**
correspondence between human and macaque systems of, 34–38, **36**
Hof's, 34, **35**
Walker's, 34–38, **36**
in Parkinson's disease, 172
posterior agranular, 36
in pseudopsychopathic personality, 53, 118, 209
in recognition of reinforcing stimuli, 47–49
satiety and, 49, 57, 59
in schizophrenia, 21, 56–57
sensory innervation of, **38,** 38–41
polymodal, 40–41
and smell/odor discrimination, 131
somatosensory input to, **38,** 39
in stimulus-reinforcer learning, 50–52
in stimulus-reward associations, 50–51
in substance abuse, 46, 54–57
visceral input to, **38,** 39–40, 45
visual input to, **38,** 39, **40**
Orbitofrontal disinhibition syndrome, 4, **117,** 117–118, 131–133, 139
psychopharmacotherapy for, 156
Orbitofrontal gyrus, 33
Organization skills, 7
dorsolateral prefrontal circuit and, 17, **20**
temporal, frontal lobe injury and, 206–207, **208**
Othello syndrome, 215–216, 221–222, 227

Pain, indifference to, anterior cingulate circuit and, 22, **22**
Paleocortex, 22–23, **23,** 27, 38, 41
Papez circuit, in obsessive-compulsive disorder, 241
Parafascicular thalamus, 24, **24**
Parahippocampal cortex, associations of, with orbitofrontal cortex, 44, **44**
Paralimbic areas, in depression, 168–170, 177–179
with Parkinson's disease, 171
Paralimbic belts, 23, **23,** 27, 41–42
Paramedian thalamic artery infarction, 141
Paranoid disorder, content-specific delusions versus, 217–218
Parasitophobia, 216
Parasitosis, delusional, 216–217, 222–228
Parietal cortex
associations of
with motor subsystem, 126
with orbitofrontal cortex, 41
with prefrontal cortex, 75, **75**
in visual processing, 75, **75**
Parkinson's disease
apathy with, 8, 22
assessment of, 127
depression with, 21, 91, 167, 169–172, **173,** 176–179
biochemical mechanisms in, 172
neuroimaging in, 170–172, **171**
dopamine in, 28, 170–172
executive cognitive dysfunction in, 8, 120–121
neurotransmitter dysfunction in, 28
orbitofrontal dysfunction with, 21
Pars compacta of substantia nigra, 24, **24, 26**
Pars magnocellularis
association of, with orbitofrontal cortex, 38, 43, 45–46, **46,** 50, 60
in obsessive-compulsive disorder, 60
Parvocellular thalamus, 22–24
Pathological doubt, 240–241
Pathological laughter and crying, 168
Patient history, 139, 150
Perceptual disorders, content-specific delusions versus, 217
Periaqueductal gray, association of, with orbitofrontal cortex, 45
Perirhinal cortex, associations of, with orbitofrontal cortex, **44,** 44–45

Perseveration, 88
age and, 134
in assessment of dorsolateral prefrontal cortex and executive cognitive functions, 128–130
between-task, 129
cross-task, 130
in dorsal convexity dysexecutive syndrome, 117
frontal lobe injury and, 202, **202**
inferior convexity lesions and, 51
neurosurgical treatment of obsessive-compulsive disorder and, 240
in obsessive-compulsive disorder, 58
right hemisphere and, 88
within-task, 129–130
Persistent vegetative state, 104
Personality change
with frontal lobe injury, 209
with neurosurgical treatment of obsessive-compulsive disorder, 239–240
with orbitofrontal dysfunction, 20, **21**
PET. *See* Positron emission tomography
Phasic attention, 104
Phobia, orbitofrontal cortex in, 54
Phosphodiesters, in schizophrenia, 192
Phosphoinositide
in frontal subcortical circuits, 28–29
and lithium, 29
in schizophrenia, 192
Phosphomonoesters, in schizophrenia, 192
Phrenology, 114
Physical appearance, assessment of, 133
Physical therapists, for patients with frontal system dysfunction, 10
Pick's disease, 120
Pimozide, for content-specific delusions, 228
Place, disorientation for, 216
Planning, frontal lobe injury and, 205–206, **206–207**
Planning skills, 7
Platter, Felix, 113
Pleasure-seeking behavior, orbitofrontal cortex and, 53
Positron emission tomography (PET)
in depression, 168–170, **170**
after stroke, **171,** 175, **175–177**